Falls in Older People

Risk factors and strategies for prevention

Second Edition

Stephen R. Lord
Prince of Wales Medical Research Institute, Australia, Sydney

Catherine Sherrington
Prince of Wales Medical Research Institute, Sydney, Australia and University of Sydney, Australia

Hylton B. Menz
Prince of Wales Medical Research Institute, Sydney, Australia and La Trobe University, Melbourne

Jacqueline C. T. Close
Prince of Wales Medical Research Institute, Sydney, Australia and Prince of Wales Hospital, Sydney

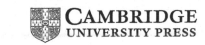

CAMBRIDGE
UNIVERSITY PRESS

CAMBRIDGE
UNIVERSITY PRESS

University Printing House, Cambridge CB2 8BS, United Kingdom

Published in the United States of America by Cambridge University Press, New York

Cambridge University Press is part of the University of Cambridge.

It furthers the University's mission by disseminating knowledge in the pursuit of education, learning and research at the highest international levels of excellence.

www.cambridge.org
Information on this title: www.cambridge.org/9780521680998

© Cambridge University Press 2007

First published 2007
3rd printing 2011

A catalogue record for this publication is available from the British Library

ISBN 978-0-521-68099-8 Paperback

Contents

Preface

In the preface to the first edition of this book published in 2001, we remarked on the enormous amount of work on risk factors for falling in older people and falls prevention strategies published in the last two decades of the twentieth century. As shown in Figure 1.0, an even larger body of research has been published in the international literature in the subsequent five years. Much has happened in this time and there have been many substantial gains in the evidence base that has increased our understanding of falls risk factors and prevention strategies. Listed below are some highlights of progress and encouraging findings.

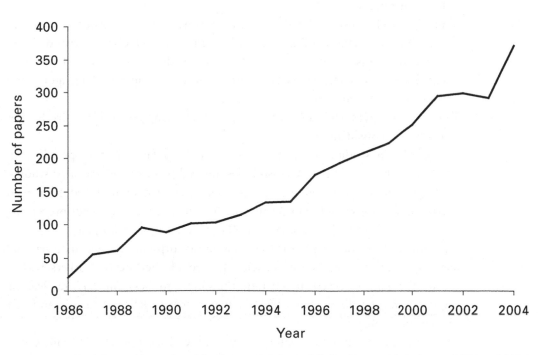

Fig. 1.0   Research publications pertaining to falls in older people between 1986 and 2004 (Source: Medline).

- Studies aimed at understanding balance have evolved more to using paradigms such as tripping, slipping and stepping that more accurately reflect situations in which people fall.
- Several studies have found that contrast sensitivity and depth perception are the most important visual risk factors for falls. It has also been shown that multifocal glasses may add to this risk because near-vision lenses impair distance contrast sensitivity and depth perception in the lower visual field.
- A large body of neuropsychological research has shown that balance activities that were generally considered to be reflex or automatic require attention, and that older people who have difficulties undertaking dual tasks are at increased risk of falls.
- There is increased evidence of the role that syncope plays in unexplained falls.
- The rationale for vitamin D supplementation as a falls prevention strategy for older people has been strengthened by cohort and intervention studies.
- A well designed randomized controlled trial has found that maximizing vision through cataract surgery is an effective falls prevention strategy.
- The role of environmental assessment/modification and safety education undertaken by trained professionals has been strengthened.
- Two randomized controlled trials have shown that falls can be prevented in hospital patients.
- Finally, and most strikingly, a raft of randomized controlled trials has examined the effects of a range of contrasting exercise interventions in preventing falls. From this large body of evidence it is now possible to conclude that effective exercise programmes comprise challenging and progressive, weight-bearing balance exercises.

Two areas of investigation have been less encouraging and will require further research and consideration.

- Intervention studies aimed at the prevention of falls in older people with dementia have not been successful, despite well planned and executed studies.
- Despite initial encouraging findings, well conducted randomized controlled trials have found that hip protectors are not an effective strategy for preventing fractures, with much of the lack of efficacy due to poor compliance.

The aim of this second edition is to review and incorporate the new material that has been published in journal articles, to provide healthcare workers with a means for gaining access to current thinking and best clinical practice. As suggested in the title, the book has two major themes: falls risk factors and falls prevention strategies.

Part I includes an initial chapter on the epidemiology of falls and fall-related injuries in older people. Chapters 2 to 8 present critical appraisals of the many posited falls risk factors, addressed under the headings of postural stability, gait, sensory and neuromuscular, psychological, medical, medication and environmental risk factors. In Chapter 9, the importance of the risk factors in each of the above domains is weighted as weak, moderate or strong, using evidence from published studies.

Part II addresses falls prevention strategies. An initial overview provides an outline of falls prevention strategies which address the multitude of falls risk factors. The first two chapters (Chapters 10 and 11) summarize the very large body of published findings on the role exercise can play in preventing falls and improving physical function in older people. Chapter 12 presents guidance for a systematic approach to the medical management of older persons at risk of falling, including management of medication use. Chapters 13 and 14 examine the role of specific intervention strategies such as the use of safe footwear, aids and appliances, and environmental modifications for preventing falls and fall injury. In Chapter 15, suggested strategies for preventing falls in institutions are summarized and discussed. Chapter 16 describes a novel profile system for quantifying an individual's risk of falling and targeting intervention strategies. The final chapter (Chapter 17) synthesizes the evidence on successful falls prevention strategies and collates the information in a format that can be used to facilitate the translation of research findings into routine clinical practice.

Part III contains a single chapter which reviews the research issues that still need to be addressed in this field.

In each chapter we have attempted to be analytical in nature. Thus, we have not simply presented lists of the many and varied factors that have been suggested as possible (but unproven) risk factors for falls and the suggested (but untested) falls prevention strategies. Instead, we have attempted to evaluate the evidence for each factor implicated with falls to determine whether they constitute important areas for consideration and intervention. For example, we present arguments that challenge some traditional approaches to the management of older persons at risk of falls. We question the utility of falls risk assessment based solely on diagnoses of disease processes and the value of standard clinical tests of vision, sensation, strength and balance. We also discuss the role of particular medications in predisposing older people to falls and why factors such as alcohol use, vestibular disorders and postural hypotension (which are considered important risk factors in clinical practice) have not been demonstrated to be significant risk factors for falls in well planned epidemiological studies. With regard to interventions, we examine the effectiveness of suggested strategies for preventing falls and question the value of certain exercise interventions and prevention strategies that do not take participant compliance issues into account.

As neurophysiological factors have been found to be key factors in the prediction and prevention of falls, this book places a major emphasis on these. Findings from our own studies have highlighted tests that have great utility in that they are reliable and highly predictive of falls. As outlined in Chapter 16, these tests can be used in a 'profile' based approach to falls risk which is aimed at identifying specific impairments in the major sensorimotor systems that contribute to balance, i.e. vision, peripheral sensation, strength and reaction time as well as measures of sway and stability. This enables intervention strategies to be tailored to address an individual's specific deficits.

The length of the chapters in this book varies considerably. The longer chapters are in areas in which there is a greater amount of available evidence on which to base falls risk factor assessment and the development of prevention strategies.

We hope this book will be of interest to medical and allied health care undergraduate and postgraduate students, medical practitioners, nurses, physiotherapists, occupational therapists, podiatrists, research workers in the fields of gerontology and geriatrics, health service managers, and scientists and health care workers in the disciplines of public health, injury and occupational health. We feel that this book is of relevance to those working in community, hospital and residential aged care settings.

Acknowledgements

The authors would like to acknowledge Anne Tiedemann and Julie Whitney for their contributions. We would also like to thank Dr Daina Sturnieks, Ms Rebecca St George and Ms Judy Sherrington for their thoughtful comments and contributions to various chapters of this book. Dr Jos Verbaken gave permission to reproduce the MET visual contrast chart.

Finally we would like to thank our partners and families for their support and tolerance throughout the writing process.

Part I

Epidemiology and risk factors for falls

Epidemiology of falls and fall-related injuries

In this chapter, we examine the epidemiology of falls in older people. We review the major studies that have described the incidence of falls, the locations where falls occur and falls sequelae. We also examine the costs and services required to treat and manage falls and fall-related injuries. Before addressing these issues, however, it is helpful to briefly discuss four important methodological considerations that are pertinent to all research studies of falls in older people: how falls are defined, how falls are counted, how injurious falls are defined and what constitutes an older person.

The definition of a fall

In 1987, the Kellogg International Working Group on the Prevention of Falls in the Elderly defined a fall as 'unintentionally coming to the ground or some lower level and other than as a consequence of sustaining a violent blow, loss of consciousness, sudden onset of paralysis as in stroke or an epileptic seizure' [1]. Since then, many researchers have used this or very similar definitions of a fall. The Kellogg definition is appropriate for studies aimed at identifying factors that impair sensorimotor function and balance control, whereas broader definitions that include dizziness and loss of consciousness are appropriate for studies that also address cardiovascular and neurological causes of falls such as syncope, postural hypotension and transient ischaemic attacks. More recently, the Prevention of Falls Network Europe (ProFaNE) collaborators, in conjunction with international experts in the field and using consensus methodology, have adopted a simpler definition to include falls that occur from all causes, i.e. 'an unexpected event in which the participant comes to rest on the ground, floor or lower level' [2]. A comparable definition has also been adopted by the World Health Organization.[1] This simple definition is appropriate for

---

[1] www.who.int/violence_injury_prevention/unintentional_injuries/falls/falls1/en/

multi-centre studies requiring a core data set or for situations where details of falls are unrecorded (routine surveillance data/accident records), or where a high proportion of subjects cannot provide reliable information about their falls (i.e. those with delirium or cognitive impairment).

Although falls are often referred to as accidents, it has been shown statistically that falls incidence differs significantly from a Poisson distribution [3]. This implies that causal processes are involved in falls and that they are not merely random events.

Falls ascertainment

The earliest published studies on falls were retrospective in design, in that they asked subjects whether and/or how many times they had fallen over in a defined period of time – usually 12 months. This approach has limitations in that subjects have limited accuracy in remembering falls over a prolonged period [4]. More recent studies have used prospective designs, in which subjects are followed up for a period, again usually 12 months, to more accurately determine the incidence of falling. Not surprisingly, these studies have usually reported higher rates of falling. In community studies, the only feasible method of ascertaining falls is by self report and a number of methods have been used to record falls in prospective follow-up periods. These include monthly or bi-monthly mail-out questionnaires [5, 6], weekly [7] or monthly falls calendars [8] and monthly telephone interviews [9].

The ProFaNE collaborators recommend that falls should be recorded using prospective daily recording and a notification system with a minimum of monthly reporting [2]. Telephone or face to face interview should be used to chase missing data and to ascertain further details of falls and injuries. Specific information about the circumstances of any falls can also be ascertained with additional questions on the falls diary forms. An example of a monthly falls calendar is shown in Figure 1.1a, with additional questions in Figure 1.1b. Telephone interviews gain the same information as mail-out questionnaires and falls diaries, but may require many calls to contact active older people. In research studies, fall data should be summarized as: number of falls; number of fallers/non-fallers/frequent fallers; and fall rate per person years [2].

However, even with the most rigorous reporting methodology, it is quite likely that falls are under-reported and that data regarding circumstances surrounding falls are sometimes incomplete or inaccurate. After a fall, older people are often shocked and distressed and may not remember the predisposing factors that led to the fall. Denial is also a factor in under-reporting, as it

SUN	MON	TUES	WED	THURS	FRI	SAT
		1	2	3	4	5
6	7	8	9	10	11	12
13	14	15	16	17	18	19
20	21	22	23	24	25	26
27	28	29	30	31		

Fig. 1.1a   Example of a monthly falls diary.

is common for older people to lay the blame on external factors for their fall, and not count it as a 'true' one. Simply forgetting falls leads to further under-reporting, especially in those with cognitive impairment.

In residential aged care settings, the use of falls record books maintained by nursing staff can provide an ancillary method for improving the accuracy of recording falls. In a study of intermediate care (hostel) residents in Sydney, we found that systematic recording of falls by nurses increased the number of falls reported by 32% [5]. In hospitals, falls incident forms are now commonly used.

The definition of a fall-related injury

The definitions of injurious falls have differed considerably in the literature, due primarily to whether or not minor injuries such as bruises, cuts and abrasions have been classified as fall-related injuries. The ProFaNE collaborators recommend that due to difficulties in standardizing definitions and classifications of fall injury type, the most rigorous definition of a serious fall-related injury is radiologically confirmed peripheral fracture, i.e. fractures of the limbs and limb girdles [2].

The definition of the older person

There is no consistency among studies as to what demographic group constitutes older people. The term is used for age-groups starting from as low as 50 years. However, the most frequently used definition is people aged 65 years and over. Within this age-band, commonly accepted subgroups are those aged 65–74 years, 75–84 years and 85 years and older.

If you have had <u>no falls</u> please stop here, otherwise please continue

1. WHERE HAVE YOU FALLEN?

<u>Inside:</u>

On the one level	Yes [ ]	No [ ]
Getting out of bed	Yes [ ]	No [ ]
Getting out of a chair	Yes [ ]	No [ ]
Using the shower/bath	Yes [ ]	No [ ]
Using the toilet	Yes [ ]	No [ ]
Walking up or down stairs	Yes [ ]	No [ ]

<u>Home entrances or in the garden:</u>

Walking up or down a step/stairs	Yes [ ]	No [ ]
On the one level (e.g. pathway)	Yes [ ]	No [ ]
In the garden	Yes [ ]	No [ ]

<u>Away from home:</u>

On the footpath	Yes [ ]	No [ ]
On a kerb/gutter	Yes [ ]	No [ ]
In a public building	Yes [ ]	No [ ]
Getting out of a vehicle	Yes [ ]	No [ ]
In another person's home	Yes [ ]	No [ ]

Falls not described above (please specify)

2. HOW DID YOU FALL?

(Tick more than one if necessary)

I tripped	[ ]
I slipped	[ ]
I lost my balance	[ ]
My legs gave way	[ ]

Fig. 1.1b   (Cont.)

I felt faint   [ ]

I felt giddy/dizzy   [ ]

I am not sure   [ ]

3. AS A RESULT OF THIS FALL OR FALLS DID YOU SUFFER ANY INJURIES?   Yes [ ]   No [ ]

4. IF YES WHAT TYPE OF INJURIES DID YOU SUFFER?

Bruises   [ ]

Cuts/grazes   [ ]

Broken wrist   [ ]

Broken hip   [ ]

Broken ribs   [ ]

Back pain   [ ]

Thank you very much for your co-operation. Please return it to us by using the enclosed envelope

Fig. 1.1b   Example of additional questions seeking specific information about the circumstances of falls.

The incidence of falls in older people

Community-dwelling older people

In 1977, Exton-Smith examined the incidence of falls in 963 people over the age of 65 years living in England [10]. He found that in women, the proportion that fell increased with age from 30% in the 65–9 year age group to over 50% in those over the age of 85. In men, the proportion that fell increased from 13% in the 65–9 year age group to levels of approximately 30% in those aged 80 years and over.

Retrospective community studies in primarily White populations undertaken since Exton-Smith's work have reported similar findings – that approximately 30% of older persons experience one or more falls per year [11–13]. Campbell *et al.* [11] analysed a stratified population sample of 533 subjects aged 65 years and over, and found that 33% experienced one or more falls in the previous year. Blake *et al.* [13] reported a similar incidence (35%) in a study of 1042 subjects aged 65 years and over. In a large study of 2793 subjects aged 65 years and over, Prudham and Grimley-Evans [12] estimated an annual incidence for accidental falls of 28%, a figure identical to that found in

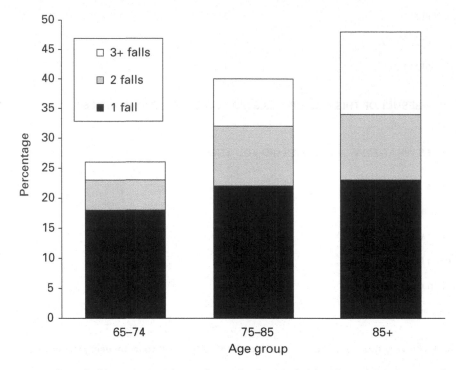

Fig. 1.2   Proportion of older women who took part in the Randwick Falls and Fractures Study who reported falling once, twice, or three or more times in a 12 month period. Diagram adapted from Lord *et al*. [15].

the Australian Dubbo Osteoporosis Epidemiology Study of 1762 older people aged 60 years and over [14].

More recent prospective studies undertaken in community settings have found higher falls incidence rates. In the Randwick Falls and Fractures Study conducted in Australia, we found that 39% of 341 community-dwelling women aged 65 years and over reported one or more falls in a one-year follow-up period [15]. In a large study of 761 subjects aged 70 years and over undertaken in New Zealand, Campbell *et al*. [16] found that 40% of the 465 women and 28% of the 296 men fell at least once in the study period of one year, an overall incidence rate of 35%. In the United States, Tinetti *et al*. [8] found an incidence rate of one or more falls of 32% in 336 subjects aged 75 years and over. Similar rates have been reported in Canada by O'Loughlin *et al*. [9] in a 48-week prospective study of a random sample of 409 community-dwelling people aged 65 years and over (29%), and in Finland community-dwelling people aged 70 years and over by Luukinen *et al*. in 833 from five rural districts (30%) [17].

Fall rates also increase beyond the age of 65 years. Figure 1.2 shows the proportion of women who took part in the Randwick Falls and Fractures Study [15] who reported falling once, twice, or three or more times in a 12 month period.

The prospective studies that have reported the incidence of multiple or recurrent falls are also in agreement. The incidence of two or more falls in a follow-up year reported in five studies ranges between 11% and 21% (average 15%). Three studies have reported data for three or more falls and all report an incidence of 8%.

Rigorous data regarding falls incidence in older people from non-White populations is limited. However, studies of fall rates in Japanese people living in both Japan and Hawaii reveal a contrasting picture to that of White populations. Aoyaga *et al.* [18] studied falls among 1534 (624 men, 910 women) community-dwelling people aged 65 years and over in Japan. They found that only 9% of the men and 19% of the women reported one or more falls in the previous year. Similarly low incidence rates have also been found in seven other large community studies undertaken in Japan [19]. As part of the Hawaii Osteoporosis Study, Davis *et al.* prospectively assessed falls incidence among older Japanese men and women living in Hawaii [20]. The falls incidence rates were 13.9 per 100 person years for men and 27.6 per 100 person years for women, representing about half the fall rates of comparable studies in predominantly White populations.

In a subsequent study, Davis *et al.* attempted to identify neuromuscular performance measures and functional disabilities that could account for such differences in fall rates [21]. They found that the Japanese women had faster walking speeds, chair stands and performed better on a series of balance tests. On the other hand, the White women had greater strength, particularly of the quadriceps, and faster hand and foot reaction times. After adjusting for the neuromuscular test results and the number of functional disabilities, the odds ratio for the risk of falls remained essentially the same. It is possible that the better performances in the more functional strength and balance tests that translate more directly to activities of daily living could explain the lower risk of falls among Japanese women.

Finally, Ellis and Trent compared risks for falls and their consequences among 104 902 people from four major race/ethnic groups who were admitted to non-federal hospitals in California from 1995 to 1997 [22]. Rates per 100 000 for the same level hospitalized fall injuries for Whites (161) were distinctively higher than for Blacks (64), Hispanics (43) and Asian/Pacific Islanders (35). Whites were also more likely to have suffered a fracture and to be discharged to long term care, suggesting poorer outcomes and greater injury severity. It is possible that differing levels of bone density, medical insurance and family support may account for some of these differences observed among the groups.

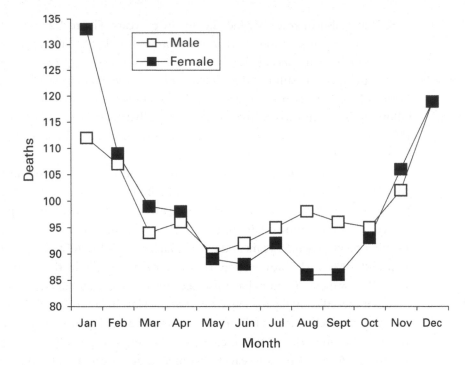

Fig. 1.3   Deaths from accidental falls – annualized monthly ratios; 1993–7 [23].

Seasonal variations in falls frequency

It is possible that the ambient temperature may lead to a seasonal variation in the incidence of falls. People tend to hurry more in colder weather, and mild hypothermia and slowed responses are more common. Equally, people tend to be less active in winter, the hours of daylight are shorter and vitamin D deficiency is more likely. There appears to be a seasonal variation in deaths from accidental falls as illustrated in Figure 1.3 which shows annualized monthly ratios in England and Wales for 1993–7 [23].

In a Finnish study, Luukinen *et al.* found that the incidence of outdoor falls was higher in periods of extreme cold [24]. However, there was no association between indoor falls and temperature which they attributed to adequately heated houses. A similar study in the UK found that apart from the presence of ground frost, there was no significant association between the prevailing weather conditions and the incidence of hip fractures [25]. The precise effect of seasonal change on the epidemiology of falls is therefore somewhat unclear.

Secular trends in falls injuries

Two recent studies have examined routinely collected fall injury data as a means of assessing secular trends in falls incidence. In Finland, Kannus *et al.* analysed data from the National Hospital Discharge Register and found that the number of older people with fall-induced injuries increased between 1970 and 1995 at a rate that could not be explained simply by demographic changes [26]. The age-standardized incidence increased by 127% in women (from 648 in 1970 to 1469 in 1995) and by 124% in men (from 434 in 1970 to 972 in 1995). Secular changes in falls hospitalization rates have also been examined in the Australian states of Victoria and South Australia [27]. Between 1988 and 1997, age-standardized falls hospitalization rates increased significantly – by 32% in Victoria and 5% in South Australia. Such increases may partially account for the commonly found secular increases in hip and other fractures reported in several Western countries [28, 29].

Residents of residential aged care facilities

Studies on the prevalence of falls have also been conducted in residential aged care facilities, where the reported frequency of falling is considerably higher than among those living in their own homes. For example, Luukinen *et al.* [30] estimate that among people aged 70 and over in Finland, the rate of falling in the residential care population is three times higher than that among those living independently in the community.

Prospective studies conducted in nursing homes have found 12-month falls incidence rates ranging from 30% to 56%. In an early study, Fernie *et al.* [31] monitored 205 nursing home residents for 12 months and found 30% of the men and 42% of the women had one or more falls. More recently, studies have reported higher falls incidence rates in older people living in residential care facilities. Lipsitz *et al.* [32] found that 40% of 901 ambulatory nursing home residents fell two or more times in six months, and Yip and Cumming [33] found that 56% of 126 nursing home residents fell at least once in a year.

Two other studies have calculated falls incidence rates across a number of nursing homes. Rubenstein *et al.* [34] summarized the findings from five published and two unpublished studies on the incidence of falls in long term care facilities. They calculated that the incidence rate ranged between 60% to 290% per bed, with a mean fall incidence rate of 170% or 1.7 falls per person per year. Thapa *et al.* [35] conducted a 12-month prospective study in 12 nursing homes involving 1228 residents. They report that during the 1003 person years of follow up, 548 residents suffered 1585 falls.

Fall rates are also high in residents living in intermediate-care hostels. We found a yearly falls incidence rate for one or more falls of 52%, and for two or more falls of 39% in a hostel population of older people [5]. Tinetti *et al.* [36] also found a high incidence of falling in 79 persons admitted consecutively to intermediate-care facilities – 32% fell two or more times in a three month period.

In the Fracture Risk Epidemiology in the Elderly (FREE) study, 1000 residents from 26 nursing homes and 17 intermediate-care hostels were followed prospectively for a mean period of 15 months to ascertain risk factors for falls [37]. In this period, 621 residents fell at least once: 214 fell once only, 102 fell twice, 77 fell three times, 55 fell four times and 173 fell five or more times. There were 2554 falls in all (5.45 falls/1000 resident bed days), with 786 falls (30.9%) resulting in an injury. Interestingly, there were non-linear associations between physical functioning and falls in this group, and the falling rate was significantly higher in intermediate-care residents (65%) compared with the nursing home residents (58%).

Finally two studies have examined falls incidence in residents of apartment-style retirement villages. Liu *et al.* [38] found a relatively high proportion (61%) of 96 residents fell over a 12 month period. In a randomized controlled trial examining the effects of group exercise on falls incidence, we found that 44% of 199 residents of self-care apartments in the control arm of the study fell on one or more occasions during the one-year trial [39] – a rate that is comparable to community-dwelling people of similar age (age range 62–92, mean = 77 years).

Particular groups

Older people who have suffered a fall are at increased risk of falling again. In a prospective study of 325 community-dwelling persons who had fallen in the previous year, Nevitt *et al.* [7] found that 57% experienced at least one fall in a 12-month follow-up period and 31% had two or more falls. Not surprisingly, falls are also more prevalent in frail older people, in those who have difficulties undertaking activities of daily living, and in those with particular medical conditions that affect posture, balance and gait. Northridge *et al.* [40] reported that when community-dwelling persons were classified as either frail or vigorous, frailer people were more than twice as likely to fall as vigorous people. Similarly, Speechley and Tinetti [41] reported 52% of a frail group fell in a one-year prospective period compared with only 17% of a vigorous group.

Falls are a common presenting condition in hospital emergency departments. Close *et al.* found 20% of patients aged 65 years and over attending an emergency department had a primary diagnosis of a fall [42], and Davies and Kenny reported an even higher percentage (44%) for this age group [43]. Falls also occur frequently when older people are in hospital. Rates vary from approximately 2% in general hospitals where lengths of stay are relatively short [44, 45] to 27% in an acute hospital geriatrics ward [46].

With regard to medical conditions, Mahoney *et al.* [47] found that 14% of older patients fell in the first month after discharge from hospital following a medical illness. Fall rates are also increased in those with stroke, Parkinson's disease and amputations. Forster and Young [48] found that 73% of elderly stroke patients fell within six months of hospital discharge. Jorgensen *et al.* also present evidence that fall rates remain high in this group [49]. In a prospective study, they found that 23% of 111 community-dwelling people with long-standing stroke fell one or more times in a four month period, and that this rate was double that found in 143 age- and sex-matched controls. Annual falls incidence rates above 60% in community-dwelling people with idiopathic Parkinson's disease have been reported in several studies [50–52]. It has also been noted that frequent falls are a problem in Parkinson's disease patients, with 13% reporting falling more than once a week [53]. Falls incidence is also high in older people following lower limb amputation. Kulkarni *et al.* [54] found that 58% of people with a unilateral amputation had at least one fall within a 12 month period before their survey.

Two studies have reported falls incidence rates in people with identified vestibular disorders. In a study of 247 people with vestibular pathology (mean age = 63 years), Whitney *et al.* found a six-month retrospective falls incidence of 37% [55]. Interestingly, subjects aged less than 65 years reported more falls than those aged 65 years and over. In the second study, Herdman *et al.* measured falls incidence in people aged 24 to 89 years with unilateral (n = 70) and bilateral (n = 45) vestibular hypofunction confirmed by vestibular function testing [56]. In those with unilateral vestibular loss, fall incidence was not different from that expected in an aged matched community-based population. In those with bilateral vestibular loss, falls incidence was 51% in those aged 65–74 years but only 18% in those aged 75 years and over. Taken together, the findings of these studies indicate that falls incidence is not particularly elevated in people with identified vestibular disorders, despite these conditions having a marked impact on balance. It appears that people with vestibular impairments are aware of their manifestly poor balance and adopt appropriate corrective strategies. Both Whitney *et al.* and Herdman *et al.* also suggest that the lower incidence of falls in older people with vestibular disorders may be due, at least in part, to a decrease in risk-taking behaviours.

Fall rates have been reported for small samples of older people with cognitive impairment. Tinetti *et al.* reported a 12-month incidence rate of 67% in 24 community-dwellers with cognitive impairment as part of a larger trial [8], and van Dijk [57] found a 12-month falls incidence of 85% in 71 nursing home residents with dementia. In a recent randomized controlled trial examining the effectiveness of a multifactorial falls prevention strategy in older people with cognitive impairment and dementia presenting to an accident and emergency department, Shaw *et al.* found that 80% of the 114 subjects randomized to the conventional care control group fell within a prospective period of one year [58]. These high incidence rates appear to be accurate estimates as cognitive impairment has been found to be a strong independent risk factor for falls in many prospective studies (see Chapter 6).

Increased falls incidence is also evident in persons with arthritis and diabetes. We recently conducted a study of 684 community-dwelling men and women aged 75–98 years, of which 283 reported lower limb osteoarthritis [59]. A total of 137 subjects with arthritis (48.4%) fell in the previous year, compared with 157 (39.2%) subjects without arthritis (sex-adjusted RR = 1.22, 95% CI = 1.03–1.46). Similarly those with arthritis reported significantly more injurious falls than those without arthritis, 94 subjects (33.2%) and 104 subjects (25.9%) respectively (sex-adjusted RR = 1.27, 95% CI = 1.01–1.60).

Finally, falls incidence in older people with diabetes has been reported as part of the Study of Osteoporotic Fractures [60]. This prospective cohort study included 9249 women aged 67 years and over, of which 629 (6.8%) had diabetes, including 99 who used insulin. During an average of 7.2 years, 1640 women (18%) fell more than once a year. Fall rates were lowest in those without diabetes (17%), intermediate in those with non-insulin treated diabetes (26%) and highest in those with insulin-treated diabetes (34%). The authors found that women with diabetes were at an increased risk of falling due in part to increased rates of known fall risk factors, such as poor lower limb sensation and balance.

Falls location

In older community-dwelling people, about 50% of falls occur within their homes and immediate home surroundings (Figure 1.4) [17, 61]. Most falls occur on level surfaces within commonly used rooms such as the bedroom, lounge and kitchen. Comparatively few falls occur in the bathroom, on the stairs, or from ladders and stools. While a proportion of falls involve a hazard such as a loose rug or a slippery floor, many do not involve obvious environmental hazards [61]. The remaining falls occur in public places and other people's homes. Commonly reported environmental factors involved in falls in public places include pavement cracks and misalignments, gutters, steps, construction works, uneven ground, and slippery surfaces.

The location of falls is related to age, sex and frailty. In community-dwelling older women, we found that the number of falls occurring outside the home decreased with age, with a corresponding increase in the number of falls occurring inside the home on a level surface (Figure 1.5) [15]. Campbell *et al.*

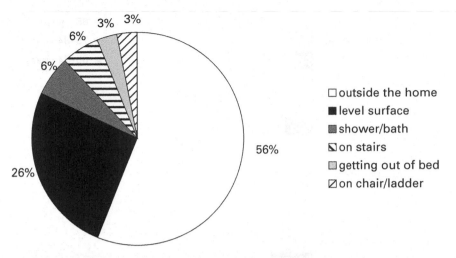

3% 3%

6%

6%

56%

26%

☐ outside the home
■ level surface
▨ shower/bath
◩ on stairs
☐ getting out of bed
▨ on chair/ladder

Fig. 1.4   Location of falls. Some 56% of falls occur outside the home (in the garden, street, footpath or shops), with the remainder (44%) occurring at various locations in the home [15].

[61] found that fewer men than women fell inside the home (44% vs. 65%) and more men fell in the garden (25% vs. 11%). Frailer groups with limited mobility suffer most falls within the home. These findings indicate that the occurrence of falls is strongly related to exposure, that is, they occur in situations where older people are undertaking their usual daily activities. Furthermore, most falls occur during periods of maximum activity in the morning or afternoon, and only about 20% occur between 9 p.m. and 7 a.m. [61].

Consequences of falls

Falls are the leading cause of injury-related hospitalization in persons aged 65 years and over, and account for 14% of emergency admissions [42] and 4% of all hospital admissions in this age group [62]. Hospital admissions resulting from falls are uncommon in young adulthood but with advancing age, the incidence of fall-related admissions increases at an exponential rate. Beyond 65 years, the admission rate due to falls increases exponentially for both sexes, with a nine-fold increase in the rate in males and females between the ages of 65 and 85 years (Figure 1.6) [63]. Falls also account for 40% of injury-related deaths and 1% of total deaths in this age group [64].

Depending on the population studied, anywhere between 22%–60% of older people suffer injuries from falls, 10%–15% suffer serious injuries, 2%–6% suffer fractures and 0.2%–1.5% suffer hip fractures. The most commonly self-reported injuries include superficial cuts and abrasions, bruises, and sprains. The most common injuries that require hospitalization comprise hip fractures, pelvic

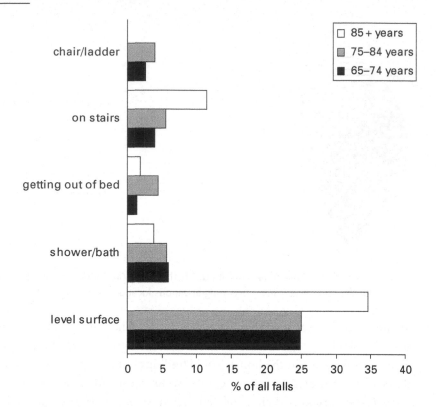

Fig. 1.5   Indoor falls location according to age. Adapted from Lord *et al.* [15].

fractures, other fractures of the leg, fractures of the radius, ulna and humerus, and fractures of the neck and trunk [1, 63, 64].

In terms of morbidity and mortality, one of the most serious fall-related injuries is fracture of the hip. Elderly people often recover slowly from hip fractures and are vulnerable to post-operative complications. In many cases, hip fractures result in death and of those who survive, many never regain complete mobility. Marottoli *et al.* [65] analysed the outcomes of 120 subjects from a cohort study who suffered a hip fracture over a six year period. They found that before their fractures, 86% could dress independently, 75% could walk independently and 63% could climb a flight of stairs. Six months after their injuries, these percentages had fallen to 49%, 15% and 8%, respectively.

Another consequence of falling is the 'long lie' – remaining on the ground or floor for more than an hour after a fall. The long lie is a marker of weakness, illness and social isolation, and is associated with high mortality rates among older people. Time spent on the floor is associated with fear of falling, muscle damage, pneumonia, pressure sores, dehydration and hypothermia [7, 66, 67]. Wild *et al.* [68] found that half of those who lie on the floor for an hour or

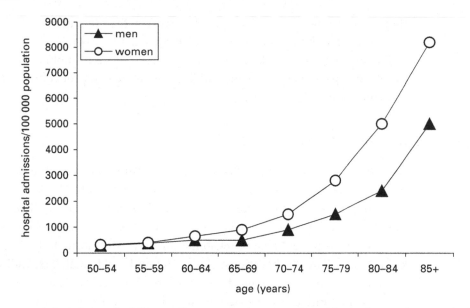

Fig. 1.6   Hospital admissions for falls according to age and gender. Adapted from Cripps and Carman [63].

longer die within six months, even if there is no direct injury from the fall. Vellas *et al.* [69] found that more than 20% of patients admitted to hospital as a result of a fall had been on the ground for an hour or more. Such a figure could be expected as Tinetti *et al.* [70] found that up to 47% of non-injured fallers are unable to get up off the floor without assistance.

Falls can result in restriction of activity and fear of falling (see Chapter 5), reduced quality of life, and loss of independence. In a study of 5093 older people, Kiel *et al.* [71] found that fallers, especially recurrent fallers, were at a greater risk of reporting subsequent difficulties with activities of daily living, instrumental activities of daily living and more physically demanding activities, after controlling for age, sex, self-perceived health status and pre-existing difficulties with activities of daily living. Tinetti and Williams found similar associations in a study involving 957 community-dwelling persons over the age of 71 years [72]. They found that after adjusting for potential confounding factors, both non-injurious and injurious falls were associated with declines in basic and instrumental activities of daily living over a three year prospective period. Furthermore, those who suffered two or more non-injurious falls reported declines in social activities and those who suffered one or more injurious falls reported reduced physical activity levels.

Falls can lead to an excessive fear of falling, sometimes referred to as the 'post-fall syndrome' which is manifest as a loss of confidence, hesitancy, tentativeness, with a resultant loss of mobility and independence. It has been found that after falling, many older people report a fear of falling [72, 73] and a curtailing of activities due to a fear of further falls [7, 74].

Finally, falls can also lead to disability and decreased mobility which often results in dependency on others, and hence an increased probability of requiring residential care [75, 76].

The economic cost of falls

As indicated above, falls in older people are common and can lead to numerous disabling conditions, extensive hospital stays and death. It is therefore not surprising that falls constitute a significant health care cost. Fall-related costs can include the direct costs such as doctor visits, acute hospital and nursing home care, outpatient clinics, rehabilitation stays, diagnostic tests, medications, home care, home modifications, equipment and residential care. Indirect costs include carer and patient morbidity and mortality costs. There are many difficulties and limitations involved in estimating the economic cost of any disease or condition. Problems exist because cost data are only estimates, and many costs are only relevant to the country in which they are incurred. Furthermore, because of inflation and other economic and health care factors, costs are outdated soon after they are published.

A number of researchers have estimated the hospital costs of an injurious fall in absolute terms and as a proportion of health budgets [58, 77–84]. In a report to the US Congress in 1989, Rice and MacKenzie [80] calculated that in 1985, nearly US$10 billion, or 6% of the lifetime cost of injury in the United States, was attributable to falls in older people. Furthermore, falls account for 70% of all injury-related costs in elderly people. The cost per injured person in 1985 was US$4226, which was nearly double that of the average cost per injured person for all age groups. Englander et al. [81] updated the costs of falls as presented by Rice and MacKenzie [80] from 1985 US dollars to 1994 US dollars. They projected the cost of falls in 1994 to total US$20.2 billion, with a cost per injured person being US$7399. The authors further extrapolated these figures to the year 2020 and estimated the cost of falls injuries at US$32.4 billion.

A study in the United Kingdom found the total cost to the UK government from accidental falls was nearly £1 billion in 1999 [82]. The major component was hospital admissions which accounted for nearly half (49.4%) of the total costs. Long term care costs were the second highest, accounting for 41%, primarily in those aged 75 years and over.

Two recent reports have examined the current and projected costs of fall injury in Australia. A report examining all injury categories found that falls injuries were the most costly of any injury mechanism [83]. For the year of the study (1998–9) the direct costs resulting from falls (hospitalization, ambulance, emergency department presentation, non-hospital medical care, non-hospital allied health care and non-hospital pharmaceutical costs) totalled AUD$333 million. This represented 62.8% of direct costs of all unintentional injury categories. Direct injury costs for the 11 most common injury categories are shown in Figure 1.7.

The second report prepared for the Australian Government [84] found that ageing of the Australian population will have a significant impact on the Australian health system due to the increased number of older people suffering fall-related injuries. By 2051, the total health cost attributable to fall-related injury will increase almost three-fold from current levels to AUD$1375 million per annum if age-specific fall rates remain unchanged. Some 886 000 additional hospital bed days or the equivalent of 2500 additional beds permanently allo-cated to fall injury treatment will be required for the increased demand and 3320 additional nursing home places will be required. The report concluded that to maintain cost parity over this period, prevention strategies will need to deliver approximately a 66% reduction in falls incidence.

To complement the population-aggregated costs presented above, we recently conducted an analysis of the cost of individual injurious falls that occurred in a sample of 578 community-dwelling people aged 75 years and over. For each fall we ascertained costs for hospitalization, ambulance use, emergency department presentation, non-hospital medical care, non-hospital allied health care, and non-hospital pharmaceutical and diagnostic investigations. In addition, we sought information on out-of-pocket expenses, including the repair of broken spectacles, the purchase of non-prescription analgesics, installation of safety rails in the home, and the purchase of bandages and other items for wound care. In the 12-month surveillance period, 275 subjects suffered 534 falls. We found that 225 falls required medical attention. Of these falls, the average cost of a fall not requiring a hospital visit was AUD$205, the average cost of a fall requiring a visit to a hospital emergency department was AUD$1040 (AUD$420 hospital costs and AUD$620 post-hospital costs) and the average cost of a fall which required admission to hospital was AUD$12 300 (AUD$10 000 hospital costs and AUD$2300 post-hospital costs) per person. Overall, hospital costs accounted for 67% of the total cost of falls.

Conclusion

Despite the disparate methodologies of falls ascertainment used in the above studies, the incidence rates reported are remarkably similar. Approximately one-third of older White people living in the community fall at least once a year, with many suffering multiple falls. Fall rates are lower in Japanese, Black

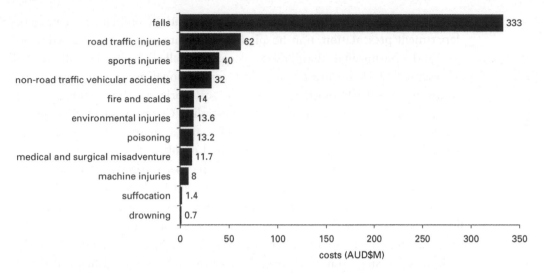

Fig. 1.7   Direct costs for 11 unintentional fall injury categories. Falls injuries account for 62.8% of total direct costs. Adapted from Potter-Forbes and Aisbett [83].

Americans, Hispanics and Asian/Pacific Islanders. There appears to be a seasonal variation in the rate of falls in countries with cold climates and there is some evidence that falls incidence has been increasing over the past one or two decades. Fall rates are higher in older community-dwelling women (40%) than in older men (28%) and continue to increase with age above 65 years. The incidence of falls is increased in people living in retirement villages, hostels and nursing homes, in those who have fallen in the past year, and in those with particular medical conditions that affect muscle strength, balance and gait. In community-dwelling older people, about 50% of falls occur within the home and 50% in public places. Falls account for 4% of hospital admissions, 40% of injury-related deaths and 1% of total deaths in persons aged 65 years and over. The major serious injuries that result from falls include fractures of the wrist, pelvis and hip. Falls can also result in disability, restriction of activity and fear of falling, which can reduce quality of life and independence, and contribute to an older person being admitted to a nursing home. Finally, as many fall-related injuries require medical treatment including hospitalization, falls constitute a condition requiring considerable healthcare expenditure.

REFERENCES

1. M. J. Gibson, R. O. Andres, B. Isaacs, T. Radebaugh & J. Worm-Petersen, The prevention of falls in later life. A report of the Kellogg International Work Group on the Prevention of Falls by the Elderly. *Danish Medical Bulletin*, **34**(Suppl 4) (1987), 1–24.

2. S. E. Lamb, E. C. Jørstad-Stein, K. Hauer & C. Becker, Prevention of Falls Network Europe and Outcomes Consensus Group. Development of a common outcome data set for fall injury prevention trials: the Prevention of Falls Network Europe consensus. *Journal of the American Geriatrics Society,* **53** (2005), 1618–22.

3. J. Grimley-Evans, Fallers, non-fallers and Poisson. *Age and Ageing,* **19** (1990), 268–9.

4. S. R. Cummings, M. C. Nevitt & S. Kidd, Forgetting falls. The limited accuracy of recall of falls in the elderly. *Journal of the American Geriatrics Society,* **36** (1988), 613–16.

5. S. R. Lord, R. D. Clark & I. W. Webster, Physiological factors associated with falls in an elderly population. *Journal of the American Geriatrics Society,* **39** (1991), 1194–200.

6. S. R. Lord, J. A. Ward, P. Williams & K. J. Anstey, Physiological factors associated with falls in older community-dwelling women. *Journal of the American Geriatrics Society,* **42** (1994), 1110–17.

7. M. C. Nevitt, S. R. Cummings, S. Kidd & D. Black, Risk factors for recurrent nonsyncopal falls. A prospective study. *Journal of the American Medical Association,* **261** (1989), 2663–8.

8. M. E. Tinetti, M. Speechley & S. F. Ginter, Risk factors for falls among elderly persons living in the community. *New England Journal of Medicine,* **319** (1988), 1701–7.

9. J. L. O'Loughlin, Y. Robitaille, J. F. Boivin & S. Suissa, Incidence of and risk factors for falls and injurious falls among the community-dwelling elderly. *American Journal of Epidemiology,* **137** (1993), 342–54.

10. A. N. Exton-Smith, Functional consequences of ageing: clinical manifestations. In *Care of the Elderly: Meeting the Challenge of Dependency,* ed. A. N. Exton-Smith & J. Grimley-Evans. (London: Academic Press, 1977).

11. A. J. Campbell, J. Reinken, B. C. Allan & G. S. Martinez, Falls in old age: a study of frequency and related clinical factors. *Age and Ageing,* **10** (1981), 264–70.

12. D. Prudham & J. Grimley-Evans, Factors associated with falls in the elderly: a community study. *Age and Ageing,* **10** (1981), 141–6.

13. A. Blake, K. Morgan, M. Bendall *et al.,* Falls by elderly people at home – prevalence and associated factors. *Age and Ageing,* **17** (1988), 365–72.

14. S. R. Lord, P. N. Sambrook, C. Gilbert *et al.,* Postural stability, falls and fractures in the elderly: results from the Dubbo Osteoporosis Epidemiology Study. *Medical Journal of Australia,* **160** (1994), 684–5, 688–91.

15. S. R. Lord, J. A. Ward, P. Williams & K. J. Anstey, An epidemiological study of falls in older community-dwelling women: the Randwick Falls and Fractures Study. *Australian Journal of Public Health,* **17** (1993), 240–5.

16. A. J. Campbell, M. J. Borrie & G. F. Spears, Risk factors for falls in a community-based prospective study of people 70 years and older. *Journal of Gerontology,* **44** (1989), M112–17.

17. H. Luukinen, K. Koski, P. Laippala & S. L. Kivela, Predictors for recurrent falls among the home-dwelling elderly. *Scandinavian Journal of Primary Health Care,* **13** (1995), 294–9.

18. K. Aoyagi, P. D. Ross, J. W. Davis *et al.,* Falls among community-dwelling elderly in Japan. *Journal of Bone and Mineral Research,* **13** (1998), 1468–74.

19. S. Yasumara, Frequency of falls and fractures in the elderly. *Japanese Medical Association Journal,* **44** (2001), 192–7.

20. J. W. Davis, P. D. Ross, M. C. Nevitt & R. D. Wasnich, Incidence rates of falls among Japanese men and women living in Hawaii. *Journal of Clinical Epidemiology*, **50** (1997), 589–94.

21. J. W. Davis, M. C. Nevitt, R. D. Wasnich & P. D. Ross, A cross-cultural comparison of neuromuscular performance, functional status, and falls between Japanese and white women. *Journal of Gerontology*, **54** (1999), M288–92.

22. A. A. Ellis & R. B. Trent, Hospitalized fall injuries and race in California. *Injury Prevention*, **7** (2001), 316–20.

23. Office for National Statistics, 1997 Mortality Statistics: Injury and Poisons. Number: 0 11 621259 4. (London: The Stationery Office, 1999).

24. H. Luukinen, K. Koski & S. L. Kivela, The relationship between outdoor temperature and the frequency of falls among the elderly in Finland. *Journal of Epidemiology and Community Health*, **50** (1996), 107.

25. M. J. Parker & S. Martin, Falls, hip fractures and the weather. *European Journal of Epidemiology*, **10** (1994), 441–2.

26. P. Kannus, J. Pakkari, S. Koskinen *et al.*, Fall-induced injuries and deaths among older adults. *Journal of the American Medical Association*, **281** (1999), 1895–9.

27. K. Hill, N. Kerse, F. Lentini *et al.*, Falls: a comparison of trends in community, hospital and mortality data in older Australians. *Aging – Clinical and Experimental Research*, **14** (2002), 18–27.

28. P. Kannus, S. Niemi, J. Parkkari *et al.*, Hip fractures in Finland between 1970 and 1997 and predictions for the future. *The Lancet*, **353** (1999), 802–5.

29. T. Spector, C. Cooper & A. F. Lewis, Trends in admission for hip fractures in England and Wales. *British Medical Journal*, **300** (1990), 1173–4.

30. H. Luukinen, K. Koski, L. Hiltunen, S. L. Kivela, Incidence rate of falls in an aged population in northern finland. *Journal Of Clinical Epidemiology*, **47** (1994), 843–50.

31. G. R. Fernie, C. I. Gryfe, P. J. Holliday & A. Llewellyn, The relationship of postural sway in standing to the incidence of falls in geriatric subjects. *Age and Ageing*, **11** (1982), 11–16.

32. L. A. Lipsitz, P. V. Jonsson, M. M. Kelley & J. S. Koestner, Causes and correlates of recurrent falls in ambulatory frail elderly. *Journal of Gerontology*, **46** (1991), M114–122.

33. Y. B. Yip & R. G. Cumming, The association between medications and falls in Australian nursing-home residents. *Medical Journal of Australia*, **160** (1994), 14–18.

34. L. Z. Rubenstein, A. S. Robbins, B. L. Schulman *et al.*, Falls and instability in the elderly [clinical conference]. *Journal of the American Geriatrics Society*, **36** (1988), 266–78.

35. P. B. Thapa, K. G. Brockman, P. Gideon, R. L. Fought & W. A. Ray, Injurious falls in nonambulatory nursing home residents: a comparative study of circumstances, incidence, and risk factors. *Journal of the American Geriatrics Society*, **44** (1996), 273–8.

36. M. E. Tinetti, T. F. Williams & R. Mayewski, Fall risk index for elderly patients based on number of chronic disabilities. *American Journal of Medicine*, **80** (1986), 429–34.

37. S. R. Lord, L. M. March, I. D. Cameron *et al.*, Differing risk factors for falls in nursing home and intermediate-care residents who can and cannot stand unaided. *Journal of the American Geriatrics Society*, **51** (2003), 1645–50.

38. B. A. Liu, A. K. Topper, R. A. Reeves, C. Gryfe & B. E. Maki, Falls among older people: relationship to medication use and orthostatic hypotension. *Journal of the American Geriatrics Society*, **43** (1995), 1141–5.

39. S. R. Lord, S. Castell, J. Corcoran *et al.*, The effect of group exercise on physical functioning and falls in frail older people living in retirement villages: a randomised controlled trial. *Journal of the American Geriatrics Society*, **51** (2003), 1685–92.

40. M. E. Northridge, M. C. Nevitt, J. L. Kelsey & B. Link, Home hazards and falls in the elderly: the role of health and functional status. *American Journal of Public Health*, **85** (1995), 509–15.

41. M. Speechley & M. Tinetti, Falls and injuries in frail and vigorous community elderly persons. *Journal of the American Geriatrics Society*, **39** (1991), 46–52.

42. J. Close, M. Ellis, R. Hooper *et al.*, Prevention of falls in the elderly trial (PROFET): a randomised controlled trial. *The Lancet*, **353** (1999), 93–7.

43. A. J. Davies and R. A. Kenny, Falls presenting to the accident and emergency department: types of presentation and risk factor profile. *Age and Ageing*, **2** (1996), 362–6.

44. G. A. Clark, A study of falls among elderly hospitalized patients. *Australian Journal of Advanced Nursing*, **2** (1985), 34–44.

45. J. Donham, C. Sadewhite & M. Seltzer, Identifying characteristics of the fall-prone medical-surgical patient. *Kansas Nurse*, **62** (1977), 5–6.

46. D. Oliver, M. Britton, P. Seed, F. C. Martin & A. H. Hopper, Development and evaluation of evidence based risk assessment tool (STRATIFY) to predict which elderly inpatients will fall: case-control and cohort studies. *British Medical Journal*, **315** (1997), 1049–53.

47. J. Mahoney, M. Sager, N. C. Dunham & J. Johnson, Risk of falls after hospital discharge. *Journal of the American Geriatrics Society*, **42** (1994), 269–74.

48. A. Forster & J. Young, Incidence and consequences of falls due to stroke: a systematic inquiry. *British Medical Journal*, **311** (1995), 83–6.

49. L. Jorgensen, T. Engstad & B. K. Jacobsen, Higher incidence of falls in long-term stroke survivors than in population controls. *Stroke*, **33** (2002), 542–7.

50. A. Schrag, Y. Ben-Shlomo & N. Quinn, How common are complications of Parkinson's disease? *Journal of Neurology*, **249** (2002), 419–23.

51. B. H. Wood, J. A. Bilclough, A. Bowron & R. W. Walker, Incidence and prediction of falls in Parkinson's disease: a prospective multidisciplinary study. *Journal of Neurology, Neurosurgery and Psychiatry*, **72** (2002), 721–5.

52. A. Ashburn, E. Stack, R. M. Pickering & C. D. Ward, A community-dwelling sample of people with Parkinson's disease: characteristics of fallers and non-fallers. *Age and Ageing*, **30** (2001), 47–52.

53. W. C. Koller, S. Glatt, B. Vetere-Overfield & R. Hassanein, Falls and Parkinson's disease. *Clinical Neuropharmacology*, **12** (1989), 98–105.

54. J. Kulkarni, C. Toole, R. Hirons, S. Wright & J. Morris, Falls in patients with lower limb amputations: prevalence and contributing factors. *Physiotherapy*, **82** (1996), 130–6.

55. S. L. Whitney, M. T. Hudak & G. F. Marchetti, The dynamic gait index relates to self-reported fall history in individuals with vestibular dysfunction. *Journal of Vestibular Research*, **10** (2000), 99–105.

56. S. J. Herdman, P. Blatt, M. C. Schubert & R. J. Tusa, Falls in patients with vestibular deficits. *American Journal of Otology*, **21** (2000), 847–51.

57. P. T. M. van Dijk, O. R. G. M. Meulenberg, H. J. van del Sande & J. D. F. Habbema, Falls in dementia patients. *Gerontologist*, **33** (1993), 200–4.

58. F. E. Shaw, J. Bond, D. A. Richardson *et al.*, Multifactorial intervention after a fall in older people with cognitive impairment and dementia presenting to the accident and emergency department: randomised controlled trial. *British Medical Journal*, **326** (2003), 73–8.

59. D. Sturnieks, S. R. Lord, A. Tiedemann *et al.*, Physiological risk factors for falls in older people with lower limb arthritis. *Journal of Rheumatology*, **31** (2004), 2272–9.

60. A. V. Schwartz, T. A. Hillier, D. E. Sellmeyer *et al.*, Older women with diabetes have a higher risk of falls: a prospective study. *Diabetes Care*, **25** (2002), 1749–54.

61. A. J. Campbell, M. J. Borrie, G. F. Spears *et al.*, Circumstances and consequences of falls experienced by a community population 70 years and over during a prospective study. *Age and Ageing*, **19** (1990), 136–41.

62. S. P. Baker & A. H. Harvey, Fall injuries in the elderly. *Clinics in Geriatric Medicine*, **1** (1985), 501–12.

63. R. Cripps, & J. Carman, Falls by the elderly in Australia: trends and data for 1998. Injury Research and Statistics Series. (AIHW cat. no. INJCAT 35). (Adelaide: Australian Institute of Health and Welfare, 2001).

64. New South Wales Health Department, The epidemiology of falls in older people in NSW, 1994.

65. R. A. Marottoli, L. F. Berkman & L. M. Cooney, Decline in physical function following hip fracture. *Journal of the American Geriatrics Society*, **40** (1992), 861–6.

66. W. Mallinson & M. Green, Covert muscle injury in aged persons admitted to hospital following falls. *Age and Ageing*, **14** (1985), 174–8.

67. M. B. King & M. E. Tinetti, Falls in community-dwelling older persons. *Journal of the American Geriatrics Society*, **43** (1995), 1146–54.

68. D. Wild, U. S. Nayak & B. Isaacs, How dangerous are falls in old people at home? *British Medical Journal*, **282** (1981), 266–8.

69. B. Vellas, F. Cayla, H. Bocquet, F. De Pemille & J. L. Albarede, Prospective study of restriction of activity in old people after falls. *Age and Ageing*, **16** (1987), 189–93.

70. M. E. Tinetti, W. L. Liu & E. B. Claus, Predictors and prognosis of inability to get up after falls among elderly persons. *Journal of the American Medical Association*, **269** (1993), 65–70.

71. D. P. Kiel, P. O. O'Sullivan, J. M. Teno & V. Mor, Health care utilization and functional status in the aged following a fall. *Medical Care*, **29** (1991), 221–8.

72. M. E. Tinetti & C. S. Williams, The effect of falls and fall injuries on functioning in community-dwelling older persons. *Journal of Gerontology*, **53** (1998), M112–19.

73. M. E. Tinetti, D. E. Mendes, C. F. Leon, J. T. Doucette & D. I. Baker, Fear of falling and fall-related efficacy in relationship to functioning among community-living elders. *Journal of Gerontology*, **49** (1994), M140–147.

74. B. J. Vellas, S. J. Wayne, L. J. Romero, R. N. Baumgartner & P. J. Garry, Fear of falling and restriction of mobility in elderly fallers. *Age and Ageing*, **26** (1997), 189–93.

75. S. R. Lord, Predictors of nursing home placement and mortality of residents in intermediate care. *Age and Ageing,* **23** (1994), 499–504.
76. M. E. Tinetti & C. S. Williams, Falls, injuries due to falls, and the risk of admission to a nursing home. *New England Journal of Medicine,* **337** (1997), 1279–84.
77. B. H. Alexander, F. P. Rivara & M. E. Wolf, The cost and frequency of hospitalization for fall-related injuries in older adults. *American Journal of Public Health,* **82** (1992), 1020–3.
78. D. L. Covington, J. G. Maxwell & T. V. Clancy, Hospital resources used to treat the injured elderly at North Carolina trauma centers. *Journal of the American Geriatrics Society,* **41** (1993), 847–52.
79. H. Sjogren & U. Bjornstig, Unintentional injuries among elderly people: incidence, causes, severity, and costs. *Accident Analysis and Prevention,* **21** (1989), 233–42.
80. D. P. Rice & E. J. MacKenzie, *Cost of Injury in the United States: a Report to Congress* (San Francisco: Institute for Health and Ageing, University of California, 1989).
81. F. Englander, T. J. Hodson & R. A. Terregrossa, Economic dimensions of slip and fall injuries. *Journal of Forensic Sciences,* **41** (1996), 733–46.
82. P. Scuffham, S. Chaplin & R. Legood, Incidence and costs of unintentional falls in older people in the United Kingdom. *Journal of Epidemiology and Community Health,* **57** (2003), 740–4.
83. M. Potter-Forbes & C. Aisbett, *Injury Costs! A Valuation of the Burden of Injury in New South Wales in 1998–1999* (Sydney: NSW Injury Risk Management Research Centre, University of New South Wales, 2003).
84. J. Moller, Projected costs of fall related injury to older persons due to demographic change in Australia. (Publication 3314). (Canberra: Commonwealth Government, 2003).

2

Postural stability and falls

Postural stability can be defined as the ability of an individual to maintain the position of the body, or more specifically, its centre of mass, within specific boundaries of space, referred to as *stability limits*. Stability limits are boundaries in which the body can maintain its position without changing the base of support [1]. This definition of postural stability is useful as it highlights the need to discuss stability in the context of a particular task or activity. For example, the stability limit of normal relaxed standing is the area bounded by the two feet on the ground, whereas the stability limit of unipedal stance is reduced to the area covered by the single foot in contact with the ground. Due to this reduction in the size of the stability limit, unipedal stance is an inherently more challenging task requiring greater postural control.

Regardless of the task being performed, maintaining postural stability requires the complex integration of sensory information regarding the position of the body relative to the surroundings and the ability to generate forces to control body movement. Thus, postural stability requires the interaction of musculo-skeletal and sensory systems. The musculo-skeletal component of postural stability encompasses the biomechanical properties of body segments, muscles and joints. The sensory components include vision, vestibular function and somatosensation, which act to inform the brain of the position and movement of the body in three-dimensional space. Linking these two components together are the higher level neurological processes enabling anticipatory mechanisms responsible for planning a movement and adaptive mechanisms responsible for the ability to react to changing demands of the particular task [1].

Normal ageing is associated with changes in function of each of the subcomponents of musculo-skeletal and sensory systems which contribute to postural stability [2–5]. Consequently, ageing may manifest as a measurable deficit in any task involving maintaining postural stability, such as quiet standing, leaning, performing voluntary movements and responding to external perturbations. This chapter reviews the available literature regarding age-associated changes in postural stability for each of these tasks and their relationship to falls.

Standing

Normal relaxed standing is characterized by small amounts of *postural sway*, which has been defined by Sheldon as 'the constant small deviations from the vertical and their subsequent correction to which all human beings are subject when standing upright' [6]. Control of postural sway when standing involves continual muscle activity (primarily of the calf muscles), and requires an integrated reflex response to visual, vestibular and somatosensory inputs [7]. The relative contribution of each of these systems has been determined by experimentally blocking each of these inputs and measuring the subsequent increase in postural sway. The role of vision has been assessed by simply asking the subjects to close their eyes. Vestibular input has been minimized by tilting the head [8] or assessing the ability of subjects to balance an equivalent mechanical body [9]. Somatosensory input has been blocked by ischaemia [9], standing on compliant surfaces [10, 11] or immersing the feet in cold water [12–14]. Such investigations have revealed that if any of these inputs are removed, postural sway increases. Although the extent to which one input can compensate for the loss of another is still unclear, there is some evidence that peripheral sensation is the most important sensory system in the regulation of standing balance in older adults [11].

The generalized decline in sensory functions due to normal ageing and its contribution to increased postural sway have been widely evaluated in the literature. Although interest in the measurement of sway dates back to the classic studies on tabes dorsalis by Romberg in 1853 [15], the first attempt to assess age-related changes in postural sway was conducted by Hellbrandt and Braun in 1939 [16], who measured subjects aged from three to 86 years. The results showed that the magnitude of sway was largest in the very young and very old subjects. A similar study by Boman and Javalisto [17] measured sway with an overhead camera in subjects aged 18–30 and 61–88 years, and reported that sway was greater in the elderly group, particularly in those aged over 80 years. Since these early investigations, a large number of studies have reported age-associated increases in standing postural sway after the age of 30 years using various swaymeters, optical systems and force platforms, particularly when subjects close their eyes [6, 18–40]. There is no clear consensus in the literature regarding gender differences in sway; although some studies report higher postural sway values in women compared to men across a range of age groups [18, 21, 24], other authors have reported no significant differences [27, 29, 34, 41].

Factors found to be highly correlated with increased sway include reduced lower extremity muscle strength [11, 42–45], reduced peripheral sensation [22, 43, 46–49], poor near visual acuity [11, 50] and slowed reaction time [11, 51]. We have previously found that while reaction time is not associated with sway when standing on a firm surface, when subjects stand on a compliant foam rubber surface a significant association between sway and reaction time is evident [11]. This suggests that subjects can perceive large amounts of sway and therefore consciously react to control their body movements. Smaller associations between vestibular function and sway have been reported [8, 11, 22, 52]. Postural sway does not appear to be strongly associated with anthropometric measures. Danis *et al.* [53] reported that skeletal alignment was not associated with postural sway on a force plate, however, Lichtenstein *et al.* [50] and Era *et al.* [43] reported that low body mass is associated with greater sway in both men and women. More recently, Kejonen *et al.* [54] measured a broad range of anthropometric parameters in 100 people aged 31–80 years and found that few measures were strongly correlated with body displacement when standing.

Measurement of postural sway when standing has been reported to be a useful predictor of falls in older people. These investigations have taken two forms: cross-sectional studies which classify subjects as 'fallers' or 'non-fallers' based on self-reported previous history of experiencing a fall, and prospective studies which measure balance variables among a group of subjects, then follow them over a period of time to delineate fallers from non-fallers. Although the evidence is not entirely consistent, a number of cross-sectional studies have reported significantly greater sway in subjects with a history of falling compared to non-fallers [21, 41, 55, 56]. Similarly, numerous prospective studies have revealed that the measurement of an individual's sway is a useful predictor of the risk of falling during follow-up periods [57–62].

In our studies we have found that fallers show greater sway in four test conditions: standing on a firm base with the eyes open; standing on a firm base with the eyes closed; standing on a 15 cm thick high density foam rubber mat with the eyes open; and standing on the foam rubber with the eyes closed [57, 63–65]. In each of these studies, we have used a portable 'sway-meter' which records the displacements of the body at the level of the waist (see Figure 2.1). We have also noted that an inability to maintain balance on the foam at all is associated with falling.

In addition to the investigation of standing postural sway, a number of other standing tests have been developed which provide a greater challenge to the postural control system. One technique for further challenging the postural control system is simply to alter foot position, thereby decreasing the size of the

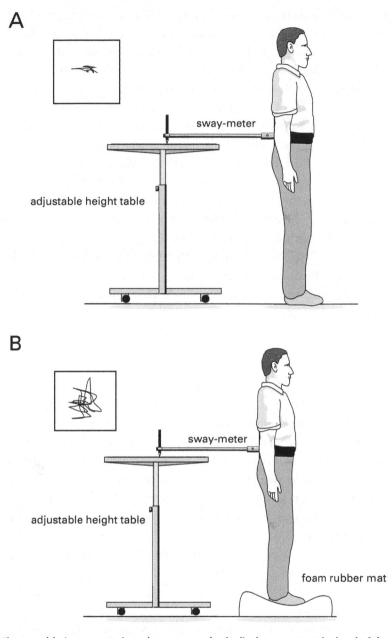

Fig. 2.1   The portable 'sway-meter' used to measure body displacements at the level of the waist. A: sway on the floor, B: sway on a foam rubber mat.

stability limit. This concept was first explored by Romberg [15], who assessed balance by observing the ability of patients to stand with their feet together. The effect of foot position on sway has more recently been evaluated in detail by numerous authors [66–69], who evaluated postural stability on a force plate with subjects standing with their feet in varying positions (i.e. toe-in, toe-out, variations in space between the heels and tandem stance). Increased sway was apparent with the more challenging conditions due to the reduction in the size of the stability limit. In accordance with investigations into normal bipedal standing, ageing is also associated with poorer performance in tandem standing [44, 70– 74] and unipedal stance [23, 24, 70–73, 75–79]. We have also found that older people with a history of falls had increased lateral sway with the eyes open and closed when undertaking a near tandem stability test. The fallers were also significantly more likely to take a protective step when undertaking the test with the eyes closed [80]. Consistent with this finding, a recent study of 439 older people in the Netherlands found that an inability to stand in the tandem position for at least ten seconds was a significant independent predictor of recurrent falls in the 12-month follow-up period [62]. Similarly, three studies have reported that performance in the unipedal standing test is also capable of predicting falls in older people [79, 81, 82], however, the utility of timed uni- pedal standing as a falls predictor is limited, as many frail elderly people are unable to complete the test.

Leaning

An alternative approach to challenge postural control is to measure sway when the subject is placed at the perimeter of their stability limit, or to measure the dimensions of the stability limit itself. Hasselkus and Shambes [20] assessed postural sway in young and older women in a normal relaxed stance, and when the subjects leaned forward at the waist by approximately 45 degrees. The results revealed that sway was greater in the older group in both conditions, but par- ticularly so when leaning forward, suggesting that the older women were less able to stabilize their posture when approaching the perimeter of their stability limit. King et al. [83] evaluated the ability of women aged 20 to 91 years to reach as far forward and backward as possible when standing, in order to establish age-related differences in the functional base of support. Decreased functional base of support was evident after the age of 60 years and declined 16% per decade thereafter.

A similar technique is the *functional reach test*, which involves the mea- surement of a subject's ability to reach forward as far as possible with the arm positioned at 90 degrees of shoulder flexion. This test was first described by Duncan et al. [84], who evaluated subjects aged 21 to 87 years and reported a significant age-related decline in functional reach. Similar results were reported by Hageman et al. [34], who reported that older subjects exhibited a smaller mean reach than younger subjects. Subsequent investigations of functional reach have shown the test to be correlated with performance in activities of daily living [85], a predictor of falls [86] and sensitive to improvements in function following rehabilitation [87]. However, a recent investigation by Wernick-Robinson et al. [88] suggested that functional reach is not a valid indicator of dynamic balance, due to the variety of strategies that can be used to extend the arm from the shoulder. More recently, two variations on this test have been proposed – the *lateral reach test* [89] and the *multi-direction reach test* [90]. The lateral reach test involves the clinical measurement of maximal excursion of the extended arm, in conjunction with laboratory measures of centre of pressure displacement, when subjects lean as far as possible to the right and left sides [89]. The multi-direction reach test involves subjects leaning forward, to the right, to the left and backwards while the excursion of their arm is measured [90]. Despite their theoretical advantages over the functional reach test, neither test has been found to be an accurate predictor of falls. In a six-month prospective study, the lateral reach test was not found to differentiate between fallers and non-fallers [91]. The multi-direction reach test has yet to be used in a prospective falls study. However, a cross-sectional investigation found performance on this test to be associated with the Berg Balance Test and Timed Up and Go test, and the backward leaning component to be associated with fear of falling [90].

We have developed two additional leaning tests as measures of postural stability [92]. The *maximum balance range* test involves the subject leaning forward and backward from the ankles as far as possible (without moving their feet or bending at the hips). Maximal antero-posterior distance moved is measured using a pen attached to a rod extending anteriorly from the subject's waist. This technique provides some benefits over the functional reach test, as it avoids problems associated with variations in shoulder movement when extending the arm. The pen records the anterior and posterior movements of the subject on a sheet of graph paper which is fastened to the top of an adjustable height table. Using a similar apparatus, an additional test of *coordinated stability* can be performed in which the subject is asked to bend and rotate their hips without moving the feet. The pen on the end of the rod follows and remains within a convoluted track which is marked on a piece of paper attached to the top of an adjustable height table. To complete the test without errors, subjects have to remain within the track, which is 1.5 cm wide, and be capable of adjusting the position of the pen 29 cm laterally and 18 cm in the antero-posterior plane. A total error score is calculated by summing the number of occasions that the pen on the sway meter failed to stay within the path. Both the maximal balance range and coordinated stability tests have been found to be reliable [92, 93], predictive of falls [94, 95] and sensitive to improvement following exercise intervention in older people [92, 96–98]. An example of the coordinated stability test is shown in Figure 2.2.

Voluntary stepping

To avoid a fall, a three-stage response is required [99, 100]. This involves: (i) perception of a postural threat; (ii) selection of an appropriate corrective response; and (iii) proper response execution. To gain a single measure of this complex, multi-system response, our group has devised the choice stepping reaction time test that requires subjects to perform quick, correctly targeted steps in response to visual cues. We used this test in a study involving 510 retirement village residents aged 62–95 years [101]. These subjects stood on the choice stepping reaction time apparatus, which comprised a $0.8\,m^2$ non-slip black platform containing four white rectangular panels ($32\,cm \times 13\,cm$). Two panels were situated in front of the subject (one in front of each foot) and one panel was situated on each side of the subject (adjacent to each foot). Participants were given practice trials where they were instructed to step on to the two left panels (front and side) with the left foot only and the two right panels (front and side) with the right foot only. The panels were then illuminated in a random order and subjects were instructed to step on to the illuminated panel as quickly as possible, but in a safe manner so as not to lose balance. A total of 20 trials were conducted with five trials for each of the four stepping responses. The choice stepping reaction time test is shown in Figure 2.3. Each subject also underwent assessments of visual contrast sensitivity, lower limb proprioception, lower limb strength, simple reaction time, standing balance (postural sway) and leaning balance (maximal balance range) [102], and completed a questionnaire on falls in the past year. We found that those with a history of falls had significantly increased choice stepping reaction times compared with those who reported no falls. Furthermore, ability to perform this test well was dependent upon adequate visual contrast sensitivity, lower limb extension strength, simple reaction time, and standing and leaning balance control. These measures, which have all been shown to be important risk factors for falls in previous studies [102], accounted for much of the variance in choice stepping reaction time (multiple $r^2 = 0.42$). This suggests that this new test may provide a composite measure of falls risk in older people.

Other voluntary stepping tests have also been suggested. Medell and Alexander [103] assessed the ability of young and old subjects to take the longest forward step possible (referred to as *maximal step length*), as well as to take rapid steps in three directions (front, side and back). Performance on both tests was correlated with a balance confidence scale and was significantly impaired in the older subjects. A follow-up study of 167 older people found that maximal step

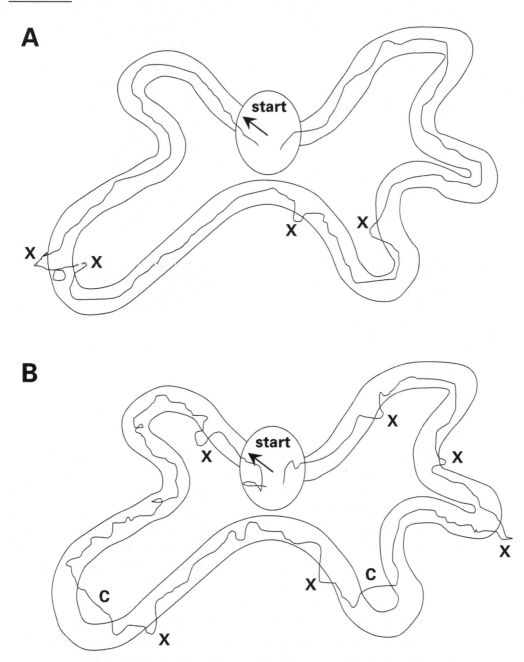

Fig. 2.2   The coordinated stability test. The subject is asked to adjust balance by bending or rotating the body without moving the feet. The pen on the end of the rod follows and remains within a convoluted track which is marked on a piece of paper attached to the top of an adjustable height table. Leaving the track scores one error point, while failing to navigate a corner scores five error points. A: error score is 4, B: error score is 16.

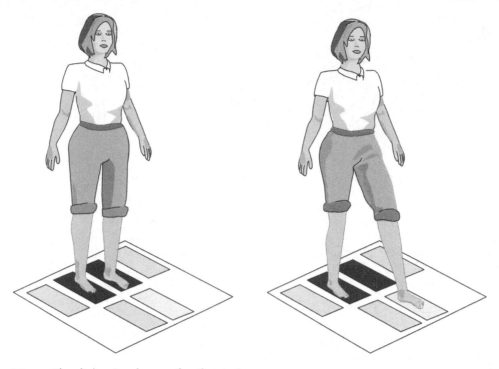

Fig. 2.3   The choice stepping reaction time test.

length was smaller in those who had fallen in the previous 12 months [103]. Luchies *et al.* [104] assessed the ability of young and old subjects to quickly step in eight directions (anterior, posterior, right, left, right and left anterior, right and left posterior) in response to a visual cue. They found that older subjects exhibited slower response, lift-off and landing times. Performances in the elderly subjects were significantly slower when asked to respond to a randomly selected step direction cue, indicating the slowing effect of the decision-making component of the response. However, no comparison between elderly fallers and non-fallers on this test has yet been undertaken. Dite and Temple [105] evaluated time taken to step to the right, backwards, to the left and forwards over walking canes placed on the floor in 81 older people. They found that those who had suffered multiple falls in the previous six months were significantly slower than non-fallers. The predictive value of the test was also found to be superior to the Timed Up and Go Test (TUGT) and the functional reach test.

Each of these voluntary stepping tests would appear to have some value in the assessment of falls risk, as they mimic the response required to avoid a fall and emphasize the reaction time component of balance preservation movements. They also have practical benefits over laboratory tests in that they require little or no equipment to undertake.

Internal perturbations generated by functional tasks

Leaning and stepping can be regarded as perturbations of an internal (i.e. self-generated) origin. A range of other functional tasks also represent internal perturbations which may result in loss of balance in a compromised postural control system. These include turning, bending, standing up from a chair and walking (see Chapter 3 for a more complete discussion of gait characteristics and falls). A wide range of clinical rating scales and functional tests have now been evaluated in older people to determine their ability to predict falls. These include sit-to-stand ability [106–110], turning [109], bending down [111], tandem walk [108], and Tinetti's Performance Oriented Balance and Mobility Assessment (POMA) [112–115] scales.

One of the most commonly used balance assessment scales, the POMA, is a simple clinical scale that grades performance on 14 balance items and ten gait items as normal, adaptive or abnormal [115]. The POMA has been shown to be correlated with the Berg Balance Scale (BBS) [116] and laboratory measures of postural sway [117, 118], and is a moderately good predictor of falls. In a recent prospective study of 225 people aged over 75, Raiche *et al.* [119] found that a cut-off score of 36 on the POMA provides falls prediction with 70% sensitivity, but only moderate specificity (52%).

The BBS consists of 14 items that are scored on a scale of 0 to 4. A score of 0 is given if the participant is unable to do the task and a score of 4 is given if the participant is able to complete the task based on the criterion that has been assigned to it. The maximum total score on the test is 56. The items include mobility tasks such as transfers, standing unsupported, sit-to-stand, tandem standing, turning 360 degrees and single-leg stance [120]. While some authors have found the BBS to be a useful predictor of falls [120–124], others have not [91, 125]. Overall, it would appear that the BBS has moderate-good specificity but low sensitivity in predicting falls [126]. However, the addition of a self-reported history of falling to the BBS score has been shown to enhance both the specificity and sensitivity of the instrument [127].

The TUGT, derived from the original Up and Go Test [128], is an indicator of basic mobility and measures the time required for a person to rise from a chair, walk three metres, turn, walk back and sit down. The tool was originally validated on 60 day hospital patients, where it was found that a poor performance was significantly correlated with slow gait speed, low BBS performance and low Barthel Index scores [129]. Subsequently, three retrospective studies have examined the relationship between TUGT performance and falls in community-dwelling people. In a study of 15 subjects with a history of two or more falls in the previous six months and 15 non-fallers, Shumway-Cook *et al.* [130]

found that a TUGT cut-off point of 14 seconds significantly discriminated between the faller and non-faller groups. Using this criterion, 13/15 subjects from both groups were correctly classified – providing a sensitivity and specificity for identifying falls outcome of 87%. Rose *et al.* [131] used a similar classification of faller status (no falls vs. two or more falls in the past year) in their study of 134 subjects. A considerably lower cut-off point (10 seconds) was identified as optimal for discriminating between non-fallers and recurrent fallers. With this criterion the overall prediction rate was 80% (specificity 86%, sensitivity 71%). The third study comprised 157 subjects classified as either fallers (one or more falls in the past year) or non-fallers [132]. In this sample, the TUGT had a very high sensitivity, with 98% of the 109 fallers being correctly classified, but considerably lower specificity, with only 15% of the 48 non-fallers being correctly classified.

The above evidence for the TUGT as a falls screening test is encouraging but could be described as still only preliminary due to the retrospective study designs. The findings are also likely to overestimate the predictive ability of the TUGT in a general community setting due to the selection of subjects with only a marked risk of falling as 'fallers'. The utility of this test may also be limited in very frail elderly subjects due to floor effects – a recent population-based study of 2305 older people in Canada found that 30% of subjects were unable to perform the test [133]. Furthermore, it is important that clinicians follow standardized testing procedures when applying the TUGT, as performance can be significantly influenced by chair height [134]. Nevertheless, the TUGT warrants further examination and validation because of its simplicity and ease of administration.

The benefit of clinical tests is that they require little or no equipment, and are quick and easy to perform. However, the predictive validity of these tests varies between studies, possibly due to differences in the interpretation of some of the more subjective items, or, in the case of the TUGT, variation in equipment used. The other limitation of this approach to falls risk assessment is that, if performed in isolation, they offer only limited insight into the specific physiological risk factors present in an individual, and as such, offer little guidance in relation to targeted falls prevention programmes. Therefore, we believe that such tests are useful as population-based screening tools, but need to be supplemented with more detailed physiological assessment procedures prior to implementing falls prevention programmes.

Responding to external perturbations

Although evaluation of standing sway, reach and functional tasks has provided useful information regarding the interaction of musculo-skeletal and sensory components of postural stability, it can only provide limited information regarding the ability to react to the changing demands of a particular task. To more closely assess this component of postural stability, a number of investigations have been performed in which the subject is mechanically perturbed by applying a direct force to their body, or by tilting or translating the surface upon which they stand. These techniques are thought to provide useful information regarding how effectively the subject's sensory and motor systems respond to external stimuli.

Perhaps the simplest technique for assessing postural responses to perturbation is by applying a direct force to the subject's body and measuring the ability of the subject to regain stability. This technique, sometimes referred to as the *postural stress test,* was first described by Wolfson *et al.* [135] and involves a simple pulley-weight apparatus which displaces the centre of mass behind the subject's stability limit. Performance on this task is rated on a nine-point ordinal scale which ranges from 'covert reactions' (score 9), in which the subject remains stable with little observable body displacement, and 'absent reactions' (score 0), in which the subject experiences a backwards fall. Wolfson *et al.* [135] reported that older nursing home-dwelling subjects scored much lower on the postural stress test than younger subjects and that elderly fallers performed significantly worse on the test than non-fallers. Subsequent investigations by Chandler *et al.* [136] and Studenski *et al.* [81] achieved similar results in community-dwelling individuals with respect to fallers versus non-fallers. A clinical version of this test, in which the clinician directly exerts a force on the subject and observes their postural response, has also been found to be associated with falls in several prospective studies [109, 113, 137]. However, it is difficult to compare results across studies due to the inability to accurately standardize the force applied.

More recent investigations into responses to perturbation have utilized specialized platforms which translate in the antero-posterior and medio-lateral planes or rotate co-axially with the subjects' ankle joints. The use of platform rotation as a postural perturbation was first described by Nashner [138] and was subsequently developed into the *sensory organization test.* This technique involves the modification of visual and support surface conditions. For the visual perturbation, the enclosure in which the subject is tested is rotated, while for the support surface perturbation, the platform upon which the subject stands is rotated according to the degree of the subject's postural sway [139]. Numerous investigations utilizing this technique have reported that older subjects are less able to compensate for the altered visual and support surface conditions compared to younger adults [139–141]. This has been explained by the observation that older people have significantly slower lower limb muscle reflex responses to rotational perturbation [139, 142, 143].

In addition to rotational perturbation, a number of authors have assessed age-related changes in response to unexpected antero-posterior and medio-lateral translation of the supporting surface. Pioneering work into translational postural perturbations was undertaken by Nashner [138, 144, 145], who established normal electromyographic responses to perturbation, referred to as *muscle synergies*, in addition to describing three stereotypical postural *strategies* to compensate for different velocity perturbations. The *ankle strategy*, thought to be the most common response to standing perturbation, describes the reaction in which the subject leans forward from the ankle in response to small antero-posterior translations of the supporting surface. The *hip strategy* involves forward trunk leaning at the level of the hip joint and occurs in response to larger perturbations. The *stepping strategy* is characterized by rapid steps, hops or stumbles which occur in order to shift the base of support under the falling centre of mass when the ankle or hip strategies have failed to compensate for very large or rapid perturbations [146].

As with rotational perturbation, older people are less able to maintain stability in response to translational perturbation compared to younger adults [26, 51, 58, 147–149]. This has been explained by the observation that older people have slower muscle reflex responses to translational perturbation [37, 150], a slower choice reaction time [100], and tend to utilize the hip strategy rather than the ankle strategy to maintain balance [148, 151]. Due to the increased challenge to the postural control system, translational perturbation reveals more pronounced age-related differences than unperturbed postural sway [26]. However, although differences in responses to translational perturbation have also been used to predict falls in older people [26, 58, 100], two investigations have revealed that measures of unperturbed sway may be better able to distinguish fallers from non-fallers than measures of response to perturbation [26, 58]. This may be because sway is a better overall indicator of physiological decline, or that platform perturbation is an unnatural movement unrelated to the context of falls in most real-life circumstances.

More recently, the *stepping strategy* has been investigated in more detail, based on the suggestion that the ability to control the centre of mass when the stability limit is moved is likely to be quite distinct from the ability to maintain balance within a stationary stability limit [152]. Luchies *et al.* [153] assessed the responses of young and older people when they were subjected to a sudden backwards pull at the waist. Young subjects responded to the perturbation by taking a single step, while older subjects took multiple shorter steps, suggesting a decreased ability to re-establish postural stability in response to centre of mass displacement. Similarly, McIlroy and Maki [154] assessed stepping responses in young and old subjects when an antero-posterior perturbation was applied to the platform on which they stood. Although both groups of subjects performed similarly with regard to the characteristics of the first step, older subjects were twice as likely to take additional steps to maintain stability. Furthermore, the additional steps in older subjects were laterally directed in 30% of cases, suggesting the need to control for lateral instability arising after the first compensatory stepping manoeuvre. A subsequent study utilizing medio-lateral platform perturbation revealed that older subjects not only took more steps, but were also more likely to contact the contralateral limb when doing so, possibly increasing the risk of a fall [155].

Rogers *et al.* [156] used a waist-pull apparatus to displace the subject's centre of mass in an anterior direction at different velocities. Compared to young people and older people without a history of falling, older people with recurrent falls exhibited increased lateral motion and increased lateral foot placement when taking a first protective step. These results were consistent with a number of previous studies indicating that older people with balance problems have difficulty stabilizing the body in the medio-lateral direction when standing [58, 157, 158] and when responding to antero-posterior perturbations [154]. Another study utilizing both anterior and posterior waist pulls found that young subjects tended to resist the perturbation by extending or flexing their torso, whereas older subjects were more likely to initiate a compensatory step. Furthermore, the compensatory step initiated by balance-impaired older subjects failed to properly arrest their momentum due to inadequate control of torso inclination before the step and inadequate control of linear momentum once the step was initiated, partly due to the more lateral foot placement [159].

A slightly different model was employed by Owings *et al.* [160]. In this study, subjects stood on a motorized treadmill and were instructed to maintain their balance in response to a posterior translation of the treadmill, then continue walking forwards. The magnitude of the backwards translation was sufficient to cause some subjects to fall. In this way, the subject's responses more accurately represented those that occur when recovering from a trip when walking. Subjects who failed to recover from the perturbation had slower reaction times, shorter step lengths and greater trunk flexion.

These perturbation studies have allowed greater insight into postural responses compared to unperturbed sway. However, the sample sizes for these studies have generally been relatively small and the ability of these tests to predict falls in older people is yet to be confirmed.

Conclusion

The maintenance of postural stability is a highly complex skill which is dependent on the coordination of a vast number of neurophysiological and biomechanical variables. Normal ageing is associated with decreased ability to maintain postural stability in standing (both bipedally and unipedally), when responding to unexpected perturbations and during voluntary stepping. This decrease in postural stability in older people may be explained by deficits in muscle strength, peripheral sensation, visual acuity, vestibular function and central processing of afferent inputs. Although numerous studies have reported impaired performance on a range of balance tests in fallers compared to non-fallers, the ability of balance tests to predict falls when used in isolation is limited. For this reason, we recommend falls screening tools incorporate a range of physiological tests in addition to a balance component.

REFERENCES

1. A. Shumway-Cook & M. Woollacott, *Motor Control: Theory and Practical Applications* (Baltimore: Williams and Wilkins, 1995).
2. E. Kokmen, R. W. Bossemeyer, Jr, J. Barney & W. J. Williams, Neurological manifestations of aging. *Journal of Gerontology*, **32** (1977), 411–19.
3. J. M. Thornbury & C. M. Mistretta, Tactile sensitivity as a function of age. *Journal of Gerontology*, **36** (1981), 34–9.
4. F. S. Kaplan, J. E. Nixon, M. Reitz, L. Rindfleish & J. Tucker, Age-related changes in proprioception and sensation of joint position. *Acta Orthopaedica Scandinavica*, **56** (1985), 72–4.
5. S. R. Lord & J. A. Ward, Age-associated differences in sensori-motor function and balance in community dwelling women. *Age and Ageing*, **23** (1994), 452–60.
6. J. H. Sheldon, The effect of age on the control of sway. *Gerontology Clinics*, **5** (1963), 129–38.
7. R. Fitzpatrick, D. K. Rogers & D. I. McClosky, Stable human standing with lower-limb muscle afferents providing the only sensory input. *Journal of Physiology*, **480** (1994), 395–403.
8. G. G. Simoneau, H. W. Leibowitz, J. S. Ulbrecht, R. A. Tyrrell & P. R. Cavanagh, The effects of visual factors and head orientation on postural steadiness in women 55 to 70 years of age. *Journal of Gerontology*, **47** (1992), M151–8.
9. R. Fitzpatrick & D. McCloskey, Proprioceptive, visual and vestibular thresholds for the perception of sway during standing in humans. *Journal of Physiology*, **478** (1994), 173–86.
10. A. Shumway-Cook & F. B. Horak, Assessing the influence of sensory interaction on balance: suggestion from the field. *Physical Therapy*, **66** (1986), 1548–50.
11. S. R. Lord, R. D. Clark & I. W. Webster, Postural stability and associated physiological factors in a population of aged persons. *Journal of Gerontology*, **46A** (1991), M69–76.
12. E. J. Orma, The effects of cooling the feet and closing the eyes on standing equilibrium: different patterns of standing equilibrium in young men and women. *Acta Physiologica Scandinavica*, **38** (1957), 288–97.
13. M. Magnusson, H. Enbom, R. Johansson & J. Wiklund, Significance of pressor input from the human feet in lateral postural control. *Acta Otolaryngologica*, **110** (1990), 321–7.

14. M. Magnusson, H. Enbom, R. Johansson & I. Pyykko, Significance of pressor input from the human feet in anterior-posterior postural control. *Acta Otolaryngologica*, **110** (1990), 182–8.

15. M. Romberg, A manual of the nervous diseases of man. *Sydenham Transactions*, **2** (1853), 396.

16. F. A. Hellbrandt & G. L. Braun, The influence of sex and age on the postural sway of man. *American Journal of Physical Anthropology*, **XXIV** (1939), 347–60.

17. K. Boman & E. Jalavisto, Standing steadiness in old and young persons. *Annales Medicinae Eperimentalis et Biologiae Fenniae*, **31** (1953), 447–55.

18. A. R. Fregly & A. Graybiel, An ataxia test battery not requiring rails. *Aerospace Medicine*, **39** (1968), 277–82.

19. M. P. Murray, A. A. Seireg & S. B. Sepic, Normal postural stability and steadiness: quantitative assessment. *Journal of Bone and Joint Surgery*, **57A** (1975), 510–16.

20. B. R. Hasselkus & E. M. Shambes, Aging and postural sway in women. *Journal of Gerontology*, **30** (1975), 661–7.

21. P. W. Overstall, A. N. Exton-Smith, F. J. Imms & A. L. Johnson, Falls in the elderly related to postural imbalance. *British Medical Journal*, **1** (1977), 261–4.

22. J. C. Brocklehurst, D. Robertson & P. James-Groom, Clinical correlates of sway in old age – sensory modalities. *Age and Ageing*, **11** (1982), 1–10.

23. P. Era & E. Heikkinen, Postural sway during standing and unexpected disturbance of balance in random samples of men of different ages. *Journal of Gerontology*, **40** (1985), 287–95.

24. C. Ekdahl, E. B. Jarnlo & S. I. Andersson, Standing balance in healthy subjects. *Scandinavian Journal of Rehabilitative Medicine*, **21** (1989), 187–95.

25. C. Ring, U. S. Nayak & B. Isaacs, The effect of visual deprivation and proprioceptive change on postural sway in healthy adults. *Journal of the American Geriatrics Society*, **37** (1989), 745–9.

26. B. E. Maki, P. J. Holliday & G. R. Fernie, Aging and postural control. A comparison of spontaneous- and induced-sway balance tests. *Journal of the American Geriatrics Society*, **38** (1990), 1–9.

27. I. Pyykko, P. Jantti & H. Aalto, Postural control in elderly subjects. *Age and Ageing*, **19** (1990), 215–21.

28. R. J. Peterka & F. O. Black, Age-related changes in human posture control: sensory organization tests. *Journal of Vestibular Research*, **1** (1990), 73–85.

29. N. R. Colledge, P. Cantley, I. Peaston et al., Ageing and balance: the measurement of spontaneous sway by posturography. *Gerontology*, **40** (1994), 273–8.

30. R. W. Baloh, T. D. Fife, L. Zwerling et al., Comparison of static and dynamic posturography in young and older normal people. *Journal of the American Geriatrics Society*, **42** (1994), 405–12.

31. H. Okuzumi, A. Tanaka, K. Haishi et al., Age-related changes in postural control and locomotion. *Perceptual and Motor Skills*, **81** (1995), 991–4.

32. J. J. Collins, C. J. De Luca, A. Burrows & L. A. Lipsitz, Age-related changes in open-loop and closed-loop postural control mechanisms. *Experimental Brain Research*, **104** (1995), 480–492.

33. B. McClenaghan, H. Williams, J. Dickerson *et al.*, Spectral characteristics of ageing postural control. *Gait and Posture*, **3** (1995), 123–31.

34. P. A. Hageman, J. M. Leibowitz & D. Blanke, Age and gender effects on postural control measures. *Archives of Physical Medicine and Rehabilitation*, **76** (1995), 961–5.

35. G. Kamen, C. Patten, C. D. Du, S. Sison, An accelerometry-based system for the assessment of balance and postural sway. *Gerontology*, **44** (1995), 40–5.

36. L. Hay, C. Bard, M. Fleury & N. Teasdale, Availability of visual and proprioceptive afferent messages and postural control in elderly adults. *Experimental Brain Research*, **108** (1996), 129–39.

37. P. P. Perrin, C. Jeandel, C. A. Perrin & M. C. Bene, Influence of visual control, conduction, and central integration on static and dynamic balance in healthy older adults. *Gerontology*, **43** (1997), 223–31.

38. S. M. Slobounov, S. A. Moss, E. S. Slobounova & K. M. Newell, Aging and time to instability in posture. *Journal of Gerontology*, **53A** (1998), B71–8.

39. R. W. Baloh, S. Corona, K. M. Jacobson, J. A. Enrietto & T. Bell, A prospective study of posturography in normal older people. *Journal of the American Geriatrics Society*, **46** (1998), 438–43.

40. N. L. Choy, S. Brauer & J. Nitz, Changes in postural stability in women aged 20 to 80 years. *Journal of Gerontology*, **58A** (2003), 525–30.

41. G. R. Fernie, C. I. Gryfe, P. J. Holliday & A. Llewellyn, The relationship of postural sway in standing to the incidence of falls in geriatric subjects. *Age and Ageing*, **11** (1982), 11–16.

42. J. O. Judge, M. B. King, R. Whipple, J. Clive & L. I. Wolfson, Dynamic balance in older persons: effects of reduced visual and proprioceptive input. *Journal of Gerontology*, **50A** (1995), M263–70.

43. P. Era, M. Schroll, H. Ytting *et al.*, Postural balance and its sensory-motor correlates in 75-year-old men and women: a cross-national comparative study. *Journal of Gerontology*, **51A** (1996), M53–63.

44. W. A. Satariano, G. N. DeLorenze, D. Reed & E. L. Schneider, Imbalance in an older population: an epidemiological analysis. *Journal of Aging and Health*, **8** (1996), 334–58.

45. N. D. Carter, K. M. Khan, A. Mallinson & P. A. Janssen, Knee strength is a significant determinant of static and dynamic balance as well as quality of life in older community-dwelling women with osteoporosis. *Gerontology*, **48** (2002), 360–8.

46. W. J. MacLennan, J. I. Timothy & M. R. P. Hall, Vibration sense, proprioception and ankle reflexes in old age. *Journal of Clinical and Experimental Gerontology*, **2** (1980), 159–71.

47. G. Duncan, J. A. Wilson, W. J. MacLennan & S. Lewis, Clinical correlates of sway in elderly people living at home. *Gerontology*, **38** (1992), 160–6.

48. S. L. Anacker & R. P. Di Fabio, Influence of sensory inputs on standing balance in community-dwelling elders with a recent history of falling. *Physical Therapy*, **72** (1992), 575–81.

49. E. K. Kristinsdottir, G. B. Jarnlo & M. Magnusson, Aberrations in postural control, vibration sensation and some vestibular findings in healthy 64–92-year-old subjects. *Scandinavian Journal of Rehabilitation Medicine*, **29** (1997), 257–65.

50. M. J. Lichtenstein, S. L. Shields, R. G. Shiavi & M. C. Burger, Clinical determinants of biomechanics platform measures of balance in aged women. *Journal of the American Geriatrics Society*, **36** (1988), 996–1002.

51. G. E. Stelmach, J. Phillips, R. P. DiFabio & N. Teasdale, Age, functional postural reflexes, and voluntary sway. *Journal of Gerontology*, **44** (1989), B100–6.

52. H. Cohen, L. G. Heaton, S. L. Congdon & H. A. Jenkins, Changes in sensory organization test scores with age. *Age and Ageing*, **25** (1996), 39–44.

53. C. G. Danis, D. E. Krebs, K. M. Gill-Body & S. Sahrmann, Relationship between standing posture and stability. *Physical Therapy*, **78** (1998), 502–517.

54. P. Kejonen, K. Kauranen & H. Vanharanta, The relationship between anthropometric factors and body-balancing movement in postural balance. *Archives of Physical Medicine and Rehabilitation*, **84** (2003), 17–22.

55. S. M. Woolley, S. J. Czaja & C. G. Drury, An assessment of falls in elderly men and women. *Journal of Gerontology*, **52A** (1997), M80–7.

56. C. Y. Cho & G. Kamen, Detecting balance deficits in frequent fallers using clinical and quantitative evaluation tools. *Journal of the American Geriatrics Society*, **46** (1998), 426–30.

57. S. R. Lord, R. D. Clark & I. W. Webster, Physiological factors associated with falls in an elderly population. *Journal of the American Geriatrics Society*, **39** (1991), 1194–2000.

58. B. E. Maki, P. J. Holliday & A. K. Topper, A prospective study of postural balance and risk of falling in an ambulatory and independent elderly population. *Journal of Gerontology*, **49** (1994), M72–84.

59. S. R. Lord, D. G. Lloyd & S. K. Li, Sensori-motor function, gait patterns and falls in community-dwelling women. *Age and Ageing*, **25** (1996), 292–9.

60. S. R. Lord & R. D. Clark, Simple physiological and clinical tests for the accurate prediction of falling in older people. *Gerontology*, **42** (1996), 199–203.

61. P. B. Thapa, P. Gideon, K. G. Brockman, R. L. Fought & W. A. Ray, Clinical and biomechanical measures of balance as fall predictors in ambulatory nursing home residents. *Journal of Gerontology*, **51A** (1996), M239–46.

62. V. S. Stel, J. H. Smit, S. M. F. Pluijm & P. Lips, Balance and mobility performance as treatable risk factors for recurrent falling in older persons. *Journal of Clinical Epidemiology*, **56** (2003), 659–68.

63. S. R. Lord, P. N. Sambrook, C. Gilbert *et al.*, Postural stability, falls and fractures in the elderly: results from the Dubbo Osteoporosis Epidemiology Study. *Medical Journal of Australia*, **160** (1994), 684–5, 688–91.

64. S. R. Lord, D. McLean & G. Stathers, Physiological factors associated with injurious falls in older people living in the community. *Gerontology*, **38** (1992), 338–46.

65. S. R. Lord, J. A. Ward, P. Williams & K. J. Anstey, Physiological factors associated with falls in older community-dwelling women. *Journal of the American Geriatrics Society*, **42** (1994), 1110–17.

66. R. L. Kirby, N. A. Price & D. A. MacLeod, Influence of foot position on standing balance. *Journal of Biomechanics*, **20** (1987), 423–7.

67. P. A. Goldie, T. M. Bach & O. M. Evans, Force platform measures for evaluating postural control: reliability and validity. *Archives of Physical Medicine and Rehabilitation*, **70** (1989), 510–17.

68. H. Kollegger, C. Wober, C. Baumgartner & L. Deecke, Stabilizing and destabilizing effects of vision and foot position on body sway of healthy young subjects: a posturographic study. *European Neurology*, **29** (1989), 241–5.

69. B. L. Day, M. J. Steiger, P. D. Thompson & C. D. Marsden, Effect of vision and stance width on human body motion when standing: implications for afferent control of lateral sway. *Journal of Physiology*, **469** (1993), 479–99.

70. A. R. Fregly, M. J. Smith & A. Graybiel, Revised normative standards of performance of men on a quantitative ataxia test battery. *Acta Otolaryngologica*, **75** (1973), 10–16.

71. R. W. Bohannon, P. A. Larkin, A. C. Cook, J. Gear & J. Singer, Decrease in timed balance test scores with aging. *Physical Therapy*, **64** (1984), 1067–70.

72. D. K. Heitmann, M. R. Gossman, S. A. Shaddeau & J. R. Jackson, Balance performance and step width in noninstitutionalized, elderly, female fallers and nonfallers. *Physical Therapy*, **69** (1989), 923–31.

73. B. D. Iverson, M. R. Gossman, S. A. Shaddeau & M. E. Turner, Jr., Balance performance, force production, and activity levels in noninstitutionalized men 60 to 90 years of age. *Physical Therapy*, **70** (1990), 348–55.

74. R. A. Speers, J. A. Ashton-Miller, A. B. Schultz & N. B. Alexander, Age differences in abilities to perform tandem stand and walk tasks of graded difficulty. *Gait and Posture*, **7** (1998), 207–13.

75. W. J. Crosbie, M. A. Nimmo, M. A. Banks, M. G. Brownlee & F. Meldrum, Standing balance responses in two populations of elderly women: a pilot study. *Archives of Physical Medicine and Rehabilitation*, **70** (1989), 751–4.

76. R. C. Briggs, M. R. Gossman, R. Birch, J. E. Drews & S. A. Shaddeau, Balance performance among noninstitutionalized elderly women. *Physical Therapy*, **69** (1989), 748–56.

77. B. E. Maki, P. J. Holliday & A. K. Topper, Fear of falling and postural performance in the elderly. *Journal of Gerontology*, **46** (1991), M123–31.

78. J. A. Balogun, K. A. Akindele, J. O. Nihinlola & D. K. Marzouk, Age-related changes in balance performance. *Disability and Rehabilitation*, **16** (1994), 58–62.

79. B. J. Vellas, S. J. Wayne, L. Romero *et al.*, One-leg balance is an important predictor of injurious falls in older persons. *Journal of the American Geriatrics Society*, **45** (1997), 735–738.

80. S. R. Lord, M. W. Rogers, A. Howland & R. Fitzpatrick, Lateral stability, sensorimotor function and falls in older people. *Journal of the American Geriatrics Society*, **47** (1999), 1077–81.

81. S. Studenski, P. W. Duncan & J. Chandler, Postural responses and effector factors in persons with unexplained falls: results and methodologic issues. *Journal of the American Geriatrics Society*, **39** (1991), 229–34.

82. E. Hurvitz, J. Richardson, R. Werner, A. Ruhl & M. Dixon, Unipedal stance testing as an indicator of fall risk among older outpatients. *Archives of Physical Medicine and Rehabilitation*, **81** (2000), 587–91.

83. M. B. King, J. O. Judge & L. Wolfson, Functional base of support decreases with age. *Journal of Gerontology*, **49** (1994), M258–63.

84. P. W. Duncan, D. K. Weiner, J. Chandler & S. Studenski, Functional reach: a new clinical measure of balance. *Journal of Gerontology*, **45** (1990), M192–7.

85. D. K. Weiner, P. W. Duncan, J. Chandler & S. A. Studenski, Functional reach: a marker of physical frailty. *Journal of the American Geriatrics Society*, **40** (1992), 203–7.

86. P. W. Duncan, S. Studenski, J. Chandler & B. Prescott, Functional reach: predictive validity in a sample of elderly male veterans. *Journal of Gerontology*, **47** (1992), M93–8.

87. D. K. Weiner, D. R. Bongiorni, S. A. Studenski, P. W. Duncan & G. G. Kochersberger, Does functional reach improve with rehabilitation? *Archives of Physical Medicine and Rehabilitation*, **74** (1993), 796–800.

88. M. Wernick-Robinson , D. E. Krebs & M. M. Giorgetti, Functional reach: does it really measure dynamic balance? *Archives of Physical Medicine and Rehabilitation*, **80** (1999), 262–9.

89. S. Brauer, Y. Burns, P. Galley, Lateral reach: a clinical measure of medio-lateral postural stability. *Physiotherapy Research International*, **4** (1999), 81–8.

90. R. Newton, Validity of the multi-directional reach test: a practical measure for limits of stability in older adults. *Journal of Gerontology*, **56A** (2001), M248–52.

91. S. Brauer, Y. Burns & P. Galley, A prospective study of laboratory and clinical measures of postural stability to predict community dwelling fallers. *Journal of Gerontology*, **55A** (2000), M469–76.

92. S. R. Lord, J. A. Ward & P. Williams, Exercise effect on dynamic stability in older women: a randomized controlled trial. *Archives of Physical Medicine and Rehabilitation*, **77** (1996), 232–6.

93. S. R. Lord & H. B. Menz, Physiologic, psychologic and health predictors of 6-minute walk performance in older people. *Archives of Physical Medicine and Rehabilitation*, **83**, (2002), 907–11.

94. H. B. Menz & S. R. Lord, The contribution of foot problems to mobility impairment and falls in older people. *Journal of the American Geriatrics Society*, **49** (2001), 1651–6.

95. D. L. Sturnieks, S. R. Lord, A. Tiedemann *et al.*, Physiological risk factors for falls in older people with lower limb arthritis. *Journal of Rheumatology*, **31** (2004), 2272–9.

96. L. Day, B. Fildes, I. Gordon, A randomized factorial trial of falls prevention among older people living in their own homes. *British Medical Journal*, **325** (2002), 128–33.

97. A. Barnett, B. Smith, S. R. Lord, M. Williams & A. Bauman, Community-based group exercise improves balance and reduces falls in at-risk older people: a randomised controlled trial. *Age and Ageing*, **32** (2003), 407–14.

98. S. R. Lord, S. Castell, J. Corcoran *et al.*, The effect of group exercise on physical functioning and falls in frail older people living in retirement villages: a randomised controlled trial. *Journal of the American Geriatrics Society*, **51** (2003), 1685–92.

99. G. E. Stelmach & C. J. Worringham, Sensorimotor deficits related to postural stability. Implications for falling in the elderly. *Clinics in Geriatric Medicine*, **1** (1985), 679–94.

100. M. D. Grabiner & D. W. Jahnigen, Modeling recovery from stumbles: preliminary data on variable selection and classification efficacy. *Journal of the American Geriatrics Society*, **40** (1992), 910–13.

101. S. R. Lord & R. C. Fitzpatrick, Choice stepping reaction time: a composite measure of falls risk in older people. *Journal of Gerontology*, **56A** (2001), M627–32.

102. S. R. Lord, H. B. Menz & A. Tiedemann, A physiological profile approach to falls risk assessment and prevention. *Physical Therapy*, **83** (2003), 237–52.

103. J. L. Medell & N. B. Alexander, A clinical measure of maximal and rapid stepping in older women. *Journal of Gerontology*, **55A** (2000), M424–8.

104. C. Luchies, J. Schiffman, L. Richards *et al.*, Effects of age, step direction, and reaction condition on the ability to step quickly. *Journal of Gerontology*, **57A** (2002), M246–9.

105. W. Dite & V. Temple, A clinical test of stepping and change of direction to identify multiple falling older adults. *Archives of Physical Medicine and Rehabilitation*, **83** (2002), 1566–71.

106. J. W. Davis, P. D. Ross, M. C. Nevitt & R. D. Wasnich, Risk factors for falls and for serious injuries on falling among older Japanese women in Hawaii. *Journal of the American Geriatrics Society*, **47** (1999), 792–8.

107. A. J. Campbell, M. J. Borrie & G. F. Spears, Risk factors for falls in a community-based prospective study of people 70 years and older. *Journal of Gerontology*, **44** (1989), M112–17.

108. M. Nevitt, S. Cummings, S. Kidd & D. Black, Risk factors for recurrent non-syncopal falls. *Journal of the American Medical Association*, **261** (1989), 2663–8.

109. L. A. Lipsitz, P. V. Jonsson, M. M. Kelley & J. S. Koestner, Causes and correlates of recurrent falls in ambulatory frail elderly. *Journal of Gerontology*, **46** (1991), M114–22.

110. A. V. Schwartz, M. L. Villa, M. Prill *et al.*, Falls in older Mexican American women. *Journal of the American Geriatrics Society*, **47** (1999), 1371–8.

111. J. L. O'Loughlin, Y. Robitaille, J. F. Boivin & S. Suissa, Incidence of and risk factors for falls and injurious falls among the community-dwelling elderly. *American Journal of Epidemiology*, **137** (1993), 342–54.

112. M. E. Tinetti, T. F. Williams & R. Mayewski, Fall risk index for elderly patients based on number of chronic disabilities. *American Journal of Medicine*, **80** (1986), 429–34.

113. M. E. Tinetti, M. Speechley & S. F. Ginter, Risk factors for falls among elderly persons living in the community. *New England Journal of Medicine*, **319** (1988), 1701–7.

114. M. J. Faber, R. J. Bosscher & P. C. Van Wieringen, Clinimetric properties of the performance-oriented mobility assessment. *Physical Therapy*, **86** (2006), 944–54.

115. M. E. Tinetti, Performance-oriented assessment of mobility problems in elderly patients. *Journal of the American Geriatrics Society*, **34** (1986), 119–26.

116. K. O. Berg, B. E. Maki, J. I. Williams, P. J. Holliday & S. L. Wood-Dauphinee, Clinical and laboratory measures of postural balance in an elderly population. *Archives of Physical Medicine and Rehabilitation*, **73** (1992), 1073–80.

117. M. J. Lichtenstein, M. C. Burger, S. L. Shields & R. G. Shiavi, Comparison of biomechanics platform measures of balance and videotaped measures of gait with a clinical mobility scale in elderly women. *Journal of Gerontology*, **45** (1990), M49–54.

118. C. A. Laughton, M. Slavin, K. Katdare *et al.*, Aging, muscle activity, and balance control: physiologic changes associated with balance impairment. *Gait and Posture*, **18** (2003), 101–8.

119. M. Raiche, R. Hebert, F. Prince & H. Corriveau, Screening older adults at risk of falling with the Tinetti balance scale. *The Lancet*, **356** (2000), 1001–2.

120. K. O. Berg, S. L. Wood-Dauphinee, J. I. Williams & B. Maki, Measuring balance in the elderly: validation of an instrument. *Revue Canadienne de Sante Publique*, **83** (1992), S7–11.

121. L. D. Thorbahn & R. A. Newton, Use of the Berg Balance Test to predict falls in elderly persons. *Physical Therapy*, **76** (1996), 576–83.

122. A. Shumway-Cook, M. Baldwin, N. L. Polissar & W. Gruber, Predicting the probability for falls in community-dwelling older adults. *Physical Therapy*, **77** (1997), 812–19.

123. K. O'Brien, E. Culham & B. Pickles, Balance and skeletal alignment in a group of elderly female fallers and nonfallers. *Journal of Gerontology*, **52A** (1997), B221–6.

124. A. Y. Chiu, S. S. Au-Yeung & S. K. Lo, A comparison of four functional tests in discriminating fallers from non-fallers in older people. *Disability and Rehabilitation*, **25** (2003), 45–50.

125. M. E. Daubney & E. G. Culham, Lower-extremity muscle force and balance performance in adults aged 65 years and older. *Physical Therapy*, **79** (1999), 1177–85.

126. D. L. Riddle & P. W. Stratford, Interpreting validity indexes for diagnostic tests: an illustration using the Berg balance test. *Physical Therapy*, **79** (1999), 939–48.

127. A. Shumway-Cook, M. Woollacott, K. A. Kerns & M. Baldwin, The effects of two types of cognitive tasks on postural stability in older adults with and without a history of falls. *Journal of Gerontology*, **52A** (1997), M232–40.

128. S. Mathias, U. S. L. Nayak & B. Isaacs, Balance in elderly patients: the "Get-up and Go" test. *Archives of Physical Medicine and Rehabilitation*, **67** (1986), 387–9.

129. D. Podsiadlo & S. Richardson, The timed "Up and Go": a test of basic functional mobility for frail elderly persons. *Journal of the American Geriatrics Society*, **39** (1991), 142–8.

130. A. Shumway-Cook, S. Brauer & M. Woollacott, Predicting the probability for falls in community-dwelling older adults using the Timed Up and Go Test. *Physical Therapy*, **80** (2000), 896–903.

131. D. J. Rose, C. J. Jones & N. Lucchese, Predicting the probability of falls in community-residing older adults using the 8-foot up-and-go: a new measure of functional mobility. *Journal of Aging and Physical Activity*, **10** (2002), 466–75.

132. K. Gunter, K. White, W. C. Hayes & C. M. Snow, Functional mobility discriminates nonfallers from one-time and frequent fallers. *Journal of Gerontology*, **55** (2000), M672–6.

133. K. Rockwood, E. Awalt, D. Carver & C. MacKnight, Feasibility and measurement properties of the Functional Reach and the Timed Up and Go tests in the Canadian Study of Health and Aging. *Journal of Gerontology*, **55A** (2000), M70–3.

134. K. Siggeirsdottir, B. Jonsson, H. Jonsson & S. Iwarsson, The timed Up and Go is dependent on chair type. *Clinical Rehabilitation*, **16** (2002), 609–16.

135. L. I. Wolfson, R. Whipple, P. Amerman & A. Kleinberg, Stressing the postural response. A quantitative method for testing balance. *Journal of the American Geriatrics Society*, **34** (1986), 845–50.

136. J. M. Chandler, P. W. Duncan & S. A. Studenski, Balance performance on the postural stress test: comparison of young adults, healthy elderly, and fallers. *Physical Therapy*, **70** (1990), 410–15.

137. R. D. Clark, S. R. Lord & I. W. Webster, Clinical parameters associated with falls in an elderly population. *Gerontology*, **39** (1993), 117–23.

138. L. M. Nashner, Adaptation of movement to altered environments. *Trends in Neuroscience*, **5** (1982), 358–61.

139. M. H. Woollacott, A. Shumway-Cook & L. M. Nashner, Aging and posture control: changes in sensory organization and muscular coordination. *International Journal of Aging and Human Development*, **23** (1986), 97–114.

140. L. Wolfson, R. Whipple, C. A. Derby *et al.*, A dynamic posturography study of balance in healthy elderly. *Neurology*, **42** (1992), 2069–75.

141. R. Whipple, L. Wolfson, C. Derby, D. Singh & J. Tobin, Altered sensory function and balance in older persons. *Journal of Gerontology*, **48** (1993), 71–6.

142. E. A. Keshner, J. H. Allum & F. Honegger, Predictors of less stable postural responses to support surface rotations in healthy human elderly. *Journal of Vestibular Research*, **3** (1993), 419–29.

143. A. Nardone, R. Siliotto, M. Grasso & M. Schieppati, Influence of aging on leg muscle reflex responses to stance perturbation. *Archives of Physical Medicine and Rehabilitation*, **76** (1995), 158–65.

144. L. M. Nashner, Fixed patterns of rapid postural responses among leg muscles during stance. *Experimental Brain Research*, **30** (1977), 13–24.

145. L. M. Nashner, M. Woollacott & G. Tuma, Organization of rapid responses to postural and locomotor-like perturbations of standing man. *Experimental Brain Research*, **36** (1979), 463–76.

146. F. B. Horak, C. L. Shupert & A. Mirka, Components of postural dyscontrol in the elderly: a review. *Neurobiology of Aging*, **10** (1989), 727–38.

147. B. E. Maki, P. J. Holliday & G. R. Fernie, A posture control model and balance test for the prediction of relative postural stability. *Transactions on Biomedical Engineering*, **34** (1987), 797–810.

148. D. Manchester, M. Woollacott, N. Zederbauer-Hylton & O. Marin, Visual, vestibular and somatosensory contributions to balance control in the older adult. *Journal of Gerontology*, **44** (1989), M118–27.

149. R. Camicioli, V. P. Panzer & J. Kaye, Balance in the healthy elderly: posturography and clinical assessment. *Archives of Neurology*, **54** (1997), 976–81.

150. R. J. Peterka & F. O. Black, Age-related changes in human posture control: motor coordination tests. *Journal of Vestibular Research*, **1** (1990), 87–96.

151. M. J. Gu, A. B. Schultz, N. T. Shepard & N. B. Alexander, Postural control in young and elderly adults when stance is perturbed: dynamics. *Journal of Biomechanics*, **29** (1996), 319–29.

152. B. E. Maki, W. E. McIlroy, The role of limb movements in maintaining upright stance: the "change-in-support" strategy. *Physical Therapy*, **77** (1997), 488–507.
153. C. W. Luchies, N. B. Alexander, A. B. Schultz & J. Ashton-Miller, Stepping responses of young and old adults to postural disturbances: kinematics. *Journal of the American Geriatrics Society*, **42** (1994), 506–12.
154. W. E. McIlroy & B. E. Maki, Age-related changes in compensatory stepping in response to unpredictable perturbations. *Journal of Gerontology*, **51A** (1996), M289–96.
155. B. E. Maki, M. A. Edmonstone & W. E. McIlroy, Age-related differences in laterally directed compensatory stepping behavior. *Journal of Gerontology*, **55A** (2000), M270–7.
156. M. Rogers, L. Hedman, M. Johnson, T. Cain & T. Hanke, Lateral stability during forward-induced stepping for dynamic balance recovery in young and older adults. *Journal of Gerontology*, **56A** (2001), M589–94.
157. H. G. Williams, B. A. McClenaghan & J. Dickerson, Spectral characteristics of postural control in elderly individuals. *Archives of Physical Medicine and Rehabilitation*, **78** (1997), 737–44.
158. S. R. Lord, M. W. Rogers, A. Howland & R. Fitzpatrick, Lateral stability, sensorimotor function and falls in older people. *Journal of the American Geriatrics Society*, **47** (1999), 1077–81.
159. B. W. Schulz, J. A. Ashton-Miller & N. B. Alexander, Compensatory stepping in response to waist pulls in balance-impaired and unimpaired women. *Gait and Posture*, **22** (2005), 198–209.
160. T. M. Owings, M. J. Pavol & M. D. Grabiner, Mechanisms of failed recovery following postural perturbations on a motorised treadmill mimic those associated with an actual forward trip. *Clinical Biomechanics*, **16** (2001), 813–19.

3

Gait characteristics and falls

'Human walking is a unique activity during which the body, step by step, teeters on the brink of catastrophe...only the rhythmic forward movement of first one leg and then the other keeps man from falling flat on his face.'
(JR Napier, 1967 [1].)

Habitual upright walking is a characteristically human trait that provides a unique set of physiological challenges. When standing erect, two-thirds of the body's mass is located two-thirds of the body height from the ground, precariously balanced on two narrow legs with the only direct contact with the ground provided by the feet [2]. Such a structure challenges the basic principles of mechanical engineering and requires a highly developed postural control system to ensure that the body remains upright. However, in order to progress forwards, it is necessary to repeatedly initiate a forward fall and then 're-capture' this momentum by the appropriate placement of the leading limb. The potential for a loss of balance when performing an apparently simple task such as walking is considerable. It is therefore not at all surprising that between 50% and 70% of falls in older people occur when walking [3–5]. The aim of this chapter is to provide an overview of the literature pertaining to gait patterns in older people and their relationship to falls. Specifically, this chapter will address gait characteristics during level walking, stepping over and avoiding obstacles, stair walking, and the ability to respond to trips and slips.

Level walking

Many kinematic and kinetic studies have been undertaken to evaluate differences in gait patterns between young people and older people. The most consistent finding of these studies is that older people walk more slowly than young people [6–21]. This has been found to be a function of a shorter step length [6–8, 12, 13, 16, 17, 19, 20, 22–24], reduced cadence and increased time spent in double limb support [7, 8, 20, 23, 24]. These temporo-spatial differences would appear to be a direct result of variation in self-selected walking speed, as when older people and young people are instructed to walk at a specified fixed velocity, no significant differences are apparent [25]. Other gait alterations apparent in older people include reduced hip motion [7, 13, 22, 26], reduced angular velocity of the lower trunk [27], reduced ankle power generation [23, 26, 28] and range of motion [12], increased anterior pelvic tilt [23, 26], increased hip extension moment during swing phase [29], increased mechanical energy demands of lower limb musculature [30–32], and reduced toe pressure [33]. Studies which have assessed foot placement have also reported that older people walk with a larger degree of out-toeing [6, 7, 23].

Age-related changes in temporo-spatial gait parameters have generally been interpreted as indicating the adoption of a more conservative, or less destabilizing gait [34–38]. A number of investigations have revealed that certain changes in gait patterns may be predictive of falling in older people. Gait velocity has been consistently reported to differentiate between elderly fallers and non-fallers, with fallers walking significantly more slowly [9, 39–52]. A number of studies have also shown that older people who fall exhibit increased variability in cadence [20, 39, 46, 53–56] and step length [39, 53–59].

The functional importance and predictive value of step width (also referred to as base of support) is unclear. In a comparative study of young and older men, Murray et al. [7] reported that step width increases significantly with normal ageing, however, Gabell and Nayak [60] found no significant differences in mean step width between young and older adults. Guimaraes and Isaacs [39] and Weller et al. [61] both reported that older people with a history of falling walked with a significantly narrower step width than age-matched controls. However, these results are contradicted by similar investigations which reported no difference in step width [62] or an increased step width [50, 53, 63] in fallers compared to non-fallers. It is likely that different techniques have been used to measure step width that may not be directly comparable, and/or differences in the gender balance among the samples studied may explain these disparate findings.

Although these studies seem to indicate that older people who fall walk with a characteristic 'conservative' gait pattern, only recently have detailed biomechanical investigations been performed to measure variables that more directly represent instability during gait [64–66]. After controlling for walking speed, kinematic gait patterns do not differ greatly between fallers and non-fallers [67], although Kerrigan et al. [66] did find that fallers exhibited reduced peak hip extension irrespective of velocity. A kinetic study by Lee and Kerrigan [64] reported that fallers walked with decreased ankle plantarflexor torque but increased hip flexion, hip adduction, knee extension, knee varum, ankle dorsiflexion and ankle eversion torques, compared to an age-matched control group with no history of falls. However, after controlling for differences in walking speed, differences were only apparent for the sagittal plane parameters [65]. Yack and Berger [68] found that older people who reported balance problems exhibited less smooth acceleration patterns in the upper trunk. Contrary to expectations, Simoneau and Krebs [69] recently failed to show a difference in whole body momentum between non-fallers and fallers, however, this may have been due to inadequate sample size (two fallers and three non-fallers).

We have recently measured accelerations of the head and pelvis when walking on level and irregular surfaces as a means of assessing gait stability [70]. Using this technique, we have found that older people with a low risk of falling were able to maintain equivalent stability to young people by reducing their velocity and cadence [38]. However, older people with a high risk of falling, despite adopting a slower velocity, cadence and step length, demonstrate less rhythmic acceleration patterns at the head and pelvis in the vertical and antero-posterior direction, particularly when walking on an irregular surface [71]. The erratic acceleration patterns evident in high risk elderly people suggest that they have difficulty controlling the momentum of their trunk. There is also the possibility that the erratic movements of the head may interfere with normal gaze stability, as it has been shown that older people exhibit larger eye movements when the head is perturbed due to suppression of the vestibulo-ocular reflex [72, 73].

A summary of gait changes during level walking found to be associated with falls is shown in Figure 3.1. There are a range of possible explanations for the gait changes observed in elderly fallers. A number of studies have shown that reductions in the basic temporo-spatial parameters of gait (i.e. velocity and step length) are significantly associated with the same physiological factors found to be risk factors for falls, including reduced lower limb strength [20, 74–76], slow reaction time [20, 74], increased postural sway [9, 20] and impaired peripheral sensation [20]. However, as these parameters can also be modified by cognitive influences, psychological factors such as anxiety and fear of falling may also alter gait patterns, i.e. these changes may reflect a *reluctance* rather than an *inability* to walk more quickly in some people [46, 77]. In a group of older subjects with gait disorders not attributed to specific diseases or medical conditions, Herman *et al.* [78] found that stride-to-stride variations in gait cycle timing were significantly associated with fear of falling and suggested that gait changes in such subjects may be an appropriate response to unsteadiness. An alternative view is that fear of falling may actually lead to gait instability. We

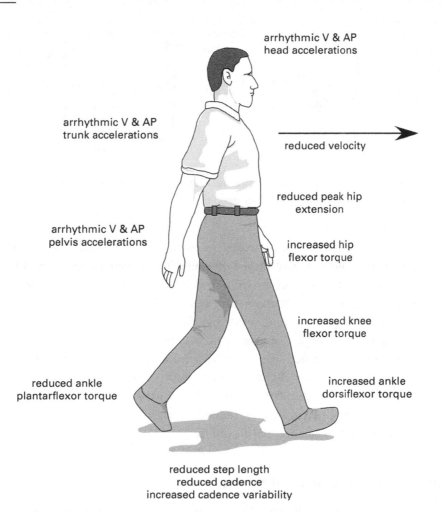

arrhythmic V & AP
head accelerations

arrhythmic V & AP
trunk accelerations

reduced velocity

reduced peak hip
extension

arrhythmic V & AP
pelvis accelerations

increased hip
flexor torque

increased knee
flexor torque

reduced ankle
plantarflexor torque

increased ankle
dorsiflexor torque

reduced step length
reduced cadence
increased cadence variability

Fig. 3.1   Changes in gait patterns during level walking that have been found to be associated with an increased risk of falling (V = vertical, AP = anterio-posterior).

recently developed a structural equation model to examine the relationships between physiological ability, fear of falling, and stability of the head and pelvis, based on gait analyses of 100 people aged 75 and over (see Figure 3.2). This model suggests that reduced sensorimotor function and fear of falling are both correlated with shorter step length, which in turn may lead to less stable pelvis accelerations and larger accelerations of the head relative to the pelvis, and these variables in turn may lead to impaired head stability [79]. This model indicates that fear of falling may make older people less stable when walking, primarily by promoting a 'guarded' stepping pattern which impairs the rhythmic movement of the upper body.

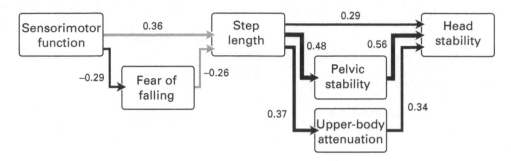

Fig. 3.2   Structural equation model of the relationship between sensorimotor function, fear of falling and gait stability in older people.

In addition to these factors, recent evidence indicates that restricted joint range of motion may play a role in altering gait patterns in elderly fallers. Escalante *et al.* [80] evaluated gait patterns in 702 older people in conjunction with a range of anthropometric measurements, and found that knee and hip flexion range of motion were significant independent predictors of walking velocity. Similarly, Kerrigan *et al.* [26, 66] have shown that hip flexion contracture is associated with reduced step length in older people who fall, but this contracture can be slightly reduced with a stretching programme [81]. Such observations suggest that the aberrant gait patterns observed in elderly fallers are not fixed, but rather are amenable to interventions aimed at improving strength, reaction time, balance and flexibility.

Stepping over and avoiding obstacles

During normal daily activities, it is not uncommon for us to step over obstacles as we walk. This poses a greater threat to the postural control system than level walking for two main reasons: first, the task of stepping over an obstacle requires a longer period of time spent standing on one leg; and second, there is a risk of the lead or trailing limb making contact with the obstacle and leading to a loss of balance. Indeed, a large proportion of falls in older people are attributed to tripping [82, 83, 84] and experiencing multiple 'stumbles' has been found to be a predictor of falls over a 12 month prospective period [85]. Assessment of level walking therefore provides only limited information regarding an individual's ability to navigate the range of environments traversed in daily activities.

Successful negotiation of an obstacle requires precise planning of the crossing step and the ability to maintain balance while allowing sufficient clearance of the leading and trailing limbs. In normal subjects, stepping over an obstacle involves reducing the normal hip flexor activity during toe-off and increasing knee flexion to enable clearance of the leading limb [86]. However, the characteristics of the crossing step are strongly influenced by the height of the obstacle. With increasing obstacle height, the speed of the crossing step decreases and the foot clearance distance increases [87]. In addition, higher obstacles require greater vertical and antero-posterior displacement of the centre of mass [88], greater muscular activity of the hip abductors, external hip rotators and ankle plantarflexors of the leading limb [89, 90], and increased knee flexion of the trailing limb [91].

Numerous studies have addressed age-related differences in obstacle crossing patterns. Chen *et al.* [87] assessed lower extremity kinematics when young and older subjects stepped over obstacles with a height of 0, 25, 51 and 152 mm, with a 4 m approach distance. Older people used a more conservative strategy when stepping over obstacles, exhibiting a slower 'crossing speed', shorter step length, and a smaller distance between the obstacle and the subsequent heel strike. Although none of the older subjects tripped over the obstacles, 25% stepped onto the obstacle itself. A subsequent study assessed age-associated differences in the ability to step over a 'virtual' obstacle (a band of light) which appeared in a variety of locations along an 8 m walkway. The virtual obstacle was designed to appear at the predicted location of the next heel strike at a range of available response times (in 50 millisecond increments). Older subjects were more likely to contact the obstacle than younger adults, particularly when the available response time was decreased [92]. More recently, Chen *et al.* [93] evaluated the effects of dividing attention on the ability to step over an obstacle in young and older people. The study utilized the same 'virtual' obstacle and walkway as in the previous study, however, in addition, subjects were asked to respond verbally when they saw a red light at the end of the room. The performance of the additional task significantly increased the likelihood of stepping on the obstacle in both groups, but was particularly evident in older people, suggesting an increased risk of tripping when attention is directed elsewhere. This is consistent with the emerging body of literature that indicates that elderly fallers have more difficulty performing balance and cognitive tasks simultaneously, which may in itself be a falls risk factor (see Chapter 5).

In addition to stepping over obstacles, successful avoidance of obstacles may also play a role in preventing falls. Cao *et al.* [94] assessed the ability of young and older subjects to suddenly turn 90 degrees when presented with a visual stimulus along a walkway, and reported that older subjects were less able to complete the turn when provided with smaller response times. A similar study by Gilchrist [95] assessed the ability of young and older women to side step to the left or right when walking after they were presented with a visual stimulus at the end of a walkway. A total of 58% of young subjects could perform the task with a single sideways step, compared to only 26% of the older subjects. In addition, older subjects' walking speed decreased significantly after the side step manoeuvre, suggesting that even when avoidance of an obstacle is successful, the older subjects were less able to incorporate the manoeuvre into their normal over-ground walking pattern. More recently, Tirosh and Sparrow [96] found that despite walking more slowly, older people took relatively longer to stop walking in response to a visual cue than younger people and their 'braking' response was more likely to involve more than one step. These results indicate that some elderly people may be at greater risk of falls as they have difficulty establishing proactive and reactive strategies to avoid obstacles altogether.

The underlying mechanisms responsible for these age-related differences have not been evaluated. However, it is likely that visual processing plays an important role in implementing avoidance strategies and en route planning of preparatory steps [97], while reaction time and lower limb strength contribute to the ability to maintain balance when stepping over the obstacle [89, 91, 98]. Thus, deficits in vision, reaction time and lower limb strength associated with ageing or disease may be responsible for impaired obstacle navigation or avoidance. Interestingly, a recent study also suggests that the use of anti-depressants may also detrimentally affect obstacle crossing in older people. A total of 12 elderly people were given single doses of amitriptyline or a placebo four hours before being asked to step over an obstacle. When under the influence of the antidepressant, subjects reduced their velocity, cadence and angular velocity of knee flexion of the trailing limb, indicating that the use of these medications may increase the risk of tripping [99].

Stair walking

Elderly people frequently report difficulties in stair walking [100]. Approximately 10% of fatal falls in older people occur when walking on stairs [101], indicating that age-related declines in physical ability may predispose elderly people to quite severe fall-related accidents when performing this common task. There are two likely mechanisms for falls on stairs; slipping (typically during stair descent) and inappropriate foot placement on the edge of the step (either during stair ascent or descent). Falls studies indicate that stair descent poses a greater risk of falling than stair ascent [102, 103] and it is clear that the movement patterns associated with these two tasks are quite different [101, 104–107]. Slipping is probably an uncommon cause of falls when descending stairs without surface contaminants, as the required coefficient of friction when walking on stairs has been found to be no different to level walking [108]. Loss of balance due to inappropriate foot placement appears more likely, as the margin for error is very small – the clearance between the swing foot and the step edge can be as little as 4 mm in young subjects [109].

A number of studies have recently been performed in an attempt to delineate the mechanical parameters that may predispose older people to falling when negotiating stairs. Williams [110, 111] found only small differences in limb movement patterns between young and older women when descending stairs. Christina and Cavanagh [108] reported less vigorous push-off and heel strike in elderly people descending stairs compared to young subjects, indicating the adoption of a more cautious gait pattern in the elderly group. Hortobagyi and DeVita [112, 113] found that older subjects demonstrated greater lower limb stiffness of the landing limb when stepping down, due to a more vertical lower limb alignment at contact and greater anticipatory muscle activation. Lark *et al.* [114] focused on the mechanics of the single support limb prior to step descent. They reported that older people remained in a flat-foot position for a longer period of time before rising onto the ball of the foot and exhibited less dynamic ankle stiffness than younger subjects. Finally, Begg and Sparrow [115] assessed limb movement patterns in young and older adults when stepping up onto a raised surface, and found that the older subjects positioned both the leading and trailing feet further from the edge of the step. Due to the larger distance between the step edge and the trailing foot, the leading foot must be placed on the step at a later period of the stride. This may be a more hazardous strategy, as in the event of obstacle contact or other postural disturbance, there would be less time for a corrective response.

Researchers have also addressed the role of vision when negotiating stairs, as it is likely that visual impairment contributes to inappropriate selection of foot placement. A kinematic analysis of stair descent on older women by Simoneau *et al.* [109] found that impaired visual acuity was associated with increased foot clearance, and a decreased distance between the descending foot and the previous step. Buckley *et al.* [116] evaluated the mechanics of older people stepping down from a range of step heights with and without light-scattering lenses, which altered contrast sensitivity to a level similar to dense cataracts. When wearing the lenses, subjects adopted a more cautious stepping down strategy, characterized by increased step execution time, increased knee flexion and ankle plantarflexion, and increased weight-bearing in the contralateral limb. The authors attributed this altered strategy to the subjects 'feeling' their way to the floor in an attempt to increase sensory input from the lower limb. A subsequent study [117] provided further explanation as to how this altered strategy could be detrimental to balance. Medio-lateral stability (assessed by comparing the position of the centre of mass relative to the centre of pressure) was found to be impaired in both step ascent and descent when wearing the lenses, but this was particularly evident when stepping down. These results help to explain findings from a recent prospective study [118] in which we found that older subjects who wore bi- and multifocal glasses were more likely to fall when walking on stairs than those who did not wear these glasses. This is because the lower lenses of these glasses impair depth perception and edge-contrast sensitivity at critical distances for detecting obstacles in the environment, such as the edges of stairs [118].

Tripping responses

Epidemiological studies reveal that up to 53% of falls in older people result from tripping [83, 119–122]. Subsequently, a series of studies have been performed to elucidate the mechanisms responsible for tripping [114–116] and to determine whether ageing is associated with inadequate responses to induced trips [117–120]. Pavol *et al.* [123, 124] induced trips in older people during gait using a concealed, mechanical obstacle and found that although the majority of the perturbation trials did not cause subjects to fall, older women fell more than four times as frequently as older men. Somewhat surprisingly, women aged 70 years or younger were more likely to fall than women aged over 70 years, which may be explained by the older subjects adopting a more 'protective', less destabilizing gait pattern. However, this finding may also have been due to the small sample size (only five women were aged over 80 years).

A follow-up investigation [125] identified two different strategies to compensate for an induced trip: (i) a *lowering* strategy, in which the tripped foot is quickly lowered to the ground and the contralateral foot initiates a recovery step; and (ii) an *elevating* strategy, in which the tripped limb is elevated over the obstacle in an attempt to continue the step. Irrespective of which strategy was adopted, subjects who fell in response to the trip walked more quickly than those who did not fall, suggesting that walking speed may be more important than foot placement. However, a subsequent mathematical modelling paper by these authors reported that although reducing walking speed would decrease the likelihood of a fall, improving response times would be more effective [126]. Leg strength is also likely to play an important role in recovering from a trip. Smeesters *et al.* [127] subjected young subjects to trips of increasing duration until recovery was no longer possible using a cable attached to the lower leg. The threshold trip duration was significantly associated with both hip flexor strength and volitional step reaction time, indicating that trip-related falls may be due to slower reaction time and muscle weakness.

More recently, Pijnappels *et al.* [128] studied push-off reactions of the support limb following an induced trip in young and older subjects. They found that older subjects who fell in response to the trip exhibited insufficient reduction in angular momentum during push-off and reduced moment generation at the ankle, knee and hip joints. These findings suggested that lower limb muscle weakness may be partly responsible for inadequate trip responses. A follow-up study by these authors found that the magnitude and rate of development of lower limb muscle activity were significantly lower in elderly subjects following a trip [129], indicating that differences in motor control also play a role.

The tripping paradigms used in these studies have enabled greater insights into the mechanisms responsible for impaired responses to walking perturbations, however, more research is required to fully explain why some older people are more likely to trip. In particular, the underlying physiological contributions to maintaining stability in response to a trip (i.e. vision, sensation, strength and reaction time) are yet to be fully explained in elderly people, although there is some preliminary evidence that reaction time [127, 130] and strength [127] may play a major role in young people. Furthermore, the ability of these tests to predict falls in real life is yet to be confirmed and may be limited, as the probability of tripping depends not only on the ability to respond to the perturbation, but also on the level of exposure to tripping hazards and the probability of seeing them in advance [131].

Slipping responses

Slips are the second most common gait-related mechanism of falls in older people [122, 132], and often result in injury due to the large impact forces that are generated when falling backwards or sideways [133]. Slips are most likely to occur shortly after heel strike, as during this period of the gait cycle a large proportion of bodyweight is placed on the very small heel region and the direction of force applied to the heel promotes forward sliding unless sufficient frictional forces are generated at the foot- or shoe-ground interface [134]. Recovery from forward sliding after heel contact requires complex neural control mechanisms to detect the sliding motion, rapidly plan a response strategy and generate a corrective step or steps [135].

During normal gait on non-slippery surfaces, the heel may slide forwards between 1 and 3 cm without being perceived by the subject and without requiring any corrective postural responses [134]. On slippery surfaces, however, forward displacements of the heel are much larger and occur at a higher velocity, thereby requiring coordinated responses to avoid falling backwards. The likelihood of falling following a slip depends on both the biomechanics of the slip event itself, and the efficacy and timing of the individual's response to the slip. Falling is more likely to occur with increased gait speed [136], increased forward heel displacement [137–139], increased posterior displacement of the body's centre of mass relative to the base of support [140] and the larger the angle of the leg relative to the ground (representative of a longer step length prior to the slip)[139].

A number of studies have evaluated the biomechanics and physiology of slip responses. When exposed to an unexpected slip, young adults generate an extremely rapid (60–90 ms onset) postural response involving large bursts of muscle activity, typically consisting of early activation of tibialis anterior, biceps femoris and rectus femoris on the slipping leg [141]. These muscle activation patterns are accompanied by increased flexion torque at the knee and extensor activity at the hip 190–350 ms after heel contact [142]. In elderly people, a similar response strategy is observed, but the response is characterized by relatively slower onset, smaller magnitude and longer duration of muscle activity [137], all of which may contribute to an inability to reduce the forward sliding of the heel [138]. In addition, elderly subjects exhibit more exaggerated 'secondary' strategies such as greater trunk hyperextension, larger arm elevation and a shorter response step [143], all considered indicative of a less efficient response.

The likelihood of slipping also depends on the subject's knowledge of the surface condition prior to walking over it. When subjects are told that they will be walking on a slippery surface, they adopt a more cautious gait pattern, with shorter step lengths, reduced angular velocity at heel contact and a shift in the medio-lateral centre of mass towards the supporting limb [144, 145]. In addition, both young and older people reduce the likelihood of slipping with repeated trials of performing a sit-to-stand task on a sliding platform [141, 142, 143]. These results suggest that the unexpected nature of slippery conditions contribute to the likelihood of falling in real life, but also raise the possibility that older people could be trained to develop protective slip responses. This may be a promising area for further research, as recent evidence suggests that training older people to respond to destabilizing waist-pull perturbations leads to faster step responses [146].

Despite these advances in understanding the biomechanics and physiology of slipping, the generalizability of laboratory-based experimental findings to real-life slipping events remains unclear. During daily activities, a vast number of movements are performed on a range of surfaces when wearing a range of different shoes. Given that there are likely to be numerous subject-specific factors influencing slip responses, it is unlikely that laboratory techniques will be able to accurately predict real-life slips in older people. Further research is therefore required to elucidate the subject-specific factors that may predispose to slips, and subsequent falls and injuries.

Conclusion

Human walking places considerable demands on the body's postural control system. Despite the high prevalence of falls in older people when performing locomotor tasks, the control of stability when walking has not received the same level of attention as standing balance. It may be that the complexity of the walking task makes it difficult to develop valid measures of stability for what is an inherently unstable activity.

Techniques to assess walking stability on level ground have provided useful information, but each has limitations. Basic parameters of gait may be useful global measures of mobility but do not provide any information about the stability of the body. Selection of foot placement appears to play an important role in the control of trunk movements, however, a direct relationship is difficult to establish as both narrow and wide foot placements have been associated with instability and falls. Recent work on the movement patterns of the head and pelvis has provided a more direct indicator of body stability during gait. It suggests that older people at high risk of falling exhibit erratic, arrhythmic movement patterns which may interfere with stable vision, thereby increasing the risk of obstacle contact.

Finally, an emerging body of literature indicates that ageing is associated with suboptimal movement strategies when stepping over or avoiding obstacles, walking on stairs, and responding to trips and slips. Further research is now required to determine whether these movement patterns are capable of predicting who is likely to fall, which physiological factors are responsible for these aberrant patterns, and whether targeted interventions are effective in improving responses to postural challenges as well as preventing falls and associated injuries.

REFERENCES

1. J. Napier, The antiquity of human walking. *Scientific American,* **216** (1967), 56–66.
2. D. A. Winter, A. E. Patla & J. S. Frank, Assessment of balance control in humans. *Medical Progress Through Technology,* **16** (1990), 31–51.
3. C. M. Cali & D. P. Kiel, An epidemiologic study of fall-related fractures among institutionalized older people. *Journal of the American Geriatrics Society,* **43** (1995), 1336–40.
4. W. P. Berg, H. M. Alessio, E. M. Mills & C. Tong, Circumstances and consequences of falls in independent community-dwelling older adults. *Age and Ageing,* **26** (1997), 261–8.
5. R. Norton, A. J. Campbell, T. Lee-Joe, E. Robinson & M. Butler, Circumstances of falls resulting in hip fractures among older people. *Journal of the American Geriatrics Society,* **45** (1997), 1108–12.
6. M. P. Murray, A. B. Drought & R. C. Kory, Walking patterns of normal men. *Journal of Bone and Joint Surgery,* **46A** (1964), 335–60.

7. M. P. Murray, R. C. Kory & B. H. Clarkson, Walking patterns in healthy old men. *Journal of Gerontology*, **24** (1969), 169–78.

8. F. R. Finley, K. A. Cody & R. V. Finizie, Locomotion patterns in elderly women. *Archives of Physical Medicine and Rehabilitation*, **50** (1969), 140–6.

9. F. J. Imms & O. G. Edholm, Studies of gait and mobility in the elderly. *Age and Ageing*, **10** (1981), 147–56.

10. D. A. Cunningham, P. A. Rechnitzer, M. E. Pearce & A. P. Donner, Determinants of self-selected walking pace across ages 19 to 66. *Journal of Gerontology*, **37** (1982), 560–4.

11. M. O'Brien, K. Power, S. Sanford, K. Smith & J. Wall, Temporal gait patterns in healthy young and elderly females. *Physiotherapy Canada*, **35** (1983), 323–6.

12. P. A. Hagemon & D. J. Blanke, Comparison of gait of young women and elderly women. *Physical Therapy*, **66** (1986), 1382–7.

13. R. J. Elble, S. S. Thomas, C. Higgins & J. Colliver, Stride-dependent changes in gait of older people. *Journal of Neurology*, **238** (1991), 1–5.

14. R. J. Dobbs, D. D. Lubel, A. Charlett *et al.*, Hypothesis: age-associated changes in gait represent, in part, a tendency towards Parkinsonism. *Age and Ageing*, **21** (1992), 221–5.

15. R. J. Dobbs, A. Charlett, S. G. Bowles *et al.*, Is this walk normal? *Age and Ageing*, **22** (1993), 27–30.

16. T. Oberg, A. Karsznia & K. Oberg, Basic gait parameters: reference data for normal subjects, 10–79 years of age. *Journal of Rehabilitation Research and Development*, **30** (1993), 210–23.

17. M. Fransen, J. Heussler, E. Margiotta & J. Edmonds, Quantitative gait analysis – comparison of rheumatoid arthritic and non-arthritic subjects. *Australian Journal of Physiotherapy*, **40** (1994), 191–9.

18. D. M. Buchner, M. E. Cress, P. C. Esselman *et al.*, Factors associated with changes in gait speed in older adults. *Journal of Gerontology*, **51A** (1996), M297–302.

19. Y. Lajoie, N. Teasdale, C. Bard & M. Fleury, Upright standing and gait: are there changes in attentional requirements related to normal aging? *Experimental Aging Research*, **22** (1996), 185–98.

20. S. R. Lord, D. G. Lloyd & S. K. Li, Sensori-motor function, gait patterns and falls in community-dwelling women. *Age and Ageing*, **25** (1996), 292–9.

21. R. W. Bohannon, Comfortable and maximum walking speed of adults aged 20–79 years: reference values and determinants. *Age and Ageing*, **26** (1997), 15–19.

22. R. D. Crowinshield, R. A. Brand & R. C. Johnston, The effects of walking velocity and age on hip kinematics and kinetics. *Clinical Orthopaedics and Related Research*, **132** (1978), 140–4.

23. D. A. Winter, A. E. Patla, J. S. Frank & S. E. Walt, Biomechanical walking pattern changes in the fit and healthy elderly. *Physical Therapy*, **70** (1990), 340–7.

24. A.-M. Ferrandez, J. Pailhous & M. Durup, Slowness in elderly gait. *Experimental Aging Research*, **16** (1990), 79–89.

25. E. C. Jansen, D. Vittas, S. Hellberg & J. Hansen, Normal gait of young and old men and women. *Acta Orthpaedica Scandinavica*, **53** (1982), 193–6.

26. D. C. Kerrigan, M. K. Todd, U. D. Croce, L. A. Lipsitz & J. J. Collins, Biomechanical gait alterations independent of speed in the healthy elderly: evidence for specific limiting impairments. *Archives of Physical Medicine and Rehabilitation*, **79** (1998), 317–22.

27. J. Gill, J. Allum, M. Carpenter *et al.*, Trunk sway measures of postural stability during clinical balance tests: effects of age. *Journal of Gerontology*, **56A** (2001), M438–47.

28. J. O. Judge, R. B. Davis & S. Ounpuu, Step length reductions in advanced age: the role of ankle and hip kinetics. *Journal of Gerontology*, **51A** (1996), M303–12.

29. P. Mills & R. Barrett, Swing phase mechanics of healthy young and elderly men. *Human Movement Science*, **20** (2001), 427–46.

30. C. McGibbon & D. Krebs, Age-related changes in lower trunk coordination and energy transfer during gait. *Journal of Neurophysiology*, **85** (2001), 1923–31.

31. C. A. McGibbon, D. E. Krebs & M. S. Puniello, Mechanical energy analysis identifies compensatory strategies in disabled elders' gait. *Journal of Biomechanics*, **34** (2001), 481–90.

32. C. McGibbon, M. Puniello & D. Krebs, Mechanical energy transfer during gait in relation to strength impairment and pathology in elderly women. *Clinical Biomechanics*, **16** (2001), 324–33.

33. T. W. Kernozek & E. E. LaMott, Comparisons of plantar pressures between the elderly and young adults. *Gait and Posture*, **3** (1995), 143–8.

34. C. Prakash & G. Stern, Neurological signs in the elderly. *Age and Ageing*, **2** (1973), 24–7.

35. L. Sudarsky, Geriatrics: gait disorders in the elderly. *New England Journal of Medicine*, **322** (1990), 1441–6.

36. L. Sudarsky & M. Ronthal, Gait disorders in the elderly: assessing the risk for falls. In *Falls, Balance and Gait Disorders in the Elderly*, ed. B. Vellas, M. Toupet, L. Rubenstein *et al.* (Paris: Elsevier, 1992), pp. 117–27.

37. M. H. Woollacott & P.-F. Tang, Balance control during walking in the older adult: research and its implications. *Physical Therapy*, **77** (1997), 646–60.

38. H. B. Menz, S. R. Lord & R. C. Fitzpatrick, Age-related differences in walking stability. *Age and Ageing*, **32** (2003), 137–42.

39. R. M. Guimaraes & B. Isaacs, Characteristics of the gait in old people who fall. *International Journal of Rehabilitative Medicine*, **2** (1980), 177–80.

40. H. Luukinen, K. Koski, P. Laippala & S.-L. Kivela, Risk factors for recurrent falls in the elderly in long-term institutional care. *Public Health*, **109** (1995), 57–65.

41. L. Wolfson, J. Judge, R. Whipple & M. King, Strength is a major factor in balance, gait, and the occurrence of falls. *Journal of Gerontology*, **50** (1995), S64–7.

42. J. Woo, S. C. Ho, J. Lau, S. G. Chan & Y. K. Yuen, Age-associated gait changes in the elderly: pathological or physiological? *Neuroepidemiology*, **14** (1995), 65–71.

43. P. Dargent-Molina, F. Favier, H. Grandjean *et al.*, Fall-related factors and risk of hip fracture: the EPIDOS prospective study. *The Lancet*, **348** (1996), 145–9.

44. S. C. Ho, J. Woo, S. S. Chan, Y. K. Yuen & A. Sham, Risk factors for falls in the Chinese elderly population. *Journal of Gerontology*, **51** (1996), M195–8.

45. J. M. VanSwearingen, K. A. Paschal, P. Bonino & J. F. Yang, The modified gait abnormality rating scale for recognizing the risk of recurrent falls in community-dwelling elderly adults. *Physical Therapy*, **76** (1996), 994–1002.

46. B. E. Maki, Gait changes in older adults: predictors of falls or indicators of fear? *Journal of the American Geriatrics Society*, **45** (1997), 313–20.

47. S. M. Woolley, S. J. Czaja & C. G. Drury, An assessment of falls in elderly men and women. *Journal of Gerontology*, **52A** (1997), M80–7.

48. B. E. Klein, R. Klein, K. E. Lee & K. J. Cruickshanks, Performance-based and self-assessed measures of visual function as related to history of falls, hip fractures, and measured gait time. The Beaver Dam Eye Study. *Ophthalmology*, **105** (1998), 160–4.

49. C.-Y. Cho & G. Kamen, Detecting balance deficits in frequent fallers using clinical and quantitative evaluation tools. *Journal of the American Geriatrics Society*, **46** (1998), 426–30.

50. A. Nelson, L. Certo, L. Lembo *et al.*, The functional ambulation performance of elderly fallers and non-fallers walking at their preferred velocity. *Neuro Rehabilitation*, **13** (1999), 141–6.

51. K. Gunter, K. White, W. C. Hayes & C. M. Snow, Functional mobility discriminates nonfallers from one-time and frequent fallers. *Journal of Gerontology*, **55** (2000), M672–6.

52. S. T. Eke-Okoro, A critical point for the onset of falls in the elderly. *Gerontology*, **46** (2000), 88–92.

53. R. D. Clark, S. R. Lord & I. W. Webster, Clinical parameters associated with falls in an elderly population. *Gerontology*, **39** (1993), 117–23.

54. S. R. Lord & R. D. Clark, Simple physiological and clinical tests for the accurate prediction of falling in older people. *Gerontology*, **42** (1996), 199–203.

55. J. M. Hausdorff, H. K. Edelberg, S. L. Mitchell, A. L. Goldberger & L. Y. Wei, Increased gait unsteadiness in community-dwelling elderly fallers. *Archives of Physical Medicine and Rehabilitation*, **78** (1997), 278–83.

56. J. M. Hausdorff, D. A. Rios & H. K. Edelberg, Gait variability and fall risk in community-living older adults: a 1-year prospective study. *Archives of Physical Medicine and Rehabilitation*, **82** (2001), 1050–6.

57. T. Nakamura, K. Meguro & H. Sasaki, Relationship between falls and stride length variability in senile dementia of the Alzheimer type. *Gerontology*, **42** (1996), 108–13.

58. K. Hill, J. Schwarz, L. Flicker & S. Carroll, Falls among healthy, community-dwelling, older women: a prospective study of frequency, circumstances, consequences and prediction accuracy. *Australian and New Zealand Journal of Public Health*, **23** (1999), 41–8.

59. G. Mbourou, Y. Lajoie & N. Teasdale, Step length variability at gait initiation in elderly fallers and non-fallers, and young adults. *Gerontology*, **49** (2003), 21–6.

60. A. Gabell & U. S. L. Nayak, The effect of age on variability in gait. *Journal of Gerontology*, **39** (1984), 662–6.

61. C. Weller, S. J. E. Humphrey, C. Kirollos *et al.*, Gait on a shoestring: falls and foot separation in Parkinsonism. *Age and Ageing*, **21** (1992), 242–4.

62. D. K. Heitmann, M. R. Gossman, S. A. Shaddeau & J. R. Jackson, Balance performance and step width in noninstitutionalized, elderly, female fallers and nonfallers. *Physical Therapy*, **69** (1989), 923–31.

63. G. M. Gehlsen & M. H. Whaley, Falls in the elderly. Part I. Gait. *Archives of Physical Medicine and Rehabilitation*, **71** (1990), 735–8.

64. L. W. Lee & D. C. Kerrigan, Identification of kinetic differences between fallers and nonfallers in the elderly. *American Journal of Physical Medicine and Rehabilitation*, **78** (1999), 242–6.

65. D. C. Kerrigan, L. W. Lee, T. J. Nieto et al., Kinetic alterations independent of walking speed in elderly fallers. *Archives of Physical Medicine and Rehabilitation*, **81** (2000), 730–5.

66. D. C. Kerrigan, L. W. Lee, J. J. Collins, P. O. Riley & L. A. Lipsitz, Reduced hip extension during walking: healthy elderly and fallers versus young adults. *Archives of Physical Medicine and Rehabilitation*, **82** (2001), 26–30.

67. M. E. Feltner, P. G. MacRae & J. L. McNitt-Gray, Quantitative gait assessment as a predictor of prospective and retrospective falls in community-dwelling older women. *Archives of Physical Medicine and Rehabilitation*, **75** (1994), 447–53.

68. H. J. Yack & R. C. Berger, Dynamic stability in the elderly: identifying a possible measure. *Journal of Gerontology*, **48** (1993), M225–30.

69. G. G. Simoneau & D. E. Krebs, Whole-body momentum during gait: a preliminary study of non-fallers and frequent fallers. *Journal of Applied Biomechanics*, **16** (2000), 1–13.

70. H. B. Menz, S. R. Lord & R. C. Fitzpatrick, Acceleration patterns of the head and pelvis when walking on level and irregular surfaces. *Gait and Posture*, **18** (2003), 35–46.

71. H. B. Menz, S. R. Lord & R. C. Fitzpatrick, Acceleration patterns of the head and pelvis when walking are associated with risk of falling in community-dwelling older people. *Journal of Gerontology*, **58A** (2003), M446–452.

72. R. P. DiFabio, A. Emasithi, J. F. Greany & S. Paul, Supression of the vertical vestibulo-ocular reflex in older persons at risk of falling. *Acta Otolaryngologica*, **121** (2001), 707–14.

73. R. P. DiFabio, J. F. Greany, A. Emasithi & J. F. Wyman, Eye-head coordination during postural perturbation as a predictor of falls in community-dwelling elderly women. *Archives of Physical Medicine and Rehabilitation*, **83** (2002), 942–51.

74. P. W. Duncan, J. Chandler, S. Studenski, M. Hughes & B. Prescott, How do physiological components of balance affect mobility in elderly men? *Archives of Physical Medicine and Rehabilitation*, **74** (1993), 1343–9.

75. E. J. Bassey, M. J. Bendall & M. Pearson, Muscle strength in the triceps surae and objectively measured customary walking activity in men and women over 65 years of age. *Clinical Science*, **74** (1988), 85–9.

76. D. M. Buchner, E. B. Larson, E. H. Wagner, T. D. Koepsell & B. J. DeLateur, Evidence for a non-linear relationship between leg strength and gait speed. *Age and Ageing*, **25** (1996), 386–91.

77. L. Brown, W. Gage, M. Polych, R. Sleik & T. Winder, Central set influences on gait: age-dependent effects of postural threat. *Experimental Brain Research*, **145** (2002), 286–96.

78. T. Herman, N. Giladi, T. Gurevich & J. M. Hausdorff, Gait instability and fractal dynamics of older adults with a "cautious" gait: why do certain older adults walk fearfully? *Gait and Posture*, **21** (2005), 178–85.

79. H. B. Menz, S. R. Lord & R. C. Fitzpatrick, A structural equation model relating sensori-motor function, fear of falling and gait patterns in older people. *Gait and Posture*, (2006), in press.

80. A. Escalante, M. J. Lichtenstein & H. P. Hazuda, Walking velocity in aged persons: its association with lower extremity joint range of motion. *Arthritis Care and Research*, **45** (2001), 287–94.

81. D. Kerrigan, A. Xenopoulos-Oddsson, M. Sullivan, J. Lelas & P. Riley, Effect of a hip flexor stretching program on gait in the elderly. *Archives of Physical Medicine and Rehabilitation*, **84** (2003), 1–6.

82. P. W. Overstall, A. N. Exton-Smith, F. J. Imms & A. L. Johnson, Falls in the elderly related to postural imbalance. *British Medical Journal*, **1** (1977), 261–4.

83. A. Blake, K. Morgan, M. Bendall *et al.*, Falls by elderly people at home – prevalence and associated factors. *Age and Ageing*, **17** (1988), 365–72.

84. A. J. Campbell, M. J. Borrie, G. F. Spears *et al.*, Circumstances and consequences of falls experienced by a community population 70 years and over during a prospective study. *Age and Ageing*, **19** (1990), 136–41.

85. J. Teno, D. P. Kiel & V. Mor, Multiple stumbles: a risk factor for falls in community-dwelling elderly. A prospective study. *Journal of the American Geriatrics Society*, **38** (1990), 1321–5.

86. B. J. McFadyen & D. A. Winter, Anticipatory locomotor adjustments during obstructed human walking. *Neuroscience Research Communications*, **9** (1991), 37–44.

87. H. -C. Chen, J. A. Ashton-Miller, N. B. Alexander & A. B. Schultz, Stepping over obstacles: gait patterns of healthy young and old adults. *Journal of Gerontology*, **46** (1991), M196–203.

88. L. -S. Chou, K. R. Kaufman, R. H. Brey & L. F. Draganich, Motion of the whole body's center of mass when stepping over obstacles of different heights. *Gait and Posture*, **13** (2001), 17–26.

89. L. -S. Chou & L. F. Draganich, Increasing obstacle height and decreasing toe-obstacle distance affect the joint moments of the stance limb differently when stepping over an obstacle. *Gait and Posture*, **8** (1998), 186–204.

90. R. Begg, W. Sparrow & N. Lythgo, Time-domain analysis of foot-ground reaction forces in negotiating obstacles. *Gait and Posture*, **7** (1998), 99–109.

91. L. Chou & L. Draganich, Stepping over an obstacle increases the motions and moments of the joints of the trailing limb in young adults. *Journal of Biomechanics*, **30** (1997), 331–7.

92. H. -C. Chen, J. A. Ashton-Miller, N. B. Alexander & A. B. Schultz, Effects of age and available response time on ability to step over an obstacle. *Journal of Gerontology*, **49** (1994), M227–33.

93. H. -C. Chen, A. B. Schultz, J. A. Ashton-Miller *et al.*, Stepping over obstacles: dividing attention impairs performance of old more than young adults. *Journal of Gerontology*, **51A** (1996), M116–22.

94. C. Cao, J. A. Ashton-Miller, A. B. Schultz & N. B. Alexander, Abilities to turn suddenly while walking: effects of age, gender, and available response time. *Journal of Gerontology*, **52A** (1997), M888–93.

95. L. A. Gilchrist, Age-related changes in the ability to side-step during gait. *Clinical Biomechanics*, **13** (1998), 91–7.

96. O. Tirosh & Sparrow, Gait termination in young and older adults: effects of stopping stimulus probability and stimulus delay. *Gait and Posture*, **19** (2004), 243–51.

97. A. E. Patla, Understanding the role of vision in the control of human locomotion. *Gait and Posture*, **5** (1997), 54–69.

98. E. L. Lamoureux, W. A. Sparrow, A. Murphy & R. U. Newton, The relationship between lower body strength and obstructed gait in community-dwelling older adults. *Journal of the American Geriatrics Society*, **50** (2002), 468–73.

99. L. Draganich, J. Zacny, J. Klafta & T. Karrison, The effects of antidepressants on obstructed and unobstructed gait in healthy elderly people. *Journal of Gerontology*, **56A** (2001), M36–41.

100. J. Williamson & L F, Characterization of older adults who attribute functional decrements to "old age". *Journal of the American Geriatrics Society*, **44** (1996), 1429–34.

101. J. K. Startzell, D. A. Owens, L. M. Mulfinger & P. R. Cavanagh, Stair negotiation in older people: a review. *Journal of the American Geriatrics Society*, **48** (2000), 567–80.

102. H. H. Cohen, J. Templer & J. Archea, An analysis of occupational stair accident patterns. *Journal of Safety Research*, **16** (1985), 178–81.

103. M. E. Tinetti, Factors associated with serious injury during falls by ambulatory nursing home residents. *Journal of the American Geriatrics Society*, **35** (1987), 644–8.

104. T. P. Andriacchi, G. B. J. Andersson, R. W. Fermier, D. Stern & J. O. Galante, A study of lower-limb mechanics during stair climbing. *Journal of Bone and Joint Surgery*, **62A** (1980), 749–57.

105. K. Lyons, J. Perry, J. K. Gronley, L. Barnes & D. Antonelli, Timing and relative intensity of hip extensor and abductor muscle action during level and stair ambulation. *Physical Therapy*, **63** (1983), 1597–605.

106. B. J. McFadyen & D. A. Winter, An integrated biomechanical analysis of normal stair ascent and descent. *Journal of Biomechanics*, **21** (1988), 733–44.

107. J. E. Zachazewski, P. O. Riley & D. E. Krebs, Biomechanical analysis of body mass transfer during stair ascent and descent of healthy subjects. *Journal of Rehabilitation Research and Development*, **30** (1993), 412–22.

108. K. Christina & P. Cavanagh, Ground reaction forces and frictional demands during stair descent: effects of age and illumination. *Gait and Posture*, **15** (2002), 153–8.

109. G. G. Simoneau, P. R. Cavanagh, J. S. Ulbrecht, H. W. Leibowitz & R. A. Tyrrell, The influence of visual factors on fall-related kinematic variables during stair descent by older women. *Journal of Gerontology*, **46** (1991), M188–95.

110. K. Williams, Intralimb coordination of older adults during locomotion: stair climbing. *Journal of Human Movement Studies*, **30** (1996), 269–84.

111. K. Williams, Intralimb coordination of older adults during locomotion: stair descent. *Journal of Human Movement Studies*, **34** (1998), 96–117.

112. T. Hortobagyi & P. DeVita, Altered movement strategy increases lower extremity stiffness during stepping down in the aged. *Journal of Gerontology*, **54A** (1999), B63–70.

113. T. Hortobagyi & P. DeVita, Muscle pre- and coactivity during downward stepping are associated with leg stiffness in aging. *Journal of Electromyography and Kinesiology*, **10** (2000), 117–26.

114. S. D. Lark, J. G. Buckley, S. Bennett, D. Jones, A. J. Sargeant, Joint torques and dynamic joint stiffness in elderly and young men during stepping down. *Clinical Biomechanics*, **18** (2003), 848–55.

115. R. Begg & W. Sparrow, Gait characteristics of young and older individuals negotiating a raised surface: implications for the prevention of falls. *Journal of Gerontology*, **55A** (2000), M147–54.

116. J. G. Buckley, K. J. Heasley, P. Twigg & D. B. Elliott, The effects of blurred vision on the mechanics of landing during stepping down by the elderly. *Gait and Posture*, **21** (2005), 65–71.

117. J. G. Buckley, K. Heasley, A. Scally & D. B. Elliott, The effects of blurring vision on medio-lateral balance during stepping up or down to a new level in the elderly. *Gait and Posture*, **22** (2005), 146–53.

118. S. R. Lord, J. Dayhew & A. Howland, Multifocal glasses impair edge-contrast sensitivity and depth perception and increase the risk of falls in older people. *Journal of the American Geriatrics Society*, **50** (2002), 1760–6.

119. D. Prudham & J. G. Evans, Factors associated with falls in the elderly: a community study. *Age and Ageing*, **10** (1981), 141–6.

120. A. J. Campbell, R. Reinken, B. C. Allan & G. S. Martinez, Falls in old age: a study of frequency and related clinical factors. *Age and Ageing*, **10** (1981), 264–70.

121. M. E. Tinetti, M. Speechley & S. F. Ginter, Risk factors for falls among elderly persons living in the community. *New England Journal of Medicine*, **319** (1988), 1701–7.

122. S. R. Lord, J. A. Ward, P. Williams & K. J. Anstey, An epidemiological study of falls in older community-dwelling women: the Randwick Falls and Fractures Study. *Australian Journal of Public Health*, **17** (1993), 240–54.

123. M. J. Pavol, T. M. Owings, K. T. Foley & M. D. Grabiner, The sex and age of older adults influence the outcome of induced trips. *Journal of Gerontology*, **54A** (1999), M103–8.

124. M. J. Pavol, T. M. Owings, K. T. Foley & M. D. Grabiner, Gait characteristics as risk factors for falling from trips induced in older adults. *Journal of Gerontology*, **54A** (1999), M583–90.

125. M. J. Pavol, T. M. Owings, K. T. Foley & M. D. Grabiner, Mechanisms leading to a fall from an induced trip in healthy older adults. *Journal of Gerontology*, **56** (2001), M428–37.

126. A. vanden Bogert, M. J. Pavol, M. D. Grabiner, Response time is more important than walking speed for the ability of older adults to avoid a fall after a trip. *Journal of Biomechanics*, **35** (2002), 199–205.

127. C. Smeesters, W. C. Hayes & T. A. McMahon, The threshold trip duration for which recovery is no longer possible is associated with strength and reaction time. *Journal of Biomechanics*, **34** (2001), 589–95.

128. M. Pijnappels, M. F. Bobbert & J. H. van Dieen, Push-off reactions in recovery after tripping discriminate young subjects, older non-fallers and older fallers. *Gait and Posture*, **21** (2005), 388–94.

129. M. Pijnappels, M. F. Bobbert & J. H. van Dieen, Control of support limb muscles in recovery after tripping in young and older subjects. *Experimental Brain Research*, **160** (2005), 326–33.

130. T. M. Owings, M. J. Pavol & M. D. Grabiner, Mechanisms of failed recovery following postural perturbations on a motorized treadmill mimic those associated with an actual forward trip. *Clinical Biomechanics*, **16** (2001), 813–19.

131. R. J. Best, Tripping probability during gait: a theoretical basis for research. *Book of Abstracts from the Australian Falls Prevention Conference*, November 2004, Manly, Australia, pp. 55.

132. A. Gabell, M. A. Simons & U. S. L. Nayak, Falls in the healthy elderly: predisposing causes. *Ergonomics*, **28** (1985), 965–75.

133. C. Smeesters, W. C. Hayes & T. A. McMahon, Disturbance type and gait speed affect fall direction and impact location. *Journal of Biomechanics*, **34** (2001), 309–17.

134. M. Redfern, R. Cham & K. Gielo-Perczak *et al.*, Biomechanics of slips. *Ergonomics*, **44** (2001), 1138–66.

135. Y.-C. Pai & K. Iqbal, Simulated movement termination for balance recovery: can movement strategies be sought to maintain stability in the presence of slipping or forced sliding? *Journal of Biomechanics*, **32** (1999), 779–86.

136. T. Bhatt, J. D. Wening & Y.-C. Pai, Influence of gait speed on stability: recovery from anterior slips and compensatory stepping. *Gait and Posture*, **21** (2005), 146–56.

137. L. Strandberg & H. Lanshammar, The dynamics of slipping accidents. *Journal of Occupational Accidents*, **3** (1981), 153–62.

138. L. Strandberg, On accident analysis and slip resistance measurement. *Ergonomics*, **26** (1983), 11–32.

139. R. Brady, M. J. Pavol, T. M. Owings & M. D. Grabiner, Foot displacement but not velocity predicts the outcome of a slip induced in young subjects while walking. *Journal of Biomechanics*, **33** (2000), 803–8.

140. J.-Y. You, Y.-L. Chou, C.-J. Lin, F.-C. Su, Effect of slip on movement of body center of mass relative to base of support. *Clinical Biomechanics*, **16** (2001), 167–73.

141. P.-F. Tang, M. H. Woollacott & R. K. Y. Chong, Control of reactive balance adjustments in perturbed human walking: roles of proximal and distal postural muscle activity. *Experimental Brain Research*, **119** (1998), 141–52.

142. R. Cham & M. Redfern, Lower extremity corrective reactions to slip events. *Journal of Biomechanics*, **34** (2001), 1439–45.

143. P.-F. Tang & M. H. Woollacott, Inefficient postural responses to unexpected slips during walking in older adults. *Journal of Gerontology*, **53A** (1998), M471–80.

144. R. Cham & M. Redfern, Changes in gait when anticipating slippery floors. *Gait and Posture*, **15** (2002), 159–71.

145. D. Marigold & A. Patla, Strategies for dynamic stability during locomotion on a slippery surface: effects of prior experience and knowledge. *Journal of Neurophysiology*, **88** (2002), 339–53.

146. M. Rogers, M. Johnson, K. Martinez, M. Mille & L. Hedman, Step training improves the speed of voluntary step initiation in aging. *Journal of Gerontology*, **58A** (2003), M46–51.

4

Sensory and neuromuscular
risk factors for falls

As discussed in Chapter 2, human balance depends on the interaction of multiple sensory, motor and integrative systems. In this chapter we review the studies which have dealt with: (i) age-related changes in the sensory and motor factors that are involved in balance control; and (ii) associations between these sensory and motor factors and falls in older people. Specific areas reviewed include: vision; visual field dependence; peripheral sensation; muscle strength, power and endurance; and reaction time.

Age-related changes in sensorimotor function

Figure 4.1 shows the physiological systems that are the primary contributors to stability. Many studies have found that functioning of these sensory, motor and integration systems declines significantly with age, and that impairment in these systems is associated with falls in older people. In fact, researchers have noted many people experience age-related declines in sensorimotor function, even in the absence of any documented disease. We have also found that many older people with a history of falls have no identifiable neurological or musculo-skeletal disease yet perform poorly in tests of sensorimotor function. As shown in Figure 4.2, these people mostly cite trips, slips, loss of balance and muscle weakness as the causes of their falls.

Figure 4.3 shows the 'normal' age-related decline in function in a sensorimotor system that contributes to stability. The figure shows that up until age 55 there is little change in function, but beyond this age there is a progressive decline. This decline occurs in all persons but the variability in function becomes greater as age increases. If the criterion level for a loss of balance and subsequent fall is 50 units, it can be seen that persons on the lower band reach this level by age 65 whereas those toward the upper band are still above the criterion level at 80 years of age. The figure also depicts a situation in which the onset of chronic disease such as a stroke can rapidly change functional performance and result in performance

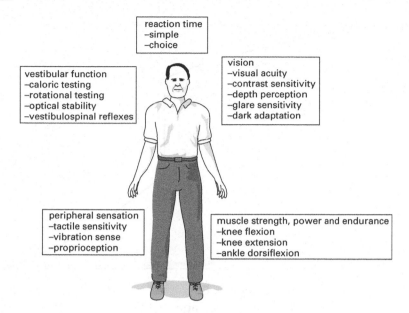

Fig. 4.1   Systems involved in the maintenance of postural stability.

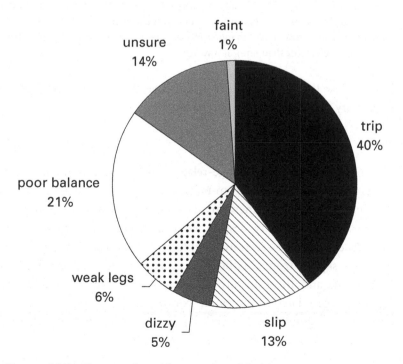

Fig. 4.2   Causes of falls. Diagram adapted from Lord *et al.* [123].

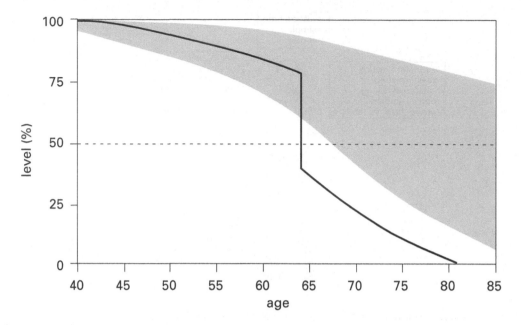

Fig. 4.3   Theoretical representation of the 'normal' age-related decline in function in a sensorimotor system that contributes to stability (grey shaded area represents upper and lower boundaries). The figure shows that up until age 55 there is little change in function, but beyond this age there is a progressive decline. This decline occurs in all persons but the range in function becomes greater as age increases. The figure also depicts a situation in which the onset of disease such as a stroke (dark line) can rapidly change functional performance and result in performance levels below the criterion (dashed line) at any age.

levels below the criterion level at any age. Acute illness may also result in a temporary decline in functional performance.

Vision

In 1864, Donders examined age-related changes in vision. He found that visual acuity decreased with age from 6/5 in people aged 20 years to 6/9 in people in their eighties [1]. Since then, many researchers have found similar age related-changes in visual acuity despite varying assessment methods. In general, the findings of large cross-sectional and longitudinal studies show that visual acuity improves slightly from childhood to 20 years of age, remains fairly constant up to 50 years and then steadily declines [2, 3]. Related research has also documented age-related declines in contrast sensitivity, glare sensitivity, dark adaptation, accommodation and depth perception, and that these changes are especially evident beyond 40 years of age [2].

A number of studies of falls risk in older people have included measures of visual impairment as a possible risk factor. Standard tests of visual acuity have been most commonly used to measure vision, however, the published findings have been inconsistent with regard to whether impaired performance in these tests increases the risk of falls. On the one hand, there are several reports that indicate impaired distant visual acuity is a risk factor for falls in community-dwelling [4–7] and institutionalized older people [8]. However, other studies have not found this to be the case, particularly when confounding factors such as age are adjusted for [9–13]. Large case control [14] and prospective studies have also assessed whether reduced visual acuity is a risk factor for hip fracture [15–17] – a serious consequence of falls in older people. Three of these have found a significant association [14–16], but the other did not [17].

In a series of studies, we have found tests of edge-contrast sensitivity to be more strongly associated with falls than visual acuity [6, 9, 18]. This was also the case in the Blue Mountains Eye Study, which compared the predictive power of a range of visual tests, including visual acuity and visual field size [4], and in two large cohorts assessing fracture risk factors [17, 19]. Edge-contrast sensitivity tests measure a person's ability to detect edges under low contrast conditions and may reflect the ability to detect ground-level hazards. Thus, a loss of edge-contrast sensitivity may predispose older people to trip over obstacles within the home as well as outdoor hazards such as steps, kerbs, and pavement cracks and misalignments.

Reduced depth perception has also consistently been found to be a significant risk factor for falls and fractures. Nevitt *et al.* [5] found that older persons who had poor stereoacuity were at a significantly higher risk of suffering recurrent falls, and Cummings *et al.* [17] and Ivers *et al.* [14] have reported that poor depth perception was an important risk factor for hip fracture. We have recently found that of nine measures of vision, impaired depth perception was the strongest risk factor for multiple falls in 156 community-dwelling older people [18]. Furthermore, subjects with good vision in both eyes had the lowest rate of falls, whereas subjects with good vision in one eye but only moderate or poor vision in the other had elevated fall rates – equivalent to those with moderate vision in both eyes. This suggests that the ability to judge distances accurately and perceive spatial relationships is important for negotiating and avoiding obstacles and hazards in the environment. Further support for impaired depth perception being a risk factor for falls comes from a study by Felson *et al.* [15], who found that older persons who had good vision in one eye, but only moderately good vision in the other, had an elevated hip fracture risk.

Although not as important as contrast sensitivity and visual acuity, Ivers *et al.* found that visual field loss was an independent risk factor for falls [4]. Klien *et al.* also reported that visual field loss was associated with both multiple falls and fractures in the Beaver Dam Eye Study [7]. In contrast, Nevitt *et al.* reported no significant association between visual field loss and recurrent falls [5], and Glyn *et al.* found that visual field loss was only weakly associated with falls in patients attending a glaucoma clinic [20].

In addition to allowing us to detect hazards in the environment, vision also plays a direct and important role in stabilizing balance by providing the nervous system with continually updated information regarding the position and movements of body segments in relation to each other and the environment. When people stand with their eyes closed, postural sway increases by between 20% and 70% [21–24]. It has also been found that moving visual fields can induce a powerful sense of self-motion, and misleading visual cues induce significant increases in sway [25]. We have found that while visual measures are not predictors of sway when older people stand on a firm surface, they are significant predictors of sway when older subjects stand on a compliant foam rubber surface [23, 24, 26], when the visual system is relied upon to detect larger movements of the body. In the most recent of these studies [26], we found that poor performances in tests of distant contrast sensitivity and stereopsis (a measure of depth perception) were independent predictors of increased sway in a multivariate regression model. This suggests that the accurate perception of visual stimuli and depth play important roles in formulating a visual reference frame for stabilization of the body relative to its surroundings.

The above findings suggest that the ability to detect low contrast hazards, judge distances and perceive spatial relationships are particularly important for maintaining balance and avoiding falls in older age groups. Tests that most closely assess these visual functions provide the best predictors of falls and fall-related fractures in this group.

Visual field dependence

In spite of the demonstrated deterioration of vision with age, it has been suggested that old people may place greater reliance on the spatial framework provided by vision in an attempt to compensate for reduced vestibular and postural sensation [27]. Thus in situations where minimal, ambiguous or misleading spatial information is provided by vision, body position may be wrongly determined and a fall may result. In test situations which place visual and postural cues in conflict (i.e. exposing older people to tilted or rolling visual stimuli) it has been found that older fallers are more reliant on the visuo-spatial framework (that is they are more field dependent) than older non-fallers [28–30].

As these studies have been undertaken in artificial situations, the findings may only partly generalize to real world situations. The implications, however, are that tilted, moving or rolling visual stimuli, such as tilted forms and landmarks, congested pedestrian or vehicular traffic, moving vehicles, structures, and shadows, may contribute to falls in older people with impaired postural control.

Peripheral sensation

Scientific interest in peripheral sensation dates back to 1830 when Mueller mentioned vibration sense briefly in a textbook of physiology [31]. At the turn of the century, a number of clinicians noted that vibration sense of older persons was inferior to that of younger ones. It was not until 1928, however, that Pearson clearly demonstrated that vibration sense decreased with age [32]. Since then many investigators, using numerous vibrating stimuli, placed on various parts of the body, have consistently found age-related declines in vibration sense to all vibration frequencies greater than 50 Hz [33–47]. It has also been found that vibration sense is poorer in the lower limb compared with the upper limb at all ages and shows a greater age-related decline [35–39, 44, 46].

Scientific interest in tactile sensitivity also dates back to the nineteenth century, although there have been comparatively fewer studies on the effect of age on this sensory modality. Like vibration sense, most reports indicate that tactile sensitivity, as measured by aesthesiometers or by two point discrimination, decreases significantly with age [24, 46, 48–52] and is reduced in the lower limb compared with the upper limb [46, 49, 51, 53].

Even fewer studies have been undertaken on the effect of age on joint position sense. Laidlaw and Hamilton were the first researchers to demonstrate an age-related decline in joint position sense [54]. They found that subjects aged 17 to 35 years had a better ability to detect direction of joint movements of the hip, knee and ankle than subjects aged 50 to 85 years. Since then, further studies have found significant age-related declines in position sense of the knee joint [55–58] and metatarsophalangeal joint [59]. However, clinical studies which have investigated whether there is a decline in joint position sense beyond 65 years of age have produced inconsistent results. This may be due at least in part to the imprecision of the tests used, which have been based on the subjects' ability to identify experimenter-induced movements of body parts [10, 60, 61].

It has also been pointed out that caution should be used in assessing joint position sense when assessments are made while subjects are in the seated position [62], as is the case in all of the above studies. This is because thresholds in the ankle and knee are much lower when measured in the standing, weight-bearing position [63, 64], where engagement of the leg muscles is greatly increased [65].

In a recent study, Bullock-Saxton *et al.* assessed the effects of age on the accuracy of knee joint-repositioning, in both full and partial weight-bearing conditions, in 60 healthy, pain-free subjects from three age groups (young: 20–35 years old, middle-aged: 40–55 years, and older: 60–75 years) [64]. They found that subjects in all three groups performed better when full weight bearing than when partial weight bearing, and significant age-related increases were found only in the partial weight-bearing condition. However, other studies assessing position sense of the ankle joint when weight bearing, have reported increased thresholds with age. Thelen *et al.* [66] compared the ability of young and older women to detect dorsiflexion and plantarflexion movements of the foot when weight bearing on a moveable platform, and reported that the threshold for movement detection was three to four times larger in the older group. High detection thresholds for inversion and eversion movements of the ankle when standing either unipedally or bipedally on a rotating platform have also been found in older people [67], and in people with a peripheral neuropathy [68]. Finally, Blaszczyk *et al.* [69] have reported that older subjects are significantly worse than young subjects in reproducing ankle joint positions when standing on a rotating platform.

It is surprising then that reduced peripheral sensation or neuropathy has only occasionally been mentioned as a cause of instability or falls. Hurley *et al.* found that reduced proprioceptive acuity at the knee was significantly associated with an increased aggregate time to perform a range of functional tasks, comprising a timed walk, the Get Up and Go Test, and stair ascent and descent, in a combined group of young, middle aged and older people [58]. Robbins *et al.* found that lower extremity 'sensory abnormalities' were associated with falls in one of two populations studied [11], and Buchner and Larson reported peripheral neuropathy to be a cause of falls in patients with Alzheimer's disease [70]. Brocklehurst *et al.*, however, reported a significant association between impaired proprioception in the ankle and/or great toe and falls in only one of three age-groups (75–84 years) above 65 years of age [10]. Nevitt *et al.* [5], Wolfsen *et al.* [71] and Grisso *et al.* [72] found no significant associations between crude measures of impaired peripheral sensation and falls.

In contrast, a recent study by Richardson *et al.* found a strong association between electromyographically documented polyneuropathy involving the lower extremities and falls [73]. Likewise, Luukinen *et al.* found that peripheral neuropathy was an independent risk factor for recurrent falling in 1016 community-dwelling persons aged 70 years or older living in Finland [74]. In a similar study, our group has found that in both men and women, older subjects with diabetes performed significantly worse in tests of body sway on firm and compliant surfaces compared with the non-diabetic subjects [75]. Richardson *et al.*

suggested that the failure to find a relationship between peripheral neuropathy and falling in previous reports may be due to the limited accuracy of clinical examinations in diagnosing neuropathy.

In many of our studies we have used quantitative assessments to measure peripheral sensation. In community [30, 76] and institutionalized settings [77, 78], we have found that tactile sensitivity at the ankle assessed with a Semmes-Weinstein aesthesiometer [6] is inferior in fallers compared with non-fallers. In a large prospective community study, we have also found that fallers demonstrated higher thresholds for detecting a 200 Hz vibration sense at the knee compared with non-fallers [6]. Impaired lower limb proprioception assessed quantitatively with a lower limb-matching task was also associated with falls in older people in the community [6], a retirement village [79] and intermediate hostel care [77].

Thus it seems that reduced peripheral sensation is associated with falls, but that such an association only emerges when the measures of peripheral sensation are accurately and quantitatively ascertained.

Vestibular sense

The vestibular system contributes to posture by maintaining the reflex arc keeping the head and neck in the vertical position, and by corrective movements elicited through the vestibulo-ocular and vestibulo-spinal pathways [62]. Ageing has been found to be associated with a diminished ability to enhance and suppress the vestibulo-ocular reflex (VOR) during horizontal rotation [80], and reduced reactivity to caloric and rotational stimulation has been reported in subjects over 60 years of age [81, 82]. Katsarkas studied over 1000 patients aged 70 years and over and found that over one-third had impaired vestibular function [83].

In spite of this apparent age-related decline in function, initial reports did not document associations between impaired vestibular function and either instability or falls in older people. Nashner [84] found that the otoliths play no role in the initial detection of body sway, and Brocklehurst et al. [10] and Woolley et al. [85] reported no significant association between vestibular sense, as measured by response to a slow tilt, and sway or falls. We have found that vestibular function, as measured by Fukuda's vertical writing [86], stepping tests [87] or a test of vestibulo-ocular stability, is not related to stability [23, 24] or falls [6, 77]. However, it is acknowledged that in these assessments the older subjects with very poor balance could not perform two of the tests, as they were unable to walk on a treadmill or walk in place unsupported with eyes closed for one minute. All of the above tests have also been indirect and possibly too insensitive to be able to detect subtle yet significant impairments in vestibular function.

More recent studies that have included more precise assessments of vestibular function have reported significant associations between vestibular impairment, and falls and fractures. In a series of studies, Kristinsdottir *et al.* have used a head-shaking stimulus applied when subjects were in a supine position to induce nystagmus – a sign indicating pathology and asymmetry of the vestibular reflexes [88, 89]. In two case-control studies they assessed whether vestibular asymmetry induced using this technique was associated with fall-related fractures in older people [88, 89]. The initial study comprised 19 subjects (mean age = 72 years) with hip fracture (which occurred 12–33 months earlier) and 28 aged-matched controls [88]. They found that 13 of the hip fracture subjects (68%) demonstrated a nystagmus following the head-shake stimulus compared with 10 of the controls (36%) – OR = 3.90 (95% CI = 0.97–16.38). The second study involved 66 subjects (mean age 68 years) who had suffered a fall-related wrist fracture during a ten month period and 49 control subjects comprising healthy community-dwelling people (mean age 75 years) [89]. Nystagmus after head shaking was found in 50 of the subjects with wrist fracture (76%) but in only 18 of the controls (37%) – OR = 5.38 (95% CI = 2.23–13.11).

In related studies, Di Fabio *et al.* have examined the contribution of VOR suppression to falls in older people [90, 91]. The control of gaze during head movement requires input from the VOR. However, during the performance of many well-practiced familiar tasks such as standing and walking the VOR needs to be suppressed when both eye and head movements are used to stabilize images on the retina [92]. In a case-control study involving 36 older people categorized as being at either high or low risk of falls (18 subjects per group), VOR suppression was assessed by measuring eye-movements using electro-oculography during a stand-walk task [90]. While the majority of subjects showed some counter-rotation of the eyes with head pitch, a greater percentage of subjects in the high-risk group did not suppress this response, and consequently gaze and gaze velocity overcompensated for head pitch. In a subsequent study of 38 women (mean age = 82 years; 11 fallers), they found that participants who failed to suppress the VOR gain when subjected to a two-handed nudge to the scapulae, were 18 times more likely to have fallen in the past year compared with participants who showed VOR suppression – OR = 18.00 (95% CI = 1.63–198.42) [91]. While these findings need to be viewed with some caution due to the small study numbers, they suggest that inadequate suppression of the VOR following a postural perturbation and during a stand-walk task may predispose older people to falls. Vestibular function is less amenable to assessment with simple screening tests compared with vision and peripheral sensation. However, recent studies provide preliminary evidence that when assessed with greater precision, impaired vestibular function may be an important risk factor for falls and fall-related fractures in older people. Further research is required to elucidate the significance of vestibular input in maintaining a stable retinal image for clear vision during head movement and otolithic functioning for balance control, and falls avoidance.

Muscle strength, power and endurance

There are numerous reports of loss of isometric and dynamic muscle strength with age [93–99]. In men, muscle strength appears to decrease only marginally between 20 and 40 years. Beyond 40 years, muscle strength declines at an accelerated pace, so that hand grip strength is reduced by 5%–15% [93, 94] and leg strength by 20%–40% [95, 98] in men aged 60–69 compared with men aged 20–29. In women, muscle strength appears to decline from an earlier age and at a greater rate, so that over the same age range, hand grip strength declines by 10%–25% [93, 94] and leg strength by 30%–50% [96, 97]. It has also been shown that muscle strength continues to decline significantly beyond the sixties in both sexes [99]. Muscle strength in women is reported to be about 50%–70% of that in men [93–99].

Leg extensor power (the product of force and the rate of force generation) appears to decline at an even greater rate with age than does isometric strength. In a cross-sectional study of 100 men and women aged 65–89 years, Skelton *et al.* [100] found a loss of isometric strength of 1%–2% per annum, whereas the loss of leg extensor power was around 3.5% per annum. Increased age is also associated with reduced isometric and dynamic endurance when measured in absolute terms. However, when endurance is measured in relation to maximal strength (i.e. 50% of maximal contraction) and therefore controlled for individual differences, no decline with age is evident [93, 101–103] – a finding suggesting that sub-maximal muscle strength is less affected by ageing than maximal muscle strength.

Muscle weakness in the lower limbs has significant practical implications for older people. Pearson *et al.* [104] found that in 14% of women aged 75 years and over living in the community, the calf muscle was not able to exert sufficient force to support the body weight. This indicates that these women would be at risk of falling in situations where they place their total body weight on one leg only, i.e. when undertaking everyday activities like stepping up a step. Vandervoort and Hayes [105] found impaired ankle plantarflexor muscle force and power in residents of geriatric care facilities who were capable of independently performing activities of daily living. They found that the ankle plantarflexor muscles in these women exhibited considerable impairment in their ability to generate stabilizing torques about the ankle joint. Reduced strength is also reflected in a difficulty in rising from a chair without the use of the hands, and it has been found that an inability to undertake this task is a significant risk factor for falls in both community [5, 12] and institutional groups of older people [106, 107].

Strength in specific lower-limb muscle groups has also been found to be reduced in fallers compared with non-fallers. In community studies, our group has found that reduced isometric knee extension strength [6, 30, 76] and isometric ankle dorsiflexion strength [6] increases the risk of falls, and reduced isometric knee extension strength increases the risk of fractures [108]. Reduced knee extension strength has also been found to be a risk factor in other samples of community-dwelling people, including participants of a large longitudinal study [109], residents of retirement villages [78], older people requiring day-care [110] and older people with vitamin D deficiency [111].

Lower-limb muscle weakness has been found to be associated with falls in nursing home and intermediate-care hostel residents. Whipple et al. [112] and Studenski et al. [113] both compared the strength of four lower-limb muscle groups: knee extensors, knee flexors, ankle plantarflexors and ankle dorsiflexors in residents of nursing homes with and without a history of falls. Both studies found that fallers were weaker than non-fallers in all four muscle groups, with ankle muscle weakness particularly evident in the faller groups. These findings are in accord with other studies which have also found that decreased ankle dorsiflexion [77], knee extension [78, 107, 114] and hip strength [11] increase the risk of falls in older people living in residential-care institutions.

Two recent retrospective studies have examined reduced muscle power and reduced muscle endurance as risk factors for falls. In a case-control study of 15 older women who had suffered three or more falls in the previous year and 15 older women who reported no falls, Skelton et al. found that the fallers demonstrated a significantly greater asymmetry in muscle strength and power, and when the less powerful legs were compared, the fallers were significantly less powerful than the non-fallers [115]. In a study assessing muscle endurance, Schwender et al. [116] used an isokinetic dynamometer to assess dynamic endurance of the quadriceps muscle in 29 young women (mean age 22 years), 26 older women who reported falls in the past 18 months (mean age 73 years) and 27 older women with no history of falls (mean age 71 years). They found that time to fatigue was shorter in the older fallers than in the young women and older non-fallers, but was not different between the young women and the older non-fallers.

The consistency of these findings indicates that lower-limb muscle weakness is a major risk factor for falling in older people.

Reaction time

Of all the studies on age-related changes in neurological and sensorimotor systems, reaction time has possibly been studied more than any other factor. Welford [117] has summarized the findings of 21 studies on the effect of age on reaction time and found a median increase of 26% in reaction time from the twenties to the sixties. Even allowing for factors such as, the amount of practice, length of preparatory interval, physical health, mode of response and level of motivation, it has been consistently found that reaction time declines with age.

In many of our studies, we have used a simple reaction time paradigm, with a simple motor response, i.e. pressing a switch with the finger, so as to emphasize the decision time component of the task. We found that increased reaction time was an independent risk factor for falls in older community-dwelling women [6], residents of retirement villages [79], and older persons living in residential care [77, 78, 107]. It has also been found that finger-press choice reaction time discriminates between older fallers and non-fallers [111], and older people who have and have not suffered fall-related fractures [118].

Fallers are also significantly slower than non-fallers in reaction time tests that involve more complex motor responses. For example, Grabiner and Jahnigen found that fallers are slower than non-fallers in simple reaction time and choice reaction time tests that require extending and flexing the knee [119]. Woolley *et al.* also found that a resisted choice reaction time task that required subjects to break contact with a heel magnet so as to generate a force equal to up to 10% of body weight and then kick one of three targets, significantly discriminated between fallers and non-fallers [120].

Reaction time has been found to be independent of body sway when subjects are standing on firm surfaces after confounding effects such as age are adjusted for [23, 119]. We have noted, however, that when subjects are standing on a compliant surface (foam rubber) which reduces proprioceptive input from the ankles, cutaneous inputs from the soles of the feet and ankle support, reaction time is moderately associated with body sway [23, 24]. Under these conditions sway is greatly exaggerated and subjects report that they detect their body movement. Thus it seems that individuals with slow reaction time may be susceptible to falls as a result of an inability to correct postural imbalances.

Integration, interaction and summation

The above studies indicate that impairment in a number of the primary physiological systems that contribute to stability is associated with falls in older people. With such an array of inputs there is also little doubt interactions occur between the various stages in the processing of a response to a fall, i.e. sensory input and feed-forward, response selection, and response execution [62, 119]. For example, much work has shown that vision can compensate for diminished peripheral input, when either experimentally induced or as a result of disease or trauma [63, 121, 122].

Our analysis suggests that while a marked impairment in just one of the physiological systems that contribute to stability is sufficient to increase the risk of falls, multiple impairments of only moderate severity are also associated with increased falls risk. For example, in the case of a trip, reduced vision and slow reaction times may both be necessary for a fall to occur. Thus it seems that adequate visual, somatosensory and vestibular acuity contribute to the detection of postural disturbances and environmental hazards, while adequate strength and reaction time permit appropriate corrections to postural imbalance.

Conclusion

There is considerable evidence that the sensorimotor factors that contribute to balance control show age-related declines. Many studies have shown that over and above the effect of ageing, older people who fall demonstrate impaired function in these measures when compared with age and sex matched non-fallers. Physiological systems identified as impaired in older fallers include visual functions such as contrast sensitivity and depth perception, visual field dependence, peripheral sensation, strength in the lower-limb muscle groups, and reaction time. There is now also preliminary evidence that impaired vestibular functioning, and reduced muscle power and endurance are also important risk factors for falls.

REFERENCES

1. F. C. Donders, *On the Anomalies of Accommodation and Refraction of the Eye. With a Preliminary Essay on Physiological Optics* (London: New Sydenham Society, 1864).
2. D. G. Pitts, The effects of aging on selected visual functions: dark adaptation, visual acuity, stereopsis, brightness contrast. In *Aging in Human Visual Functions*, ed. R. Sekuler, D. W. Kline & K. Dismukes. (New York: Liss, 1982).
3. N. S. Gittings & J. L. Fozard, Age related changes in visual acuity. *Experimental Gerontology*, **21** (1986), 423–33.
4. R. Q. Ivers, R. G. Cumming, P. Mitchell *et al.*, Visual impairment and falls in older adults: the Blue Mountains Eye Study. *Journal of the American Geriatrics Society*, **46** (1998), 58–64.
5. M. Nevitt, S. Cummings, S. Kidd & D. Black, Risk factors for recurrent non-syncopal falls. *Journal of the American Medical Association*, **261** (1989), 2663–8.

6. S. R. Lord, J. A. Ward, P. Williams & K. Anstey, Physiological factors associated with falls in older community-dwelling women. *Journal of the American Geriatrics Society*, **42** (1994), 1110–17.

7. B. E. K. Klein, S. E. Moss, R. Klein, K. E. Lee & K. J. Cruikshanks, Associations of visual function with physical outcomes and limitations 5 years later in an older population. The Beaver Dame Eye Study. *Ophthalmology*, **110** (2003), 644–50.

8. M. E. Tinetti, T. F. Williams & R. Mayewski, Falls risk index for elderly patients based on number of chronic disabilities. *American Journal of Medicine*, **80** (1986), 429–34.

9. S. R. Lord, R. D. Clark & I. W. Webster, Visual acuity and contrast sensitivity in relation to falls in an elderly population. *Age and Ageing*, **20** (1991), 175–81.

10. J. C. Brocklehurst, D. Robertson & P. James-Groom, Clinical correlates of sway in old age – sensory modalities. *Age and Ageing*, **11** (1982), 1–10.

11. A. S. Robbins, L. Z. Rubenstein, K. R. Josephson *et al.*, Predictors of falls among elderly people – results of two population-based studies. *Archives of Internal Medicine*, **149** (1989), 1628–33.

12. A. J. Campbell, M. J. Borrie & G. F. Spears, Risk factors for falls in a community-based prospective study of people 70 years and older. *Journal of Gerontology*, **44A** (1989), M112–17.

13. M. E. Tinetti, M. Speechley & S. F. Ginter, Risk factors for falls among elderly persons living in the community. *New England Journal of Medicine*, **319** (1988), 1701–7.

14. R. Q. Ivers, R. Norton, R. G. Cumming, M. Butler & A. J. Campbell, Visual impairment and hip fracture. *American Journal of Epidemiology*, **152** (2000), 663–9.

15. D. T. Felson, J. J. Anderson & M. T. Annan, Impaired vision and hip fracture. The Framingham study. *Journal of the American Geriatrics Society*, **37** (1989), 495–500.

16. P. Dargent-Mollina, F. Favier, H. Grandjean *et al.*, Fall-related factors and risk of hip fracture: the EPIDOS prospective study. *The Lancet*, **348** (1996), 145–9.

17. S. R. Cummings, M. C. Nevitt, W. S. Browner *et al.*, Risk factors for hip fracture in white women: Study of Osteoporosis Fractures Research Group. *New England Journal of Medicine*, **332** (1995), 767–73.

18. S. R. Lord & J. Dayhew, Visual risk factors for falls. *Journal of the American Geriatrics Society*, **49** (2001), 508–15.

19. M. R. De Boer, S. M. Pluijm, P. Lips *et al.*, Different aspects of visual impairment as risk factors for falls and fractures in older men and women. *Journal of Bone and Mineral Research*, **19** (2004), 1539–47.

20. R. J. Glyn, J. M. Seddon, J. H. Krug *et al.*, Falls in elderly patients with glaucoma. *Archives of Ophthalmology*, **109** (1991), 205–10.

21. M. Magnusson, H. Endom, R. Johansson & J. Wiklund, Significance of pressor input from the human feet in anterior-posterior postural control. *Acta Otolaryngologica*, **110** (1990), 182–8.

22. W. M. Paulus, A. Straube & T. Brandt, Visual stabilization of posture. Physiological stimulus characteristics and clinical aspects. *Brain*, **107** (1984), 1143–63.

23. S. R. Lord, R. D. Clark & I. W. Webster, Postural stability and associated physiological factors in a population of aged persons. *Journal of Gerontology*, **46** (1991), M69–76.

24. S. R. Lord & J. A. Ward, Age-associated differences in sensori-motor function and balance in community dwelling women. *Age and Ageing*, **23** (1994), 452–60.

25. D. N. Lee & J. R. Lishman, Visual proprioceptive control of stance. *Journal of Human Movement Studies*, **1** (1975), 87–95.

26. S. R. Lord & H. B. Menz, Visual contributions to postural stability in older adults. *Gerontology*, **46** (2000), 306–10.

27. R. Over, Possible visual factors in falls by old people. *Gerontologist*, **6** (1966), 212–14.

28. J. S. Tobis, S. Reinsch, J. M. Swanson, M. Byrd & T. Scharf, Visual perception dominance of fallers among community-dwelling older adults. *Journal of the American Geriatrics Society*, **33** (1985), 330–3.

29. S. R. Lord I. W. Webster, Visual field dependence in elderly fallers and non-fallers. *International Journal of Aging and Human Development*, **31** (1990), 269–79.

30. S. R. Lord, P. N. Sambrook, C. Gilbert *et al.*, Postural stability, falls and fractures. Results from the Dubbo Osteoporosis Epidemiology Study. *Medical Journal of Australia*, **160** (1994), 684–91.

31. J. C. Fox & W. W. Klemperer, Vibratory sensibility – a quantitative study of its thresholds in nervous disorders. *Archives of Neurology and Psychiatry*, **48** (1942), 622–45.

32. G. H. J. Pearson, Effect of age on vibratory sensibility. *Archives of Neurology and Psychiatry*, **20** (1928), 482–96.

33. R. C. Gray, A quantitative study of vibration sense in normal and pernicious anaemia cases. *Minnesota Medicine*, **15** (1932), 674–91.

34. H. W. Newman & K. B. Corbin, Quantitative determination of vibratory sensibility. *Society of Experimental Biology and Medicine*, **35** (1936), 273–6.

35. R. W. Laidlaw & M. A. Hamilton, Thresholds of vibratory sensibility as determined by the pallesthesiometer. *Bulletin of the Neurological Institute of New York*, **6** (1937), 494–503.

36. J. A. Cosh, Studies on the nature of vibration sense. *Clinical Science*, **12** (1953), 131–51.

37. I. A. Mirsky, P. Futterman & R. H. Broh-Kahn, The quantitative measurement of vibratory perception in subjects with and without diabetes mellitus. *Journal of Laboratory and Clinical Medicine*, **41** (1953), 221–35.

38. I. B. Steiness, Vibratory perception in normal subjects. *Acta Medica Scandinavica*, **158** (1957), 315–25.

39. G. Rosenberg, Effect of age on peripheral vibratory perception. *Journal of the American Geriatrics Association*, **6** (1958), 471–81.

40. F. U. Steinberg & A. L. Graber, The effect of age and peripheral circulation on the perception of vibration. *Archives of Physical Medicine and Rehabilitation*, **44** (1963), 645–50.

41. A. D. Whanger & H. S. Wang, Clinical correlates of the vibratory sense in elderly psychiatric patients. *Journal of Gerontology*, **29** (1974), 39–45.

42. C. S. Plumb & J. W. Meigs, Human vibration perception. *Archives of General Psychiatry*, **4** (1961), 103–6.

43. G. D. Goff, B. S. Rosner, T. Detre & D. Kennard, Vibration perception in normal man and medical patients. *Journal of Neurology, Neurosurgery and Psychiatry*, **28** (1965), 503–9.

44. E. Perret & F. Regli, Age and the perceptual thresholds for vibratory stimuli. *European Neurology*, **4** (1970), 65–76.

45. R. T. Verrillo, Comparison of vibrotactile threshold and suprathreshold responses in men and women. *Perception and Psychophysics*, **26** (1979), 20–4.

46. D. R. Kenshalo, Somesthetic sensitivity in young and elderly humans. *Journal of Gerontology*, **41** (1986), 732–42.

47. P. Era, J. Jokela, H. Suominen & E. Heikkinen, Correlates of vibrotactile thresholds in men of different ages. *Acta Neurologica Scandinavica*, **74** (1986), 210–17.

48. S. Axelrod & L. D. Cohen, Senescence and embedded-figure performance in vision and touch. *Perceptual and Motor Skills*, **12** (1961), 283–8.

49. P. J. Dyck, P. W. Schultz & P. C. O'Brien, Quantification of touch-pressure sensation. *Archives of Neurology*, **26** (1972), 465–73.

50. G. A. Gesheider, S. J. Bolanowski, K. L. Hall, K. E. Hoffman & R. T. Verillo, The effects of aging on information-processing channels in the sense of touch. I. Absolute sensitivity. *Somatosensory and Motor Research*, **11** (1994), 345–57.

51. C. F. Bolton, R. K. Winkelmann & P. J. Dyck, A quantitative study of Meissner's corpuscles in man. *Neurology*, **16** (1966), 1–9.

52. J. C. Stevens & K. K. Choo, Spatial acuity of the body surface over the life span. *Somatosensory and Motor Research*, **13** (1996), 153–66.

53. E. M. Halar, M. C. Hammond, E. C. LaCava, C. Camann & J. Ward, Sensory perception threshold measurement: an evaluation of semi-objective testing devices. *Archives of Physical Medicine and Rehabilitation*, **68** (1987), 499–507.

54. R. W. Laidlaw & N. A. Hamilton, A study of thresholds in appreciation of passive movement among normal control subjects. *Bulletin of the Neurological Institute*, **6** (1937), 268–73.

55. H. B. Skinner, R. L. Barrack & S. D. Cook, Age-related decline in proprioception. *Clinical Orthopaedics and Related Research*, **184** (1984), 208–11.

56. F. S. Kaplan, J. E. Nixon, M. Reitz, L. Rindfleish & J. Tucker, Age-related changes in proprioception and sensation of joint position. *Acta Orthopaedica Scandinavica*, **56** (1985), 72–4.

57. R. J. Petrella, P. J. Lattanzio & M. G. Nelson, Effect of age and activity on knee joint proprioception. *American Journal of Physical Medicine and Rehabilitation*, **76** (1997), 235–41.

58. M. V. Hurley, J. Rees & D. J. Newham, Quadriceps function, proprioceptive acuity and functional performance in healthy young, middle-aged and elderly subjects. *Age and Ageing*, **27** (1998), 55–62.

59. E. Kokmen, R. W. Bossemeyer & W. J. Williams, Quantitative evaluation of joint motion sensation in an aging population. *Journal of Gerontology*, **33** (1978), 62–7.

60. W. J. MacLennan, J. I. Timothy & M. R. P. Hall, Vibration sense, proprioception and ankle reflexes in old age. *Journal of Clinical and Experimental Gerontology*, **2** (1980), 159–71.

61. T. H. Howell, Senile deterioration of the central nervous system. *British Medical Journal*, **i** (1949), 56–8.

62. S. E. Stelmach & C. J. Worringham, Sensorimotor deficits related to postural stability. Implications for falling in the elderly. *Clinics in Geriatric Medicine*, **1** (1985), 679–94.

63. V. S. Gurfinkel, M. I. Lipshits & K. E. Popov, Thresholds for kinesthetic sensation in the vertical position. *Human Physiology*, **8** (1982), 439–45.

64. J. E. Bullock-Saxon, W. J. Wong & N. Hogan, The influence of age on weight-bearing joint reposition sense of the knee. *Experimental Brain Research*, **136** (2001), 400–6.

65. K. M. Refshauge & R. C. Fitzpatrick, Perception of movement at the human ankle: effects of leg position. *Journal of Physiology*, **488** (1995), 243–8.

66. D. G. Thelen, C. Brockmiller, J. A. Ashton-Miller, A. B. Schultz & N. B. Alexander, Thresholds for sensing foot dorsi- and plantarflexion during upright stance: effects of age and velocity. *Journal of Gerontology*, **53** (1998), M33–8.

67. M. G. Gilsing, C. G. Vanden Bosch, S. -G. Lee *et al.*, Association of age with the threshold for detecting ankle inversion and eversion in upright stance. *Age and Ageing*, **24** (1995), 58–66.

68. C. G. Vanden Bosch, M. Gilsing, S. -G. Lee, J. Richardson & J. Ashton-Miller, Peripheral neuropathy effect on ankle inversion and eversion detection thresholds. *Archives of Physical Medicine and Rehabilitation*, **76** (1995), 850–6.

69. J. W. Blaszczyk, P. D. Hansen & D. L. Lowe, Accuracy of passive ankle joint positioning during quiet stance in young and elderly subjects. *Gait and Posture*, **1** (1993), 211–15.

70. D. M. Buchner & E. B. Larson, Falls and fractures in patients with Alzheimer-type dementia. *Journal of the American Medical Association*, **257** (1987), 1492–5.

71. L. Wolfson, J. Judge, R. Whipple & M. King, Strength is a major factor in balance, gait, and the occurrence of falls. *Journal of Gerontology*, **50** (1995), S64–7.

72. J. A. Grisso, J. L. Kelsey, B. L. Strom *et al.*, Risk factors for falls as a cause of hip fracture in women. *New England Journal of Medicine*, **324** (1991), 1321–6.

73. J. Richardson, C. Ching & E. Hurvitz, The relationship between electromyographically documented peripheral neuropathy and falls. *Journal of the American Geriatrics Society*, **40** (1992), 1008–12.

74. H. Luukinen, K. Koski, P. Laippala & S. L. Kivela, Predictors for recurrent falls among the home-dwelling elderly. *Scandinavian Journal of Primary Health Care*, **13** (1995), 294–9.

75. S. R. Lord, G. A. Caplan, R. Colagiuri & J. A. Ward, Sensori-motor function in older persons with diabetes. *Diabetic Medicine*, **10** (1993), 614–18.

76. S. R. Lord, D. McLean & G. Stathers, Physiological factors associated with injurious falls in older people living in the community. *Gerontology*, **38** (1992), 338–46.

77. S. R. Lord, R. D. Clark & I. W. Webster, Physiological factors associated with falls in an elderly population. *Journal of the American Geriatrics Society*, **39** (1991), 1194–200.

78. S. R. Lord & R. D. Clark, Simple physiological and clinical tests for the accurate prediction of falling in older people. *Gerontology*, **42** (1996), 199–203.

79. S. R. Lord & R. D. Fitzpatrick, Choice stepping reaction time: a composite measure of falls risk in older people. *Journal of Gerontology*, **56A** (2001), M627–32.

80. R. W. Baloh, K. M. Jacobsen & T. M. Socotch, The effect of aging on visual vestbulo-ocular responses. *Experimental Brain Research*, **95** (1993), 509–16.

81. E. A. Karlsen, R. M. Hassanein & C. P. Goetzinger, The effects of age, sex, hearing loss and water temperature on caloric nystagmus. *The Laryngoscope*, **91** (1981), 620–7.

82. P. Ghosh, Aging and auditory vestibular response. *Ear, Nose and Throat Journal,* **64** (1985), 264–6.

83. A. Katsarkas, Dizziness in ageing: a retrospective study of 1194 cases. *Otolaryngology Head and Neck Surgery,* **110** (1994), 296–301.

84. L. M. Nashner, A model describing vestibular detection of body sway motion. *Acta Otolaryngologica,* **72** (1971), 429–36.

85. S. M. Woolley, S. J. Czaja & C. G. Drury, An assessment of falls in elderly men and women. *Journal of Gerontology,* **52A** (1997), M80–7.

86. T. Fukuda, Vertical writing with eyes covered: a new test for vestibular spinal reaction. *Acta Otolaryngologica,* **50** (1959), 26–36.

87. T. Fukuda, The stepping test: two phases of the labyrinthine reflex. *Acta Otolaryngologica,* **50** (1959), 95–108.

88. E. K. Kristinsdottir, G. B. Jarlno & M. Magnusson, Asymmetric vestibular function in the elderly might be a significant contributor to hip fractures. *Scandinavian Journal of Rehabilitation Medicine,* **32** (2000), 56–60.

89. E. K. Kristinsdottir, E. Nordell, G. B. Jarlno *et al.,* Observation of vestibular asymmetry in a majority of patients over 50 years with fall-related wrist fractures. *Acta Otolaryngologica,* **121** (2001), 481–5.

90. R. P. Di Fabio, A. Emasithi, J. F. Greany & S. Paul, Suppression of the vertical vestibulo-ocular reflex in older persons at risk of falling. *Acta Otolaryngologica,* **121** (2001), 707–14.

91. R. P. Di Fabio, J. F. Greany, A. Emasithi & J. F. Wyman, Eye-head coordination during postural perturbation as a predictor of falls in community-dwelling elderly women. *Archives of Physical Medicine and Rehabilitation,* **83** (2002), 942–51.

92. C. J. S. Collins & G. R. Barnes, Independent control of head and gaze movements during head-free pursuit in humans. *Journal of Physiology,* **515** (1999), 299–314.

93. J. S. Petrovsky, R. L. Burse & A. R. Lind, Comparison of physiological responses of men and women to isometric exercise. *Journal of Applied Physiology,* **38** (1975), 863–8.

94. H. J. Moytoye & D. E. Lamphiear, Grip and arm strength in males and females, age 10 to 69. *Research Quarterly,* **48** (1977), 109–20.

95. M. P. Murray, G. M. Gardner, L. A. Mollinger & S. B. Sepic, Strength of isometric and isokinetic contractions. Knee muscles of men aged 20 to 86. *Physical Therapy,* **60** (1980), 412–19.

96. M. P. Murray, E. H. Duthie, S. R. Gambert, S. B. Sepic & L. A. Mollinger, Age related differences in knee muscle strength in normal women. *Journal of Gerontology,* **40** (1985), 275–80.

97. W. R. Frontera, V. A. Hughes, K. L. Lutz & W. J. Evans, A cross-sectional study of muscle strength and mass in 45- to 78-year old men and women. *Journal of Applied Physiology,* **71** (1991), 644–50.

98. E. Stalberg, O. Borges, M. Ericsson *et al.,* The quadriceps femoris muscle in 20–70 year old subjects: relations between knee extensor torque, electrophysiologic parameters and muscle fiber characteristics. *Muscle and Nerve,* **12** (1989), 382–9.

99. W. J. MacLennan, M. R. P. Hall, J. I. Timothy & M. Robinson, Is weakness in old age due to muscle wasting? *Age and Ageing,* **9** (1980), 188–92.

100. D. A. Skelton, C. A. Greig, J. M. Davies & A. Young, Strength, power and related functional ability of healthy people aged 65–89 years. *Age and Ageing*, **23** (1994), 371–7.

101. L. Larsson & J. Karlsson, Isometric and dynamic endurance as a function of age and skeletal muscle characteristics. *Acta Physiologica Scandinavica*, **104** (1978), 129–36.

102. T. Johnson, Age-related differences in isometric and dynamic strength and endurance. *Physical Therapy*, **7** (1982), 985–9.

103. C. T. M. Davies & M. J. White, Effects of dynamic exercise on muscle function in elderly men, aged 70 years. *Gerontology*, **29** (1983), 26–31.

104. M. B. Pearson, E. J. Bassey, M. J. Bendall, Muscle strength and anthropometric indices in elderly men and women. *Age and Ageing*, **14** (1985), 49–54.

105. A. A. Vandervoort & K. C. Hayes, Plantarflexor muscle function in young and elderly women. *European Journal of Applied Physiology*, **58** (1989), 389–94.

106. L. A. Lipsitz, P. V. Jonsson, M. M. Kelley & J. S. Koestner, Causes and correlates of recurrent falls in ambulatory frail elderly. *Journal of Gerontology*, **46** (1991), M114–22.

107. S. R. Lord, L. M. March, I. D. Cameron *et al.*, Differing risk factors for falls in nursing home and intermediate-care residents who can and cannot stand unaided. *Journal of the American Geriatrics Society*, **51** (2003), 1645–50.

108. T. V. Nguyen, P. N. Sambrook, P. J. Kelly *et al.*, Prediction of osteoporotic fractures by postural stability and bone density. *British Medical Journal*, **307** (1993), 1111–5.

109. V. A. Stel, J. H. Smit, M. F. Pluijm *et al.*, Balance and mobility performance as treatable risk factors for recurrent falling in older people. *Journal of Clinical Epidemiology*, **56** (2003), 659–68.

110. K. Takazawa, K. Arisawa, S. Honda, Y. Shibata & H. Saito, Lower-extremity muscle forces measured by a hand-held dynamometer and the risk of falls among day-care users in Japan: using multinomial logistic regression analysis. *Disability and Rehabilitation*, **25** (2003), 399–404.

111. J. K. Dhesi, L. M. Bearne, C. Moniz *et al.*, Neuromuscular and psychomotor function in elderly subjects who fall and the relationship with vitamin D status. *Journal of Bone and Mineral Research*, **17** (2002), 891–7.

112. R. H. Whipple, L. I. Wolfson & P. M. Amerman, The relationship of knee and ankle weakness to falls in nursing home residents: an isokinetic study. *Journal of the American Geriatrics Society*, **35** (1987), 13–20.

113. S. Studenski, P. W. Duncan & J. Chandler, Postural responses and effector factors in persons with unexplained falls: results and methodologic issues. *Journal of the American Geriatrics Society*, **39** (1991), 229–34.

114. H. Luukinen, K. Koski, P. Laippala & S. -L. Kivela, Risk factors for recurrent falls in the elderly in long-term institutional care. *Public Health*, **109** (1995), 57–65.

115. D. A. Skelton, J. Kennedy & O. M. Rutherford, Explosive power and asymmetry in leg muscle function in frequent fallers and non-fallers aged over 65. *Age and Ageing*, **31** (2002), 119–25.

116. K. I. Schwender, A. E. Mikesky, W. S. Holt, M. Peacock & D. B. Burr, Differences in muscle endurance and recovery between fallers and nonfallers, and between young and older women. *Journal of Gerontology*, **52** (1997), M155–60.

117. A. T. Welford, Motor performance. In *Handbook of the Psychology of Aging*, ed. J. E. Birren & K. W. Schiae. (New York: Van Nostrand Reinhold Company, 1977).

118. S. Adelsberg, M. Pitman & H. Alexander, Lower extremity fractures: relationship to reaction time and coordination time. *Archives of Physical Medicine and Rehabilitation*, **70** (1989), 737–9.

119. M. D. Grabiner & D. W. Jahnigen, Modeling recovery from stumbles: preliminary data on variable selection and classification efficacy. *Journal of the American Geriatrics Society*, **40** (1992), 910–13.

120. S. M. Woolley, S. J. Czaja & C. G. Drury, An assessment of falls in elderly men and women. *Journal of Gerontology*, **52** (1997), M80–7.

121. H. C. Diener, J. Dichgans, B. Buschlbauer & H. Mau, The significance of proprioception on postural stabilisation as assessed by ischaemia. *Brain Research*, **296** (1984), 93–9.

122. G. R. Fernie, P. Eng & P. J. Holliday, Postural sway in amputees and normal subjects. *Journal of Bone and Joint Surgery*, **60A** (1978), 895–8.

123. S. R. Lord, J. A. Ward, P. Williams & K. J. Anstey, An epidemiological study of falls in older community-dwelling women: the Randwick Falls and Fractures Study. *Australian Journal of Public Health*, **17** (1993), 240–5.

5

Psychological factors and falls

In the preceding chapter we described how human balance and falls avoidance depend on the contributions from multiple sensory and motor systems. Considerable research has also found that psychological factors, such as attentional limitations, fear of falling, cognitive impairment and depression, are also associated with impaired stability and falling in older people. This chapter will review and discuss the implications of this work in relation to attentional limitations and fear of falling. As cognitive impairment and depression can also be viewed as medical conditions, discussion of these conditions as risk factors for falls is included in Chapter 6.

Attentional limitations

As outlined in Chapter 2, the maintenance of balance is a complex task requiring the integration of sensory information regarding the position of the body relative to its surroundings and the ability to generate forces to control body movement. This process has traditionally been considered to be automated and controlled primarily by reflex activity. However, there is an emerging body of research indicating that the control of posture also requires attentional resources, and an individual's balance may be influenced by their information processing ability when performing two or more tasks simultaneously [1]. In response to these findings, a number of investigations have been recently performed to evaluate the effect of 'dual tasking' on postural control in young people, older people and older people at risk of falls. Generally speaking, in these studies the control of posture (such as standing, responding to perturbations or walking) is considered to be the *primary* task and a cognitive task (such as responding to visual or auditory stimuli, performing tests of spatial memory, backwards counting, etc.) is considered to be the *secondary* task. An underlying assumption of these studies is that attentional resources are finite, so performing two tasks simultaneously results in a competition for limited resources, with a subsequent reduction in performance in the primary task, secondary task, or both. Clearly, the ability to adequately cope with the performance of multiple tasks has considerable implications for falls in older people if the primary task of maintaining postural stability is impaired.

The first study to indicate that standing required attentional resources was conducted by Kerr et al. [2], who asked young subjects to perform two cognitive tasks. Firstly, a visual/spatial task (involving placing numbers in imagined matrices and remembering the position of the numbers) and, secondly, a verbal memory task (remembering sentences), while they were either sitting or standing blindfolded in the tandem position. The results showed that when standing blindfolded, subjects made more errors in the visual/spatial task, indicating that some degree of attentional capacity had been allocated to the postural task. Since the publication of the Kerr et al. study, many researchers have confirmed that performing a postural task requires the re-allocation of resources away from the cognitive task [3–6]. Further, performance on the cognitive tasks has been shown to be related to the difficulty of the postural task being performed. For example, Lajoie et al. [4] reported that auditory reaction times were slower in subjects when they were walking compared to when they were sitting or standing. Similar results have been reported by Marsh and Geel [7], who found that reaction times were significantly slower when subjects stood on a platform which rotated in direct proportion to their postural sway compared to a stable platform. The reciprocal also seems to be true, i.e. the type and/or difficulty of the cognitive task influences performance on the postural task. Maylor et al. [8] assessed postural sway when subjects performed a spatial memory task and a non-spatial memory task. They found that the spatial task produced a greater increase in sway, suggesting that postural tasks may compete for visuo-spatial processing resources. Pellecchia [9] assessed standing balance in young subjects when performing three cognitive tasks of ascending difficulty – digit reversal, digit classification and counting backwards by threes – and found a linear increase in postural sway as task difficulty increased.

The effect of age on dual tasking ability has recently attracted considerable research attention. Reaction times in response to visual stimuli while walking are significantly slower in older people, particularly when they are requested to stop walking at a fixed target [10]. Compared to young subjects, while performing concurrent cognitive tasks older people exhibit: significantly greater increases in postural sway [7, 11–13]; reductions in the speed of voluntary step initiation [14]; delayed recovery of stability following voluntary arm movement [15]; impaired postural responses to platform perturbation [16–18]; increased variability in stride length and velocity when walking [19]; and increased risk of contacting obstacles when walking [20]. As with younger subjects, dual tasking appears to be more difficult when undertaking more complex postural tasks such as walking or avoiding obstacles [21]. The underlying reasons for these differences have not been fully elucidated, however, four possible explanations have been proposed: (i) older people have an inherently reduced attentional capacity; (ii) older people have difficulty shifting attention between two tasks; (iii) older people have similar attentional resources to young people but place greater demands on these resources due to their impaired postural control systems; or (iv) a combination of these factors [1]. It is also unclear as to which information processing channels are most affected by concurrent postural tasks. Although some authors argue that visuo-spatial working memory plays a major role [8, 11], the fact that many non-spatial tasks result in similar reductions in stability suggests that task difficulty is more important.

Despite the recognition of these age-related differences, few studies have adequately determined whether diminished dual tasking ability is a risk factor for falls. Several laboratory-based studies have assessed dual tasking ability in older people with either self-reported balance impairment or a history of falls. Shumway-Cook *et al.* [22] assessed postural stability when performing two cognitive tasks (sentence completion and a perceptual visual matching task) in healthy older adults and older adults with a history of falls. They found the greatest differences between the groups when standing on a compliant surface performing either of the cognitive tasks. Interestingly, the difficulty of the postural task did not affect performance on the cognitive task. A subsequent study found similar results, in that older people with a history of falls were more likely to step to maintain balance when standing on a sway-referenced platform whilst responding to an auditory stimulus [23]. Similar deficits in dual tasking in elderly fallers have been reported in response to platform perturbation. Brauer *et al.* [24] reported that elderly fallers exhibited significantly delayed responses to auditory stimuli when standing on a translating platform. However, this delay was apparently due to prioritization of the postural response, in that while elderly non-fallers could respond to the stimulus and complete a protective step simultaneously, elderly fallers completed the step before responding to the stimulus. Condron and Hill [25] assessed sway when standing on a stable or tilting platform in healthy older people and older people with increased risk of falling. Although there were only small differences in sway between the two groups of elderly subjects when standing on the stable platform, larger differences were evident when the platform tilted in an antero-posterior direction and the subjects were asked to perform a concurrent cognitive task (counting backwards by threes). Finally, Hauer *et al.* [26] found that, compared to healthy elderly subjects, geriatric patients with a history of severe falls exhibited increased sway when standing on a stable surface while performing a concurrent cognitive test (adding by twos or sevens).

The first prospective investigation to determine whether dual tasking difficulty predicts falls was conducted by Lundin-Olsson *et al.* [27]. This study involved observing whether subjects stopped walking when a conversation was initiated by their physiotherapist while accompanying them to the treatment room. Of the 58 subjects studied, 21 fell during the six month follow-up period and of these 12 stopped walking when talking at the initial assessment. Thus, 'stops walking when talking' was found to be highly sensitive (95%) in predicting falls, however, the specificity was low (48%). The test also has a number of limitations. Firstly, it is limited to those who are capable of walking at least 100 m, which makes it inappropriate for many at-risk older people. Secondly, positive classification is based on visual observation of complete stops, thereby rendering the test insensitive to more subtle postural difficulties. Thirdly, the exact nature of the attentional demands of the task are unclear, as the conversational content is not defined [28]. In response to these limitations, DeHoon *et al.* [28] have proposed a shorter version (8 m walk) and a standard question (What is your age?), and found that this modified version of the test was capable of identifying fall-prone elderly people (classified according to trunk sway measures during gait). However, the ability of the modified test to predict falls has not yet been determined.

Two other studies have found tests of dual tasking ability to be predictive of falls. Lundin-Olsson *et al.* [29] assessed the ability of older people to perform the Timed Up and Go Test (TUGT) with and without the added task of holding a glass of water. Those who took more than 4.5 seconds longer to perform the TUGT when holding the glass of water were five times more likely to fall during the six month follow-up period. However, the sample size in this study was relatively small (42 subjects) and it could be argued that holding a glass of water is merely a more difficult postural task rather than a task requiring additional cognitive resources. Finally, Verghese *et al.* [30] assessed two modifications of the stops walking while talking test: a simple version (WWT-simple), in which subjects were requested to recite the letters of the alphabet; and a complex version (WWT-complex), which required subjects to recite alternate letters of the alphabet, while the time taken to walk 40 feet was recorded. Over a 12 month follow-up period, both tests were found to be predictive of falls, with the WWT-complex test exhibiting greater predictive validity than the WWT-simple (OR of 13.7 compared to 7.02).

These studies indicate that difficulties with dual tasking may play an important role in predisposition to falls in older people. Further research is now required to determine which combination of postural and cognitive tests is the most accurate predictor of falls, and whether difficulties in dual tasking can be overcome with motor rehabilitation interventions.

Fear of falling

Interest in fear of falling in older people dates back to 1982, when Bhala *et al.* described the condition 'ptophobia' – a phobic reaction to standing or walking [31]. In the same year, Murphy and Isaacs [32] described the post-fall syndrome as a serious disabling condition that affected some older people following a fall. Since then, much research has been undertaken into determining how a fear of falling affects the lives of older people.

Definitions and measurement of fear of falling

The definitions of fear of falling used since 1982 have been quite disparate, and have often failed to differentiate between fear of falling and falls efficacy (perceived ability to confidently undertake activities of daily living without falling) [33]. For example, fear of falling has been defined as: an ongoing concern about falling that ultimately limits the performance of daily activities [34]; low fall-related efficacy and being afraid of falling [35]; being worried about falling [36]; and a loss of confidence in balance abilities [37]. Accordingly assessments used to measure fear of falling have reflected these differing definitions.

The simplest assessments are single questionnaire items such as 'are you afraid of falling?' with yes/no [34, 37–41] and graded responses [39, 42, 43]. Other single-item questions assess whether activity restrictions have resulted from a fear of falling [44].

Three scales with good psychometric properties have also been formulated to measure falls efficacy. Tinetti *et al.* [40] developed the Falls Efficacy Scale (FES) (which includes ten items that assess a person's confidence in his or her ability to avoid falling while undertaking activities such as house cleaning and dressing). The FES measures only indoor activities so it is most appropriate for frail older people who are primarily housebound. Hill *et al.* [45] have extended the FES by including four additional items that measure the degree of fear of falling while undertaking activities outside the home.

The Activities-specific Balance Confidence (ABC) Scale [46] is also appropriate for older people with higher levels of functioning. This 16-item questionnaire asks subjects to rate their balance confidence in relation to questions beginning 'How confident are you that you will not lose your balance or become unsteady while . . . ?' The scale includes activities performed outside of the home such as walking in a crowded mall and riding an escalator holding onto the railing.

The third scale – the Survey of Activities and Fear of Falling in the Elderly (SAFE) [47] – assesses the effect of fear of falling on factors such as activity restriction or poor quality of life. The SAFE examines 11 activities of daily living, mobility and social activities (e.g. taking a shower, going to the shops, using public transport and going to the cinema). Social activities were included as it was posited that restriction of these activities may indicate the onset of fear of falling. The SAFE scale has also been adapted into a self-administered form known as SAFFE [48, 49].

It is likely that asking the simple question 'are you afraid of falling' offers little understanding into the psychological status of an older person if asked in isolation. This is because a fear of falling may reflect a realistic appraisal of reduced functional abilities, and consequent increased risk of suffering a fall and fall injuries. Such a fear may result from a first hand experience (a near fall or a recent fall that resulted in pain, embarrassment or injury). For example, Howland et al. [50] found that the degree of fear of falling in their study was associated with the number and seriousness of the falls experienced. However, it is also likely that fear of falling can also result from a second-hand experience, i.e. a friend or relative with similar characteristics having fallen and suffered adverse consequences. A much more important consideration is whether or not this fear is irrational, excessive or phobic, and needlessly restricts participation in physical and social activities – a construct reflecting the original phobic condition that Bhala et al. described in 1982 [31].

Balance confidence or falls efficacy offers more insight into an older person's perceptions of their abilities to undertake various activities without falling. However, again, if falls efficacy is measured in isolation, it cannot be determined whether a low level of confidence is appropriate or excessive.

Prevalence of fear of falling

Estimates of the prevalence of fear of falling in older community-dwelling people range from 29% to 92% in those who have suffered previous falls [50, 51], and 12% to 65% in those that have not [42, 47, 50, 52, 53]. Fear of falling is more prevalent in women than in men [37, 39, 44, 52–55] and increases in prevalence with increasing age [52–54, 56]. This variability in prevalence estimates is most likely to be due to the differing definitions and assessment tools used to assess fear of falling. For example, higher prevalence rates of fear of falling are reported when graded (i.e. 'not at all afraid', 'slightly afraid', 'somewhat afraid', 'very afraid') rather than dichotomous (i.e. yes/no) responses are required and when higher risk activities such as 'going out when it is slippery' [47] are included in the questionnaires. However, despite the variation in prevalence figures, it is clear that fear of falling is a significant issue for many older people.

Factors associated with fear of falling

Factors associated with fear of falling or falls efficacy (both terms have been used in the literature, and sometimes interchangeably) are numerous. Fear of falling is associated with previous falls [44, 47, 49, 53, 56, 57], poor health status [35, 42, 50–53, 56], functional decline [35, 44, 54, 57–59] and frailty [54]. Fear of falling has been consistently correlated to restriction and curtailment of activity [50, 53, 60–62], reduced quality of life [35, 42, 47, 48, 50, 54, 57, 61], pain [63], anxiety [42, 50, 52, 63, 64], and depression and social isolation [32, 47, 50, 53].

Falls efficacy is associated with falls risk factors such as reduced leaning balance, poor strength, impaired physical performance [49] and impaired gait, as indicated by reduced stride length, reduced speed, increased double-support time and poorer clinical gait scores [41]. Measures of fear of falling have also been found to be associated with prospective falls [35, 55, 56, 65].

It is perhaps not surprising that falls efficacy measures are associated with objectively assessed measures of balance or falls. After all, most people would be quite accurate at rating their abilities across a broad spectrum of familiar or even unfamiliar activities, e.g. rising from a chair, walking, running, swimming, golf, billiards, crosswords, etc. It is probable that only sub-sets of older people have an inappropriately low level of balance confidence [33] or, on the other hand, an inappropriately high level of balance confidence, for example, those with poor insight resulting from conditions such as Alzheimer's disease [44]. Further, no studies have found that fear of falling is an independent risk factor for falls after adjusting for impaired balance and/or reduced physical functioning. This issue requires further attention in research studies.

Conclusion

The effect of attentional limitations on balance and falls has been assessed using various paradigms, including standing, an ability to withstand a perturbation, walking and obstacle avoidance. This research has shown that attention is required for balance control, even in young adults, and the amount of attention required depends on the degree of difficulty of both the balance and cognitive (secondary) tasks. With increasing age, balance tasks become more attentionally demanding and older frail people require even more attentional resources for balance control, to the extent that even simple tasks like answering a question may interfere with standing, stepping and walking. In such situations these people are likely to be at increased risk of falls. Fear of falling is prevalent in older people. This fear may in many cases reflect a realistic appraisal of falls risk. In others, however, it may be excessive and lead unnecessarily to social and physical activity restrictions. Research is required to distinguish this important difference as it has implications for both falls risk assessment and interventions.

REFERENCES

1. M. Woollacott & A. Shumway-Cook, Attention and control of posture and gait: a review of an emerging area of research. *Gait and Posture*, **16** (2002), 1–14.

2. B. Kerr, S. M. Condon & L. A. McDonald, Cognitive spatial processing and the regulation of posture. *Journal of Experimental Psychology*, **11** (1985), 617–22.

3. G. Andersson, L. Yardley & L. Luxon, A dual-task study of interference between mental activity and control of balance. *American Journal of Otology*, **19** (1998), 632–7.

4. Y. Lajoie, N. Teasdale, C. Bard & M. Fleury, Attentional demands for static and dynamic equilibrium. *Experimental Brain Research*, **97** (1993), 139–44.

5. N. Teasdale, C. Bard, J. LaRue & M. Fleury, On the cognitive penetrability of postural control. *Experimental Aging Research*, **19** (1993), 1–13.

6. Y. Lajoie, N. Teasdale, C. Bard & M. Fleury, Upright standing and gait: are there changes in attentional requirements related to normal aging? *Experimental Aging Research*, **22** (1996), 185–98.

7. A. P. Marsh & S. E. Geel, The effect of age on the attentional demands of postural control. *Gait and Posture*, **12** (2000), 105–13.

8. E. A. Maylor, S. Allison & A. M. Wing, Effects of spatial and nonspatial cognitive activity on postural stability. *British Journal of Psychology*, **92** (2001), 319–38.

9. G. L. Pellecchia, Postural sway increases with attentional demands of concurrent cognitive task. *Gait and Posture*, **18** (2003), 29–34.

10. W. A. Sparrow, E. J. Bradshaw, E. Lamoureux & O. Tirosh, Ageing effects on the attention demands of walking. *Human Movement Science*, **21** (2002), 961–72.

11. E. A. Maylor & A. M. Wing, Age differences in postural stability are increased by additional cognitive demands. *Journal of Gerontology*, **51B** (1996), P143–54.

12. I. Melzer, N. Benjuya & J. Kaplanski, Age-related changes of postural control: effect of cognitive tasks. *Gerontology*, **47** (2001), 189–94.

13. M. S. Redfern, J. R. Jennings, C. Martin & J. M. Furman, Attention influences sensory integration for postural control in older adults. *Gait and Posture*, **14** (2001), 211–16.

14. I. Melzer & L. I. E. Oddsson, The effect of a cognitive task on voluntary step execution in healthy elderly and young individuals. *Journal of the American Geriatrics Society*, **52** (2004), 1255–62.

15. G. E. Stelmach, H. N. Zelaznik & D. Lowe, The influence of aging and attentional demands on recovery from postural instability. *Aging – Clinical and Experimental Research*, **2** (1990), 155–61.

16. L. Brown, A. Shumway-Cook & M. Woollacott, Attentional demands and postural recovery: the effects of aging. *Journal of Gerontology*, **54A** (1999), M165–71.

17. J. K. Rankin, M. H. Woollacott, A. Shumway-Cook & L. A. Brown, Cognitive influence on postural stability: a neuromuscular analysis in young and older adults. *Journal of Gerontology*, **55A** (2000), M112–19.

18. M. S. Redfern, M. L. T. M. Muller, J. R. Jennings & J. F. Furman, Attentional dynamics in postural control during perturbations in young and older adults. *Journal of Gerontology*, **57A** (2002), B298–303.

19. O. Beauchet, R. W. Kressig, B. Najafi, V. Dubost & F. Mourey, Age-related decline of gait control under a dual-task condition. *Journal of the American Geriatrics Society*, **51** (2003), 1187–8.

20. H.-C. Chen, A. B. Schultz, J. A. Ashton-Miller *et al.*, Stepping over obstacles: dividing attention impairs performance of old more than young adults. *Journal of Gerontology*, **51A** (1996), M116–22.

21. B. Bloem, V. Valkenburg, M. Slabbekoorn & M. Willemsen, The multiple tasks test. Development and normal strategies. *Gait and Posture*, **14** (2001), 191–202.

22. A. Shumway-Cook, M. Woollacott, K. A. Kerns & M. Baldwin, The effects of two types of cognitive tasks on postural stability in older adults with and without a history of falls. *Journal of Gerontology*, **52** (1997), M232–40.

23. A. Shumway-Cook & M. Woollacott, Attentional demands and postural control: the effect of sensory context. *Journal of Gerontology*, **55A** (2000), M10–16.

24. S. G. Brauer, M. Woollacott & A. Shumway-Cook, The influence of concurrent cognitive task on the compensatory stepping response to a perturbation in balance-impaired and healthy elders. *Gait and Posture*, **15** (2002), 83–93.

25. J. E. Condron & K. D. Hill, Reliability and validity of a dual-task force platform assessment of balance performance: effect of age, balance impairment, and cognitive task. *Journal of the American Geriatrics Society*, **50** (2002), 157–62.

26. K. Hauer, M. Pfisterer, C. Weber *et al.*, Cognitive impairment decreases postural control during dual tasks in geriatric patients with a history of severe falls. *Journal of the American Geriatrics Society*, **51** (2003), 1638–44.

27. L. Lundin-Olsson, L. Nyberg & Y. Gustafson, "Stops walking when talking" as a predictor of falls in elderly people. *The Lancet*, **349** (1997), 617.

28. E. W. DeHoon, J. H. Allum, M. G. Carpenter *et al.*, Quantitative assessment of the stops walking while talking test in the elderly. *Archives of Physical Medicine and Rehabilitation*, **84** (2003), 838–42.

29. L. Lundin-Olsson, L. Nyberg & Y. Gustafson, Attention, frailty, and falls: the effect of a manual task on basic mobility. *Journal of the American Geriatrics Society*, **46** (1998), 758–61.

30. J. Verghese, H. Buschke, L. Viola *et al.*, Validity of divided attention tasks in predicting falls in older individuals: a preliminary study. *Journal of the American Geriatrics Society*, **50** (2002), 1572–6.

31. R. P. Bhala, J. O'Donnell & E. Thoppil, Ptophobia: phobic fear of falling and its clinical management. *Physical Therapy*, **62** (1982), 187–90.

32. J. Murphy & B. Isaacs, The post-fall syndrome: a study of 36 elderly patients. *Gerontology*, **28** (1982), 265–70.

33. K. Letgers, Fear of falling. *Physical Therapy*, **82** (2002), 264–72.

34. M. E. Tinetti & L. Powell, Fear of falling and low self-efficacy: a case of dependence in elderly persons. *Journal of Gerontology*, **48** (1993), 35–8.

35. R. G. Cumming, G. Salkeld, M. Thomas & G. Szonyi, Prospective study of the impact of fear of falling on activities of daily living, SF-36 scores, and nursing home admission. *Journal of Gerontology*, **55A** (2000), M299–305.

36. S. Tennstedt, J. Howland, M. Lachman *et al.*, A randomized, controlled trial of a group intervention to reduce fear of falling and associated activity restriction in older adults. *Journal of Gerontology*, **53B** (1998), S384–92.

37. B. E. Maki, P. J. Holliday & A. K. Topper, Fear of falling and postural performance in the elderly. *Journal of Gerontology*, **46** (1991), M123–31.

38. A. M. Myers, L. E. Powell, B. E. Maki *et al.*, Psychological indicators of balance confidence: relationship to actual and perceived abilities. *Journal of Gerontology*, **51A** (1996), M37–43.

39. E. McAuley, S. L. Mihalko & K. Rosengren, Self-efficacy and balance correlates of fear of falling in the elderly. *Journal of Aging and Physical Activity*, **5** (1997), 329–40.

40. M. E. Tinetti, D. Richman & L. Powell, Falls efficacy as a measure of fear of falling. *Journal of Gerontology*, **45** (1990), 239–43.

41. B. E. Maki, Gait changes in older adults: predictors of falls or indicators of fear? *Journal of the American Geriatrics Society*, **45** (1997), 313–20.

42. R. H. Lawrence, S. L. Tennstedt, L. E. Kasten, Intensity and correlates of fear of falling and hurting oneself in the next year: baseline findings from a Roybal Center Fear of Falling Intervention. *Journal of Aging and Health*, **10** (1998), 267–86.

43. K. Turano, G. S. Rubin, S. J. Herdman, E. Chee & L. P. Fried, Visual stabilization of posture in the elderly: fallers vs. nonfallers. *Optometry and Vision Science*, **71** (1994), 761–9.

44. P. A. Fletcher & J. P. Hirdes, Restriction in activity associated with fear of falling among community-based seniors using home care services. *Age and Ageing*, **33** (2004), 273–9.

45. K. D. Hill, J. A. Schwarz, A. J. Kalogeropoulos & S. J. Gibson, Fear of falling revisited. *Archives of Physical Medicine and Rehabilitation*, **77** (1996), 1025–9.

46. L. E. Powell & A. M. Myers, The Activities-specific Balance Confidence (ABC) Scale. *Journal of Gerontology*, **50A** (1995), M28–34.

47. M. E. Lachman, J. Howland, S. Tennstedt *et al.*, Fear of falling and activity restriction: the survey of activities and fear of falling in the elderly (SAFE). *Journal of Gerontology*, **53B** (1998), P43–50.

48. L. Yardley & H. Smith, A prospective study of the relationship between feared consequences of falling and avoidance of activity in community-living older people. *Gerontologist*, **42** (2002), 17–23.

49. K. Delbaere, G. Crombez, G. Vanderstraeten, T. Willems & D. Cambier, Fear-related avoidance of activities, falls and physical frailty. A prospective community-based cohort study. *Age and Ageing*, **33** (2004), 368–73.

50. J. Howland, E. W. Peterson, W. C. Levin *et al.*, Fear of falling among the community-dwelling elderly. *Journal of Aging and Health*, **5** (1993), 229–43.

51. K. Aoyagi, P. D. Ross, J. W. Davis *et al.*, Falls among community-dwelling elderly in Japan. *Journal of Bone and Mineral Research*, **13** (1998), 1468–74.

52. B. J. Vellas, S. J. Wayne, L. Romero *et al.*, One-leg balance is an important predictor of injurious falls in older persons. *Journal of the American Geriatrics Society*, **45** (1997), 735–8.

53. J. Howland, M. E. Lachman, E. W. Peterson *et al.*, Covariates of fear of falling and associated activity curtailment. *Gerontologist*, **38** (1998), 549–55.

54. C. L. Arfken, H. W. Lach, S. J. Birge & J. P. Miller, The prevalence and correlates of fear of falling in elderly persons living in the community. *American Journal of Public Health*, **84** (1994), 565–70.

55. S. Murphy, J. Dubin & T. Gill, The development of fear of falling among community-living older women: predisposing factors and subsequent fall events. *Journal of Gerontology*, **58A** (2003), M943–7.

56. S. M. Friedman, B. Munoz, S. K. West, G. S. Rubin & L. P. Fried, Falls and fear of falling: which comes first? A longitudinal prediction model suggests strategies for primary and secondary prevention. *Journal of the American Geriatrics Society*, **50** (2002), 1329–35.

57. F. Li, K. Fisher, P. Harmer, E. McAuley & N. Wilson, Fear of falling in elderly persons: association with falls, functional ability, and quality of life. *Journal of Gerontology*, **58B** (2003), P283–90.

58. S. Franzoni, R. Rozzini, S. Boffelli, G. B. Frisoni & M. Trabucchi, Fear of falling in nursing home patients. *Gerontology*, **40** (1994), 38–44.

59. D. L. Gill, K. Williams, L. Williams & W. A. Hale, Multidimensional correlates of falls in older women. *International Journal of Aging and Human Development*, **47** (1998), 35–51.

60. M. E. Tinetti, C. F. Mendes de Leon, J. T. Doucette & D. I. Baker, Fear of falling and fall-related efficacy in relationship to functioning among community-living elders. *Journal of Gerontology*, **49A** (1994), M140–7.

61. R. Petrella, M. Payne, A. Myers, T. Overend & B. Chesworth, Physical function and fear of falling after hip fracture rehabilitation in the elderly. *American Journal of Physical Medicine and Rehabilitation*, **79** (2000), 154–60.

62. H. Luukinen, K. Koski, S. L. Kivela & P. Laippala, Social status, life changes, housing conditions, health, functional abilities and life-style as risk factors for recurrent falls among the home-dwelling elderly. *Public Health*, **110** (1996), 115–18.

63. L. W. Drozdick & B. A. Edelstein, Correlates of fear of falling in older adults who have experienced a fall. *Journal of Clinical Geropsychology*, **7** (2001), 1–3.

64. E. J. Burker, H. Wong, P. D. Sloane *et al.*, Predictors of fear of falling in dizzy and nondizzy elderly. *Psychology and Aging*, **10** (1995), 104–10.

65. S. L. Murphy, C. S. Williams & T. M. Gill, Characteristics associated with fear of falling and activity restriction in community-living older persons. *Journal of the American Geriatrics Society*, **50** (2002), 516–20.

6

Medical risk factors for falls

It has long been recognized that frail, older people with multiple chronic illnesses experience higher rates of falls than active, healthy older people [1]. This suggests that, rather than being a non-specific accompaniment of ageing, many falls occur as a result of clinically identifiable causes. Thus, differentiating the relative contribution of pre-existing disease to the risk of falling is an important component of a falls prevention programme, as it enables clinicians involved in the management of older people to identify high risk individuals who may benefit from targeted intervention.

As discussed in Chapter 4, maintenance of the upright posture is a complex task involving many physiological systems. Sensory input from visual and vestibular pathways, muscle spindles, and joint proprioceptors is channelled centrally to the brain where it is rapidly processed to produce appropriate and coordinated motor responses [2]. The key components of this process are represented in Figure 6.1, whilst Table 6.1 lists diseases which can impact on this system to increase an individual's risk of falling.

Many diseases increase the risk of falling by impacting directly on physiological systems, i.e. cataract formation leads to impaired visual acuity and contrast sensitivity. Other intermittent pathologies are less simple to classify. Despite knowledge that treatment leads to a reduction in falls, some conditions have not been (and are never likely to be) studied in such a way as to provide evidence of being an independent predictor of falls, e.g. intermittent cardiac arrhythmias where direct cause and effect is difficult to establish in the absence of constant cardiac monitoring.

When considering medical conditions as risk factors for falls there is a significant overlap between falls, syncope and the inherent problem of limited recall or even amnesia for an event. In addition, individual disease processes can lead to an increased risk of falling via more than one physiological mechanism, e.g. Parkinson's disease causes problems with balance and gait, but can also have

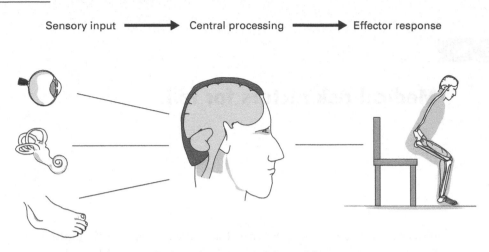

Sensory input ➡ Central processing ➡ Effector response

Fig. 6.1   Key components involved in maintenance of the upright posture.

a direct impact on the cardiovascular system leading to a fall via decreased cerebral perfusion.

Diseases affecting sensory input

Vision

With ageing, the eye undergoes physiological changes which are associated with a decline in visual acuity [3, 4]. As outlined in Chapter 4, many authors have reported visual impairment, including poor contrast sensitivity [5, 6], poor visual acuity [7, 8], impaired depth perception [9], and self-reported poor vision [10], to be a strong risk factor for falls in older people. In addition to normal age-related refractive changes, older people are particularly susceptible to developing visual deficits from common eye pathologies, including cataracts, macular degeneration and glaucoma. Older people with diabetes and hypertension can have the additional burden of associated retinopathies.

There is an increase in the incidence of structural eye disease in later life, and poor vision ranks only behind arthritis and heart disease as a cause of impaired function in those aged 70 years and above [11]. Deficits in acuity and contrast sensitivity, restriction of the visual field, increased susceptibility to glare, and poor depth perception, can result in misjudgement of distances and misinterpretation of spatial information, such as the nature of ground surfaces (see Chapter 4). Whilst there is relatively little evidence associating falls risk with specific eye pathology, it is clear that eye diseases have a direct impact on the

Table 6.1 Diseases having a direct impact on maintenance of the upright posture

Diseases affecting sensory input	*Vision*	Age-related refractive error
		Senile macular degeneration
		Glaucoma
		Cataracts
		Stroke causing visual field defect
	Proprioception	Diabetes
		Vitamin B_{12} deficiency
		Syphilis (rare)
		Degenerative joint disease, especially of neck and knees
	Vestibular	Age-related middle and inner ear changes
		Chronic ear infections
		Perforated ear drum
		Labyrinthitis
		Meniere's disease
Diseases affecting central processing	*Cerebrum*	Cerebrovascular disease (stroke)
		Dementia
		Brain tumor (benign and malignant)
	Cerebellum	Cerebrovascular disease (stroke)
		Long term alcohol misuse
		Idiopathic cerebellar degeneration
	Basal ganglia	Cerebrovascular disease (stroke)
		Parkinson's disease
	Brain stem	Cerebrovascular disease (stroke)
		Atherosclerosis
		Postural hypotension
Diseases affecting effector response	*Spinal cord and nerves*	Any condition causing narrowing of spinal cord
		Motor neurone disease
		Multiple sclerosis
		Foot drop (common peroneal nerve)
	Muscles	Cerebrovascular disease (stroke)
		Motor neurone disease
		Muscular dystrophy
		Multiple sclerosis
		Polymyalgia rheumatica
		Polymyositis
		Hypothyroidism
		Vitamin D deficiency
		Diabetes
		Muscle disuse following fracture, injury or prolonged immobility
	Joints	Osteoarthritis
		Rheumatoid arhritis
	Other	Foot deformities
		Poor fitting shoes
		Peripheral vascular disease
		Urinary incontinence

physiological domains of vision. It is these domains that have been consistently shown to increase an individual's risk of falling.

Cataracts

Cataracts affect approximately 16% of people over the age of 65 [12] and are a common cause of impaired vision in older people. The term *cataract* refers to an increase in the opacity of the lens, leading to smoky, cloudy or hazy vision. Although cataract formation is predominantly a disease of old age, the changes in molecular structure of the lens due to the ageing process itself do not fully explain the production of cataracts. There is a general consensus that cataracts form as a result of complex biochemical reactions which eventually lead to oxidation of the lens, membrane breakdown and eventual opacity, while ageing increases the susceptibility of the lens to the detrimental effects of these oxidative agents [13]. Studies have found cataracts to be associated with an increased risk of falls and fall-related injury. A ten-year prospective study of 2633 older people by Felson *et al.* [14] reported that 18% of hip fractures were associated with visual impairment, with cataracts being the most common cause. Similarly, Jack *et al.* [8] reported that older people admitted to hospital as a result of a fall were more likely to have visual impairment than those admitted for other reasons, and 37% of these patients had cataracts. More recently, cataracts have been reported to be an independent risk factor for falls in 465 community-dwelling older people [15]. A large cohort study of 3654 people over the age of 49 years in Australia reported that the presence of cataracts was significantly associated with an increased risk of suffering two or more falls in the previous 12 months [16] and hip fractures in the two years following assessment [17].

Glaucoma

Glaucoma is the name given to a group of eye diseases characterized by raised intraocular pressure leading to pathological changes in the optic disc and resultant visual field defects. Glaucoma is a common cause of blindness in older people and affects approximately 3% of people over the age of 65 [12]. The presence of glaucoma has been reported to be associated with an increased risk of falling in one retrospective study [18]. Topical treatments for glaucoma may also increase falls risk [16] although the mechanism for this is unclear, and may relate to a direct local effect of the eye drops or from systemic absorption of topical drugs such as beta blockers. Glynn *et al.* [19] reported that the use of pupil-constricting eye medications was associated with a three-fold increased risk of falling in 489 people with glaucoma, compared to people not using these medications.

Macular degeneration

Several disorders can lead to degenerative lesions in the macular region of the retina. Age-related macular degeneration is the most common and serious form, affecting approximately 9% of older people aged over 65 years [12] and up to 19% of people over 85 years of age [20]. Age-related macular degeneration is recognized as the leading cause of blindness among older people in industrialized countries [21]. Despite the recognition of macular degeneration as a common and serious eye disease, few studies have assessed the role of macular degeneration as a risk factor for falls. The Blue Mountains Eye Study in Australia found that the presence of macular degeneration was not a statistically significant risk factor for falls in a sample of 3299 older people, but only a small number of subjects in the sample had the condition documented [16].

Peripheral sensation

The proprioceptive system contributes to stability, particularly during changes of position while walking and especially on uneven surfaces. It is of most importance when other senses are impaired. Ageing is associated with reduced peripheral sensation, and several prospective studies have found that subjects who experience falls perform worse in tests of lower limb proprioception [22], vibration sense [23] and tactile sensitivity [24, 25] (see Chapter 4). Loss of peripheral sensation can also result from a wide range of causes, including diabetes mellitus, alcohol misuse, Vitamin B_{12} deficiency, chemotherapy, and overdose of pyridoxine or nitric oxide [26]. Peripheral nerve damage occurs in up to 25% of people with diabetes mellitus after ten years of being diagnosed with the disease and up to 50% of people after 20 years disease duration [27]. People with diabetic neuropathy have impaired standing stability compared to age-matched controls [28–30] and perform worse in tests of foot position sense [31, 32]. The presence of diabetes [33–35], and clinically diagnosed diabetic neuropathy [36–38] have consistently been found to be risk factors for falls and hip fractures in older people.

Degenerative joint disease is common in old age and its consequences on postural stability are manifest in a variety of ways, including disruption to postural control through its effect on cervical spine mechanoreceptors. Degeneration of the cervical spine from cervical spondylosis, injury or arthritis can disturb postural control, and predispose persons to fall because of damage to mechanoreceptors in the apophyseal joints [39].

Vestibular pathology

The function of the vestibular system is to generate information about head position and movement, and to distribute this information to sites in the nervous system involved in the maintenance of postural stability. The vestibular system contributes to spatial orientation at rest as well as during acceleration and controls visual fixation during movement.

The three main components of vestibular function are: (i) the vestibulo-ocular reflex (VOR), which is responsible for generating eye rotations to compensate for movements of the head; (ii) the vestibulocollic (VCR) and cervico-collic (CCR) reflexes, which are responsible for stabilizing the head by initiating neck movements; and (iii) the vestibulo-spinal reflexes (VSR), responsible for stabilizing the head and maintaining upright stance, by triggering muscle activity in the neck, trunk and extremities [40].

A wide range of conditions can impair the function of the vestibular system, including direct trauma, infection, calcium carbonate deposition in the semicircular canals, drug toxicity, migraine, cerebellar ataxia and auto-immune disease [41]. Depending on the site and severity of the impairment, vestibular disease may manifest as hearing loss, vertigo (an illusion of rotatory motion) and dizziness, thereby predisposing to instability and falls.

People with severe vestibular hypofunction demonstrate obvious impairments in posture and gait, characterized by postural instability and a broad-based, staggering gait pattern with unsteady turns [42], that place them at an increased risk of recurrent falls [43]. However, in cases of long term total vestibular loss, gait may appear normal and deficits will only become apparent when the subject stands in the tandem position with their eyes closed (the 'sharpened Romberg' position). This suggests that visual and somatosensory inputs are able to compensate for absence of vestibular input. Also vestibular loss may only produce overt postural instability if visual and peripheral sensation cues are altered or unavailable, or if vision and peripheral sensation are impaired.

Due to the complexity of the interaction between these three systems and the fact that vestibular function has been traditionally less amenable to assessment with simple screening tests, it has been difficult to ascertain the significance of vestibular dysfunction in relation to falls in older people. Recent studies using more direct measurement of vestibular function have shown that impaired vestibular function increases the risk of falls and fall-related fractures in older people [44, 45]. However, two other studies have found that falls incidence is not elevated in older people with identified vestibular disorders. It appears that people with these disorders are aware of their poor balance, adopt appropriate corrective strategies and reduce risk-taking behaviours [43, 46].

Diseases affecting central processing

On reaching the brain, sensory information is channelled to the cerebrum, cerebellum, basal ganglia and brain stem. Problems with balance can be experienced due to impaired central processing despite normal sensory input and normal effector organ function.

Cerebrovascular disease

Cerebrovascular disease is common in older people and represents a spectrum of symptomatology, ranging from barely detectable changes in physical or cognitive functioning through to overt multi-infarct dementia and even catastrophic cerebral events leading to death. The majority of strokes result from an occlusion of one or more cerebral vessels (infarct) brought on by accelerated atherogenesis. Cerebral haemorrhage accounts for approximately 15% of strokes and is more commonly seen in people with uncontrolled or poorly controlled hypertension. Given the complexity of the brain and the discrete functions of the various regions, a stroke can produce a wide range of abnormalities dependent on the area affected. Brain stem and cerebellar strokes may cause damage to areas of the brain closely associated with balance, while sensory and visual inattention when recovering from a stroke may produce a tendency to collide with environmental hazards. Parietal lobe damage may impair the planning and execution of locomotor activities, and in cases where the frontal lobes are damaged, there is the possibility that judgement may be affected, causing the older person to take risks when navigating obstacles in the environment [47].

A history of a stroke has been associated with a two to six-fold increased risk of falling in a number of community-based prospective investigations [9, 15, 18, 48–52]. People who have fallen following a stroke commonly attribute their fall to loss of balance, misjudgement/lack of concentration or their foot dragging on the ground causing them to trip [53]. A number of studies have been performed to elucidate the potential mechanisms responsible for balance impairment in stroke patients when standing, performing the sit-to-stand task and during walking. When lateral perturbations are applied to stroke subjects when standing, they react with a markedly abnormal postural response characterized by delayed onset latencies and amplitudes of the gluteus medius and hip adductor muscles, and increased muscle activity of the contralateral, non-paretic side [54]. During sit-to-stand, people with stroke who suffer from falls generate less force and exhibit greater medio-lateral sway than stroke patients who do not fall [55]. Following a stroke people also require more attention to control balance. Brown et al. [56] assessed verbal reaction time when people with stroke and controls performed three postural tasks (sitting, standing and standing with feet together). While the reaction times of the control subjects did not differ across the three tasks, stroke subjects demonstrated a slowing of reaction time as the postural challenge of the task increased, indicating that more attention is required for postural tasks following stroke.

A number of gait analysis studies have been performed in people who have suffered a stroke. While the changes observed depend largely on the brain region affected [57], in general, people with stroke have an inability to generate sufficient amounts of force in the lower limb muscles and difficulty coordinating the actions of agonist-antagonist muscle groups when walking [58–61]. This may result in a decreased ability to maintain the leg extended during the stance phase of walking and decreased foot clearance during the swing phase – factors that can predispose to tripping [47, 58, 59]. Stroke subjects adopt different strategies when crossing over obstacles which may be protective of tripping, such as increasing toe clearance and step time [62].

These results indicate that cerebrovascular disease is a strong predictor of falls, and that the balance and gait impairments resultant from the disease are manifold and largely determined by the site of the occlusion or haemorrhage.

Parkinson's disease

Extrapyramidal disorders lead to significant alterations in the sequencing of movement and may impair speed of a postural correction following a displacement. Parkinson's disease is characterized by the classic triad first described by Sir James Parkinson of bradykinesia, tremor and muscular rigidity, and is known to affect approximately 2% of people over the age of 65 years [63]. The disease is due to a deficiency of the neurotransmitter dopamine in the substantia nigra and associated nigra striatal pathway. It should not be confused with the symptom of 'parkinsonism' which is a manifestation of cerebrovascular disease in the same area.

Older people with Parkinson's disease commonly exhibit a flexed or stooped posture of both the trunk and limbs, and impaired postural equilibrium. The characteristic 'festinant' gait of the parkinsonian patient involves short, shuffling steps, lack of arm swing, loss of trunk movements and decreased foot clearance [64]. These changes, while not associated with increased sway when standing [65–67], are associated with impaired responses to external perturbations [68], decreased functional reach [69] and increased variability in stride length when walking [70–73].

Due to their rigid posture, abnormal gait and impaired ability to respond to external perturbations, many older people with Parkinson's disease suffer from frequent falls [74–77]. These falls may result from episodes of 'freezing', in which the individual attempts to overcome an inability to initiate movement and subsequently loses balance, or from loss of balance while turning. Paulson *et al.* [77] reported that 53% of 211 subjects with Parkinson's disease suffered from frequent falls, while a study of 100 subjects with idiopathic Parkinson's disease by Koller *et al.* [76] reported that 38% had experienced falls, with 13% falling more than once per week. Advancing age, duration of disease and disease severity are strong predictors of falls amongst people with Parkinson's disease [74, 76].

Parkinson's disease has also been found to be a strong independent risk factor for falling in epidemiological studies, in both institutionalized [78] and community-dwelling [18, 50, 79] older people.

Cerebellar disorders

The vestibulocerebellum and spinocerebellum regions of the brain are of particular importance to the maintenance of postural stability. Cerebellar disorders create grossly abnormal stepping patterns and impair corrective mechanisms. Lesions in these regions as a result of drug toxicity, alcoholism, degeneration, ischaemia or haemorrhage have been shown to increase sway when standing [80–83]. Older people with cerebellar disorders tend to have truncal ataxia, a wide-based gait and variable step length [84]. Although few authors have reported cerebellar dysfunction to be a risk factor for falls per se [1, 85], two of the characteristic gait variables associated with these syndromes – wide-based gait [86, 87] and irregular step lengths [25, 88, 89] – have been found to increase the risk of falling.

Dementia

The role of cognitive impairment and dementia in the aetiology of falls is interesting, and of particular relevance given the incidence of dementia [90] and its association not only with falls but also with hip fracture [91]. In addition, it is still far from clear as to which physiological and functional impairments contribute most to the increased risk of falls in this group.

Dementia affects approximately 6%–10% of community-dwelling older people [90], and has been reported as a strong and consistent risk factor for falls by numerous investigators [91–97]. Cognitive impairment associated with dementia and acute confusional states may increase the risk of falling by directly influencing the older person's ability to appropriately deal with environmental hazards, increasing the tendency of an older person to wander [98] and altering gait patterns [99]. In a study of 60 older women with Alzheimer's disease, Brody *et al.* [100] reported that the risk of falling was greatest in those subjects who had previously been vigorous, but had experienced marked decline over recent months.

Falls related to dementia are of particular concern in long term care facilities, as cognitive impairment is one of the most common reasons for initial nursing home admission [101]. Furthermore, it has been reported that older people with dementia have a four-fold increased risk of suffering a hip fracture as a result of a fall [100] and a three-fold increase in six-month mortality rate following hip fracture, compared to older people without dementia [102].

Of particular note is the relative lack of any evidence to support a strategy to prevent falls in a cognitively impaired population. In addition, bone health in this population is often not considered and treatment withheld because of concerns with compliance. Thus individuals with cognitive impairment are high risk in terms of both falls and hip fracture, but at present prevention of either has largely been unsuccessful in this group. More information is needed as to the relative contribution of different factors to overall risk which may in turn allow for a more evidenced-based approach to prevention.

Depression

A total of 15% of community-dwelling older people show significant depressive symptoms, with 1%–2% exhibiting major depressive disorders [103]. Numerous studies have reported an association between depression and falls. Tinetti *et al.* [104] found depression to be linked to an increased risk of falling in community-dwelling older people, as did Nevitt *et al.* [9], who reported that severe depression was associated with an increased risk of experiencing multiple falls. Subsequent investigations support these early observations, suggesting that the presence of depression is associated with an odds ratio of up to 7.5 for experiencing a fall [78, 105–108]. In nursing homes, the prevalence of depression can be as high as 25% [109].

The mechanisms underlying depressive symptoms and falls risk have not been fully evaluated. However, it has been suggested that older people who suffer from depression are less likely to be involved in physical activity, and are therefore at greater risk of falls due to reduced muscle strength, coordination and balance [1]. A recent prospective study of 7414 older women reported that those with depression exhibited significantly poorer self-reported health and functional status than those without depression, and exhibited a higher risk of hip fracture [108].

Interestingly, the use of antidepressant medications has also been reported to be a risk factor for falls in community-dwelling and institutionalized older people (see Chapter 7), and again the mechanism by which antidepressant use increases falls risk is poorly understood.

Cardiovascular problems resulting in neural failure of postural control

The hindbrain is particularly prone to alteration in perfusion and a momentary disturbance may be sufficient to impair muscle tone long enough for a fall to occur. In addition, impaired baroreceptor function may dampen the physiological response to postural change and precipitate a fall secondary to a perfusion deficit. Any condition which has the ability to temporarily impair perfusion of the hindbrain has the potential to precipitate a fall, which may or may not be associated with dizziness and/or syncope. The common causes of transient cerebral hypoperfusion relate to a drop in blood pressure or any tachy/brady arrhythmia. Local mechanical obstruction of the posterior cerebral circulation, usually through neck movement, can also cause transient hypoperfusion.

Dizziness as a symptom can be associated with many diseases, including those relating to transient cerebral hypoperfusion. The broad spectrum of diseases that may manifest in the form of dizziness often leads to a significant diagnostic challenge when looking for a direct causal relationship, and leads to the older patient being sent to several specialists, including cardiologists, geriatricians, neurologists and ENT surgeons. The confusion in the literature pertaining to dizziness in older people was the subject of an editorial [110] whereby the authors suggest that, due to the variety of ways dizziness has been classified in the literature, the results of various studies are analogous to the story of the blind men and the elephant. In this story, three blind men each feel a different part of the elephant's body and each observation provides accurate but biased information as to what the elephant is like.

Orthostatic hypotension

Orthostatic hypotension, also known as *postural hypotension*, refers to a drop in blood pressure which occurs when transferring from a supine to an erect position. It is commonly defined as a decrease in either systolic pressure of 20 mm Hg or a drop in diastolic pressure of 10 mm Hg on standing. *Symptomatic* orthostatic hypotension results when subjects reports dizziness, lightheadedness or faintness at the time of the documented drop in blood pressure.

The reported prevalence of orthostatic hypotension in older people ranges from 6%–33% [111–120]. This large variation can be attributed to variations in the population assessed, the technique of blood pressure measurement performed and the definitions used [113, 121, 122]. A major limitation of many of these studies is that they have not excluded subjects with chronic diseases or those taking medications known to cause orthostatic hypotension. In addition, many fail to differentiate between symptomatic and asymptomatic orthostatic hypotension. When confounding variables are adjusted for, the prevalence of orthostatic hypotension in community-dwelling older people is approximately 6% [116, 123]. These results suggest that orthostatic hypotension is relatively uncommon in community-dwelling healthy older people, and tends to be associated with pre-existing disease or the use of medications which have anti-hypertensive effects.

Drug induced orthostatic hypotension is the more common cause of hypotension, and includes anti-hypertensive agents, anti-anginals, antidepressants, anti-parkinsonian medication, anti-psychotics and any volume depleting drugs, e.g. diuretics [124, 125]. Numerous diseases have been found to be associated with an increased risk of developing orthostatic hypotension, including heart failure, diabetes mellitus, Parkinson's disease, stroke, dementia and depression [120, 123, 126]. A less common cause of orthostatic hypotension relates to autonomic nervous system failure [127, 128] as seen in some individuals with diseases such as diabetes or the Parkinson plus syndromes.

The association between orthostatic hypotension and falls dates back to Sheldon's 1960 study, in which 4% of 500 falls in 202 older people were attributed to 'abnormal blood pressure homeostasis' [129]. Numerous retrospective studies have since provided further evidence to support a relationship between orthostatic hypotension and falls [130–133]. Brocklehurst *et al.* [134] also suggested that 20% of hospital admissions for hip fracture could be attributed to hypotension-related loss of consciousness. In contrast to these findings, a post-fall assessment study conducted by Kirshen *et al.* [135] stated that *none* of the falls reported in two residential care facilities could be attributed to orthostatic hypotension. Similarly, Salgado *et al.* [48] did not find any difference in the prevalence of orthostatic hypotension in older people who had and had not fallen while in hospital. Other prospective studies have failed to demonstrate a link between orthostatic hypotension and falls [7, 107, 136].

A strong link between falls and orthostatic hypotension has not been documented, and relates partly to the intermittent nature of the condition, the frequent absence of symptoms and the need for continual monitoring to document blood pressure changes, including normal circadian changes [137] and post-prandial variations [138, 139].

We have used a pulse plethysmograph to measure blood pressure continuously for three minutes following a 60 degree upright tilt in a study of 70 older people. We found that subjects who fell in a 12-month follow-up period had significantly greater decreases in systolic blood pressure following the tilt than those who did not fall [140]. Furthermore, those who had unstable systolic blood pressure during the three minutes after tilting, in addition to large blood pressure drops, had a two-fold increased risk of falling compared with those with neither of these conditions. The non-fallers showed a relatively fast blood pressure change in response to the tilt, with stable levels thereafter, whereas the fallers tended to have a greater immediate decrease in blood pressure and an inconsistent response over the subsequent three minutes (see Figure 6.2).

Symptoms of dizziness were uncommon and not associated with changes in blood pressure in our study [140]. This was also the case in the cross-sectional study by Ensrud *et al.* [141]. They reported that only 23% of subjects diagnosed with orthostatic hypotension experienced feelings of dizziness and the clinical significance of such a drop is therefore uncertain. Equally, individuals can report symptoms similar to those defining symptomatic orthostatic hypotension and not have a significant drop in blood pressure [122].

Drop attacks

The term 'drop attack' was first used by Sheldon [129] and refers to a sudden, unexpected fall to the ground preceded by turning of the head or tilting of the neck. A drop attack is not associated with any loss of consciousness although there is often a transient loss of strength in the legs and trunk [142]. Since this early description, the term 'drop attack' has been variably applied to a range of neurological phenomena associated with falls and in common usage is a blanket term covering unexpected falls without a loss of consciousness.

The causative mechanism of a drop attack is still poorly understood and indeed in many cases no cause can be identified [143]. Sheldon's original description suggested that the 'sudden loss of postural alertness' associated with the condition could be attributed to brain stem dysfunction [129]. Other studies have implicated vertebro-basilar artery insufficiency [144–148], structural lesions of the cervical spine [149, 150] and carotid sinus hypersensitivity (CSH) [151–154]. While drop attacks can occur in otherwise healthy individuals, they are also commonly associated with neurological conditions including Meniere's disease [155, 156] and epilepsy [157, 158].

Drop attacks have been reported as the cause of 2%–25% of falls [129, 159–162], but the definition of a drop attack and the populations studied vary considerably in the literature. Sheldon's study attributed 25% of the 500 falls in community-dwelling women to a drop attack [129]. Clark [159], using the same definition, found that 16% of 431 fall-related hip fractures in women could be attributed to drop attacks, with an increasing prevalence of drop attacks with advancing age. Campbell *et al.* [130] also noted an increased prevalence of drop attacks with advancing age, but reported a smaller overall prevalence of 16% of all falls. An investigation of fall-related hip fractures in hospital reported that 20% of the 348 falls were due to drop attacks, however, the definition of a drop attack also included 'giddiness' and vertigo [134]. These results would seem to suggest that drop attacks are a relatively common cause of falls in older people.

Recent studies indicate that CSH, often cited as a cause of drop attacks and syncope, may be responsible for a proportion of the unexplained falls in these investigations. Prospective case-control studies have found that CSH (diagnosed by a drop in blood pressure and/or heart rate in response to massage of the carotid sinus) is present in one-third of patients admitted to hospital for

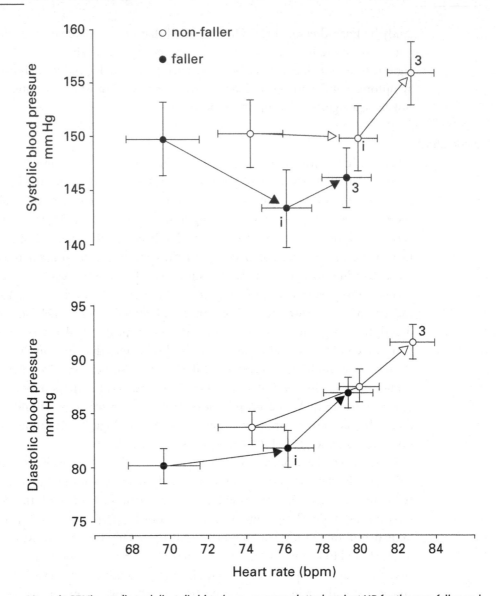

Fig. 6.2   Mean (±SEM) systolic and diastolic blood pressure are plotted against HR for the non-faller and faller groups. In each plot, the arrows progress from the resting value before tilting to the value immediately after tilting (i) and then the value three minutes after tilting (3). Figure from Heitterachi *et al.* [140].

fractured neck of femur [163] and in one-quarter to one-half of people admitted following a fall [164].

Whether a drop attack represents a single disease process for which the underlying pathophysiology is yet to be determined or a blanket term for a number of conditions presenting with a shared symptom remains to be elucidated.

Syncope

Syncope can be defined as a temporary loss of consciousness with spontaneous recovery and occurs when there is a transient decrease in cerebral blood flow. It is a symptom, not a disease, and can be precipitated by several cardiac and haemodynamic factors, including orthostatic hypotension, vasovagal syncope, transient ischaemic attacks, carotid sinus syndrome, cardiac arrhythmias and structural heart disease. Epilepsy can also manifest itself as sudden and transient loss of consciousness. However, the cause of syncope cannot be determined in up to 50% of cases [142].

The true prevalence of syncope and its contribution to falls incidence is difficult to ascertain as studies have used different definitions. Some have included transient loss of consciousness and others have specifically excluded syncope in the definition of a fall. A study of 33 patients with 'unexplained' syncope reported that 36% could be attributed to vasovagal attacks, 15% to cardiac arrhythmia, 9% to anti-hypertensive medications, 6% to orthostatic hypotension and, in one case, hyperventilation due to anxiety [165]. The relationship between cardiovascular dysfunction and syncope has also been highlighted in a recent study by Lawson *et al.* [166], who stated that the presence of syncope in patients who report severe dizziness is an accurate predictor of an eventual cardiovascular diagnosis. In addition, many studies consider falls and syncope to be two separate diagnoses with two separate sets of aetiologies, and fail to acknowledge the overlap in differential diagnoses [167]. This may explain why syncope has been reported as the cause of only 3% of falls in both nursing home [133, 168] and community-dwelling [85, 129, 134] populations.

Diseases affecting effector response

Following central processing, efferent signals are transmitted via the spinal cord and peripheral nerves to limb and trunk muscles whereby continuous muscular correction maintains postural stability. Any disease or disability that affects the bones, muscles and joints – the effector components of stability – may contribute to the risk of falling.

Osteoarthritis

Osteoarthritis is a common degenerative disease of articular cartilage which primarily affects the major weight-bearing joints of the body, leading to structural deformity, decreased range of motion and pain. An epidemiological study in Australia found osteoarthritis to be the commonest cause of musculo-skeletal disability among older people [169]. Older people with knee and hip osteoarthritis often suffer wasting of associated muscle groups. They have difficulty rising from a chair and performing daily tasks, and tend to walk more slowly than older people without the condition [170, 171]. There is also evidence to suggest that the presence of osteoarthritis impairs standing balance [172–174] and joint position sense [173, 175]. It has previously been shown that adequate joint range of movement in the lower limbs is essential to respond adequately to unexpected postural perturbations [176, 177], while the presence of pain in lower-limb joints may be a source of postural disturbance during voluntary movements. Thus, by reducing joint range of motion, reducing muscle strength and causing pain in lower-limb joints, osteoarthritis can have a detrimental effect on postural stability in older people. A medical history of osteoarthritis has been found to be a significant risk factor for falling by several prospective investigations [1, 9, 18, 50, 85, 91, 178, 179], while self-reported symptoms commonly associated with the condition, such as pain or reduced range of motion in the knees and hips, are also associated with increased falls risk [9, 50, 180].

Our group has studied 684 community-dwelling men and women aged 75–98 years (mean 80.0 ± 4.4), categorized with or without lower-limb osteoarthritis [181]. Subjects with osteoarthritis performed significantly worse than subjects without osteoarthritis in tests of knee and ankle muscle strength, lower-limb proprioception, postural sway and leaning balance, while being comparable in vision, tactile sensitivity and reaction time. The arthritis group suffered significantly more falls ($RR = 1.22$, 95% $CI = 1.03–1.46$) and injurious falls ($RR = 1.27$, 95% $CI = 1.01–1.60$) in the previous 12 months than the non-arthritis group. Within the arthritis group, reduced knee extension strength and increased sway were identified as significant predictors of falls.

Myelopathy

Degenerative change in the cervical spine (often referred to as cervical spondylosis) is a common finding in older people. With advancing age, the spinal canal in the cervical region of the spine becomes increasingly narrow due to ligamentous hypertrophy, intervertebral disc herniation and the formation of osteophytes on cervical vertebral processes. The narrowing of the spinal canal may lead to mechanical spinal cord impingement and associated postural dysfunction referred to as myelopathy [182]. Myelopathy is commonly associated with subjective reports of clumsiness, difficulty climbing stairs and experiences of the legs 'giving way', while objective findings include unsteadiness in standing and ataxic gait. No studies have reported myelopathy to be a risk factor in a large sample of older people. Nevertheless, it has been suggested that myelopathy may be under-diagnosed by clinicians, and as such, may be a more common cause of falls than is widely recognized [183].

Peripheral vascular disease

Up to 6% of people aged over 55 years suffer from symptomatic peripheral arterial disease (PAD) [184], which is a cause of mobility impairment due to its association with intermittent claudication – an intense, cramping pain in the calf muscles during exertion. People with PAD subsequently have lower levels of physical activity and may be at increased risk of falling. Gardner and Montgomery [185] conducted the first investigation into balance and falls in older people with intermittent claudication. Compared to 458 control subjects, the 367 subjects with intermittent claudication exhibited 28% shorter unipedal stance time, were 86% more likely to report gait unsteadiness and were more likely to have fallen in the last 12 months (26% vs. 15% of controls). In subjects with intermittent claudication, those with a history of falls exhibited 19% shorter unipedal stance time and took 14% longer to perform a sit-to-stand task [185]. Although these findings suggest an association between impaired circulation, instability and falls, no adjustment for potential confounders was undertaken, so the relative importance of intermittent claudication compared to other falls risk factors remains unclear. Nor is it clear whether the mechanism for increased risk is solely through the effector response or whether impaired circulation can manifest itself through altered peripheral sensation.

Prior poliomyelitis

People who have suffered from poliomyelitis in childhood may experience joint pain and muscular fatigue decades after their initial infection [186, 187]. This syndrome, referred to as 'prior poliomyelitis', 'late poliomyelitis' or 'post-polio syndrome', may lead to impaired mobility and subsequent increased risk of falls [188] and fractures of the affected limbs [189]. Silver and Aiello [188] reported a 64% incidence rate of falls and 35% rate of fractures in 233 post-polio patients, with most falls being attributed to tripping.

The likely mechanism for the high rates of falls in people with post-polio syndrome is muscle weakness and its contribution to impaired balance. In a case-control study, we compared the performance of 40 people with post-polio syndrome and age- and sex-matched controls on tests of vision, sensation, muscle strength, reaction time and balance [190]. The post-polio group demonstrated similar sensory performance, but impaired knee, hip and ankle strength, slower reaction time, and increased sway when standing. The correlation between leg strength and sway when standing on a foam rubber mat was greater in the post-polio group, indicating that decreased leg strength has a significant impact on ability to stand under challenging conditions in this group.

Foot problems

Foot problems are common in older people, affecting at least one in three community-dwelling people over the age of 65 years [191–194, 198], and up to 85% of older people in long term care facilities [195, 196]. Foot problems may result from osteoarthritic decreases in joint range of motion [197], dermatological conditions [198], detrimental effects of footwear [198–202], and systemic diseases, such as peripheral vascular disease [203], diabetes mellitus [204–206] and rheumatoid arthritis [207, 208]. The most commonly reported foot problems in older people are painful corns and calluses, hallux valgus ('bunions'), and hammer toes. Women report a higher prevalence of foot problems than men. The influence of fashion footwear has been found to contribute to foot problems due to the detrimental effect of high heels and a narrow toe-box [199–202, 209].

Foot problems are well recognized as a contributing factor to mobility impairment in older people. Older people with foot pain walk more slowly than those without and have more difficulty performing daily household tasks [210, 211]. Some 20% of older people who are housebound attribute their impaired mobility to foot problems [191]. There is some evidence that assessment of impaired foot and leg function can provide an accurate indicator of overall functional capability, and predict risk of nursing home admission [210].

As the foot provides the structural foundation for both static support and progression of the body during locomotion, it is plausible that foot problems could increase the risk of falling [212, 213]. However, few studies have directly investigated the role of foot problems in postural stability and falls. Two retrospective studies suggested that undefined foot problems were more common in older people who had fallen [180, 214] and results from prospective studies have found foot problems (including bunions, hammer toes and ulcers) to increase risk of falling [18, 23, 104, 178]. One of the limitations with the available evidence is that foot problems are generally poorly defined in epidemiological falls studies, in many cases being coded as a single variable (i.e. presence or absence) or clustered together with other leg problems. In response to this observation, we conducted detailed foot assessments of 135 older people. We found that a continuous score of overall foot impairment (including presence of lesions, hallux valgus and lesser toe deformities) was a significant independent predictor of performance in a range of balance and functional tests, and discriminated between older people with and without a history of falls [215]. Of the foot problems documented in this study, the presence of foot pain and lesser toe deformity had the greatest impact on impaired balance and functional ability [216]. More recently, we reported that hallux valgus, reduced ankle flexibility, reduced plantar tactile sensitivity and toe muscle weakness are associated with impaired balance [217] and increase the risk of falls [218].

Urinary incontinence

Incontinence is a common and often under-diagnosed problem in older people, particularly older women. In industrialized societies, up to 34% of older men and 55% of older women suffer from an inability to control urinary functions [219]. Risk factors for incontinence include multiparity, older age, obesity, previous surgery for incontinence and neurological disorders [220]. Both retrospective and prospective falls investigations have consistently reported urinary incontinence to be a risk factor for falls in community-dwelling [9, 85, 104, 106, 221–224] and institutionalized [1, 225, 226] older people.

Falls related to incontinence are generally thought to result from loss of balance when rushing to the toilet or an increased likelihood of slipping on urine. However, there is some question as to whether incontinence is a primary cause of falls or whether it is simply a marker of generalized physical frailty. While numerous falls in long term care facilities occur when going to or returning from the toilet [227], few falls in community-dwelling older people involve toileting. The close associations reported between incontinence, dementia, depression, falls and level of mobility suggests that these 'geriatric symptoms' may have shared risk factors rather than causal connections [228].

A study by Brown *et al.* [229] of 6049 community-dwelling older women followed up for three years provides the most convincing evidence of incontinence being an independent risk factor for falls and fractures. After adjusting for level of functional decline, older women with at least weekly urge incontinence were 26% more likely to fall and 34% more likely to suffer a fracture. This is presumably because urge incontinence (as opposed to stress incontinence) is associated with a sense of urgency and frequent rushed trips to the bathroom, particularly at night when environmental hazards may pose a greater threat to maintaining stability.

Conclusion

A multiplicity of medical conditions have been reported to be associated with an increased risk of falling and occur predominantly through the manifestation of physiological deficits, which have been discussed in previous chapters. It is perhaps of academic interest whether it is the specific disease or the physiological manifestations that lead to the increased risk. Many conditions have been suggested to increase the risk of falling in older people, but the literature is somewhat equivocal as to the relative importance of each of these conditions. This highlights the benefits of a functional rather than a purely disease-oriented approach to predicting falls. Attributing a degree of falls risk to a specific medical diagnosis has limitations, as the relative severity of the condition may vary considerably between individuals. Furthermore, deficits in sensory and motor function may be evident in many older people with no recorded medical illnesses. As such, the functional approach to falls risk assessment, which involves direct measurement of physical and mental capabilities, would appear to be a useful and complementary approach to assessing the risk of falling.

REFERENCES

1. M. E. Tinetti, T. F. Williams & R. Mayewski, Fall risk index for elderly patients based on number of chronic disabilities. *American Journal of Medicine*, **80** (1986), 429–34.

2. L. I. Wolfson, R. Whipple, P. Amerman, J. Kaplan & A. Kleinberg, Gait and balance in the elderly: two functional capacities that link sensory and motor ability to falls. *Clinics in Geriatric Medicine*, **1** (1985), 649–59.

3. R. Sekuler D. Kline & K. Dismukes, *Aging and Human Visual Function.* (New York: Alan R. Liss, 1982).

4. N. S. Gittings & J. L. Fozard, Age related changes in visual acuity. *Experimental Gerontology*, **21** (1986), 423–33.

5. S. R. Lord, R. D. Clark & I. W. Webster, Visual acuity and contrast sensitivity in relation to falls in an elderly population. *Age and Ageing*, **20** (1991), 175–81.

6. S. R. Lord, D. McLean & G. Stathers, Physiological factors associated with injurious falls in older people living in the community. *Gerontology*, **38** (1992), 338–46.

7. R. D. Clark S. R. Lord & I. W. Webster, Clinical parameters associated with falls in an elderly population. *Gerontology*, **39** (1993), 117–23.

8. C. I. Jack, T. Smith, C. Neoh, M. Lye & J. N. McGalliard, Prevalence of low vision in elderly patients admitted to an acute geriatric unit in Liverpool: elderly people who fall are more likely to have low vision. *Gerontology*, **41** (1995), 280–5.

9. M. C. Nevitt, S. R. Cummings, S. Kidd & D. Black, Risk factors for recurrent nonsyncopal falls. A prospective study. *Journal of the American Medical Association*, **261** (1989), 2663–8.

10. S. R. Lord, J. A. Ward, P. Williams & K. J. Anstey, An epidemiological study of falls in older community-dwelling women: the Randwick Falls and Fractures Study. *Australian Journal of Public Health*, **17** (1993), 240–5.

11. D. L. Swagerty, The impact of age-related visual impairment on functional independence in the elderly. *Kansas Medicine*, **96** (1995), 24–6.

12. H. A. Kahn, H. M. Leibowitz & J. P. Gankey, The Framingham Eye Study. I. Outline and major prevalence findings. *American Journal of Epidemiology*, **106** (1977), 17–32.

13. A. Spector, Aging of the lens and cataract formation. In *Aging and Human Visual Function*, ed. R. Sekular, D. Kline & K. Dismukes (New York: Alan R. Liss, 1982), pp. 27–43.

14. D. T. Felson, J. J. Anderson & M. T. Annan, Impaired vision and hip fracture. The Framingham study. *Journal of the American Geriatrics Society*, **37** (1989), 495–500.

15. J. G. Herndon, C. G. Helmick, R. W. Sattin *et al.*, Chronic medical conditions and risk of fall injury events at home in older adults. *Journal of the American Geriatrics Society*, **45** (1997), 739–43.

16. R. Q. Ivers, R. G. Cumming, P. Mitchell & K. Attebo, Visual impairment and falls in older adults: the Blue Mountains Eye Study. *Journal of the American Geriatrics Society*, **46** (1998), 58–64.

17. R. Q. Ivers, R. G. Cumming, P. Mitchell, J. M. Simpson & A. J. Peduto, Visual risk factors for hip fracture in older people. *Journal of the American Geriatrics Society*, **51** (2003), 356–63.

18. J. Dolinis & J. E. Harrison, Factors associated with falling in older Adelaide residents. *Australian and New Zealand Journal of Public Health*, **21** (1997), 462–8.

19. R. J. Glynn, J. M. Seddon, J. H. Krug *et al.*, Falls in elderly patients with glaucoma. *Archives of Ophthalmology*, **109** (1991), 205–10.

20. P. Mitchell, W. Smith, K. Attebo & J. J. Wang, Prevalence of age-related maculopathy in Australia: The Blue Mountains Eye Study. *Ophthalmology*, **102** (1995), 1450–60.

21. J. R. Vingerling, C. C. Klaver, A. Hofman & P. T. de Jong, Epidemiology of age-related maculopathy. *Epidemiological Reviews*, **17** (1995), 347–60.

22. S. R. Lord, J. A. Ward, P. Williams & K. J. Anstey, Physiological factors associated with falls in older community-dwelling women. *Journal of the American Geriatrics Society*, **42** (1994), 1110–17.

23. K. Koski, H. Luukinen, P. Laippala & S. L. Kivela, Risk factors for major injurious falls among the home-dwelling elderly by functional abilities. *Gerontology*, **44** (1998), 232–8.

24. G. S. Sorock & D. M. Labiner, Peripheral neuromuscular dysfunction and falls in an elderly cohort. *American Journal of Epidemiology*, **136** (1992), 584–91.

25. S. R. Lord, D. G. Lloyd & S. K. Li, Sensori-motor function, gait patterns and falls in community-dwelling women. *Age and Ageing*, **25** (1996), 292–9.

26. T. D. Sabin, Peripheral neuropathy: disorders of proprioception. In *Gait Disorders of Aging: Falls and Therapeutic Strategies*, ed. J. C. Masdeu, L. Sudarsky & L. Wolfson (Philadelphia: Lippincott-Raven, 1997).

27. J. Pirart, Diabetes mellitus and its degenerative complications: a prospective study of 4,440 patients observed between 1947 and 1973. *Diabetes Care*, **2** (1979), 168–88.

28. G. G. Simoneau, J. S. Ulbrecht, J. A. Derr, M. B. Becker & P. R. Cavanagh, Postural instability in patients with diabetic sensory neuropathy. *Diabetes Care*, **17** (1994), 1411–21.

29. L. Uccioli, P. G. Giacomini, G. Monticone *et al.*, Body sway in diabetic neuropathy. *Diabetes Care*, **18** (1995), 339–44.

30. J. K. Richardson, J. A. Ashton-Miller, S. G. Lee & K. Jacobs, Moderate peripheral neuropathy impairs weight transfer and unipedal balance in the elderly. *Archives of Physical Medicine and Rehabilitation*, **77** (1996), 1152–6.

31. C. G. Van den Bosch, M. G. Gilsing, S. G. Lee, J. K. Richardson & J. A. Ashton-Miller, Peripheral neuropathy effect on ankle inversion and eversion detection thresholds. *Archives of Physical Medicine and Rehabilitation*, **76** (1995), 850–6.

32. G. G. Simoneau, J. A. Derr, J. S. Ulbrecht, M. B. Becker & P. R. Cavanagh, Diabetic sensory neuropathy effect on ankle joint movement perception. *Archives of Physical Medicine and Rehabilitation*, **77** (1996), 453–60.

33. A. Malmivaara, M. Heliovaara, P. Knekt, A. Reunanen & A. Aromaa, Risk factors for injurious falls leading to hospitalization or death in a cohort of 19,500 adults. *American Journal of Epidemiology*, **138** (1993), 384–94.

34. R. Q. Ivers, R. G. Cumming, P. Mitchel & A. J. Peduto, Diabetes and risk of fracture: the Blue Mountains Eye Study. *Diabetes Care*, **24** (2001), 1198–203.

35. R. L. Kennedy, J. Henry, A. J. Chapman *et al.*, Accidents in patients with insulin-treated diabetes: increased risk of low-impact falls but not motor vehicle crashes – a prospective register-based study. *Journal of Trauma: Injury, Infection and Critical Care*, **52** (2002), 660–6.

36. P. R. Cavanagh, J. A. Derr, J. S. Ulbrecht, R. E. Maser & T. J. Orchard, Problems with gait and posture in neuropathic patients with insulin-dependent diabetes mellitus. *Diabetic Medicine*, **9** (1992), 469–74.

37. J. Richardson, C. Ching & E. Hurvitz, The relationship between electromyographically documented peripheral neuropathy and falls. *Journal of the American Geriatrics Society*, **40** (1992), 1008–12.

38. J. K. Richardson & E. A. Hurvitz, Peripheral neuropathy: a true risk factor for falls. *Journal of Gerontology*, **50** (1995), M211–15.

39. B. Wyke, Cervical articular contributions to posture and gait: their relation to senile disequilibrium. *Age and Ageing*, **8** (1979), 251–8.

40. S. M. Highstein, How does the vestibular part of the inner ear work? In *Disorders of the Vestibular System*, ed. R. W. Baloh and G. M. Halmagyi. (New York: Oxford University Press, 1996).

41. R. Baloh & G. Halmagyi, *Disorders of the Vestibular System* (New York: Oxford University Press, 1996).

42. T. D. Fife & R. W. Baloh, Disequilibrium of unknown cause in older people. *Annals of Neurology*, **34** (1993), 694–702.

43. S. J. Herdman, P. Blatt, M. C. Schubert & R. J. Tusa, Falls in patients with vestibular deficits. *American Journal of Otology*, **21** (2000), 847–51.

44. E. K. Kristinsdottir, E. Nordell, G. B. Jarnlo *et al.*, Observation of vestibular asymmetry in a majority of patients over 50 years with fall-related wrist fractures. *Acta Otolaryngology*, **121** (2001), 481–5.

45. R. P. Di Fabio, J. F. Greany, A. Emasithi & J. F. Wyman, Eye-head coordination during postural perturbation as a predictor of falls in community-dwelling elderly women. *Archives of Physical Medicine and Rehabilitation*, **83** (2002), 942–51.

46. S. L. Whitney, M. T. Hudak & G. F. Marchetti, The dynamic gait index relates to self reported fall history in individuals with vestibular dysfunction. *Journal of Vestibular Research*, **10** (2000), 99–105.

47. R. Tideiksaar, *Falling in Old Age: its Prevention and Treatment* (New York: Springer Publishing Company, 1989).

48. R. Salgado, S. R. Lord, J. Packer & F. Ehrlich, Factors associated with falling in elderly hospital patients. *Gerontology*, **40** (1994), 325–31.

49. J. L. O'Loughlin, Y. Robitaille, J. F. Boivin & S. Suissa, Incidence of and risk factors for falls and injurious falls among the community-dwelling elderly. *American Journal of Epidemiology*, **137** (1993), 342–54.

50. A. J. Campbell, M. J. Borrie & G. F. Spears, Risk factors for falls in a community-based prospective study of people 70 years and older. *Journal of Gerontology*, **44** (1989), M112–17.

51. D. Prudham & J. G. Evans, Factors associated with falls in the elderly: a community study. *Age and Ageing*, **10** (1981), 141–6.

52. L. Jorgensen, T. Engstad & B. K. Jacobsen, Higher incidence of falls in long-term stroke survivors than in population controls: depressive symptoms predict falls after stroke. *Stroke*, **33** (2002), 542–7.

53. D. Hyndman, A. Ashburn & E. Stack, Fall events among people with stroke living in the community: circumstances of falls and characteristics of fallers. *Archives of Physical Medical Rehabilitation*, **83** (2002), 165–70.

54. S. G. Kirker, D. S. Simpson, J. R. Jenner & A. M. Wing, Stepping before standing: hip muscle function in stepping and standing balance after stroke. *Journal of Neurology, Neurosurgery and Psychiatry*, **68** (2000), 458–64.

55. P. T. Cheng, M. Y. Liaw, M. K. Wong et al., The sit-to-stand movement in stroke patients and its correlation with falling. *Archives of Physical Medicine and Rehabilitation*, **79** (1998), 1043–6.

56. L. A. Brown, W. H. Gage, M. A. Polych, R. J. Sleik & T. R. Winder, Central set influences on gait: age-dependent effects of postural threat. *Experimental Brain Research*, **145** (2002), 286–96.

57. H. Mitoma, R. Hayashi, N. Yanagisawa & H. Tsukagoshi, Gait disturbances in patients with pontine medial tegmental lesions: clinical characteristics and gait analysis. *Archives of Neurology*, **57** (2000), 1048–57.

58. A. Moseley, A. Wales, R. Herbert, K. Shurr & S. Moore, Observation and analysis of hemiplegic gait: stance phase. *Australian Journal of Physiotherapy*, **39** (1993), 259–67.

59. S. Moore, K. Schurr, A. Wales, R. Herbert & A. Moseley, Observation and analysis of hemiplegic gait: swing phase. *Australian Journal of Physiotherapy*, **39** (1993), 271–8.

60. R. Shiavi, H. Bugle & T. Limbird, Electromyographic gait assessment. Part 2. Preliminary assessment of hemiparetic synergy patterns. *Journal of Rehabilitation Research and Development*, **24** (1987), 24–30.

61. A. Lamontagne, C. Richards & F. Malouin, Coactivation during gait as an adaptive behavior after stroke. *Journal of Electromyography and Kinesiology*, **10** (2000), 407–15.

62. C. M. Said, P. A. Goldie, A. E. Patla & W. A. Sparrow, Effect of stroke on step characteristics of obstacle crossing. *Archives of Physical Medicine and Rehabilitation*, **82** (2001), 1712–19.

63. C. M. Tanner, Epidemiology of Parkinson's disease. *Neurology Clinics*, **10** (1992), 317–29.

64. J. P. Martin, *The Basal Ganglia and Posture* (London: Pitman Medical Publishing, 1967).

65. M. Schieppati & A. Nardone, Free and supported stance in Parkinson's disease. *Brain*, **114** (1991), 1227–31.

66. J. Kitamura, H. Nakagawa, K. Iinuma et al., Visual influence on center of contact pressure in advanced Parkinson's disease. *Archives of Physical Medicine and Rehabilitation*, **74** (1993), 1107–12.

67. M. Gregoric & A. Lavric, Statokinesimetric analysis of the postural control in parkinsonism. *Agressologie*, **18** (1977), 45–8.

68. M. W. Rogers, Disorders of posture, balance, and gait in Parkinson's disease. *Clinics in Geriatric Medicine*, **12** (1995), 825–45.

69. M. Schenkman, M. Morey & M. Kuchibhatla, Spinal flexibility and balance control among community-dwelling adults with and without Parkinson's disease. *Journal of Gerontology*, **55A** (2000), M441–5.

70. M. E. Morris, R. Iansek, T. A. Matyas & J. J. Summers, Abnormalities in the stride length-cadence relation in parkinsonian gait. *Movement Disorders*, **13** (1998), 61–9.

71. M. E. Morris, R. Iansek, T. A. Matyas & J. J. Summers, Stride length regulation in Parkinson's disease. Normalization strategies and underlying mechanisms. *Brain*, **119** (1996), 551–68.

72. M. E. Morris, R. Iansek, T. A. Matyas & J. J. Summers, The pathogenesis of gait hypokinesia in Parkinson's disease. *Brain*, **117** (1994), 1169–81.

73. F. Smithson, M. E. Morris & R. Iansek, Performance on clinical tests of balance in Parkinson's disease. *Physical Therapy*, **78** (1998), 577–92.

74. A. Ashburn, E. Stack, R. M. Pickering & C. D. Ward, A community-dwelling sample of people with Parkinson's disease: characteristics of fallers and non-fallers. *Age and Ageing*, **30** (2001), 47–52.

75. R. Burns, Falling and getting up again. *Parkinson Report*, **XV** (1994), 18.

76. W. C. Koller, S. Glatt, B. Vetere-Overfield *et al.*, Falls and Parkinson's disease. *Clinical Neuropharmacology*, **12** (1989), 98–105.

77. G. W. Paulson, K. Schaefer & B. Hallum, Avoiding mental changes and falls in older Parkinsons' patients. *Geriatrics*, **41** (1986), 59–62.

78. E. Granek, S. P. Baker, H. Abbey *et al.*, Medications and diagnoses in relation to falls in a long-term care facility. *Journal of the American Geriatrics Society*, **35** (1987), 503–11.

79. S. Studenski, P. W. Duncan, J. Chandler *et al.*, Predicting falls: the role of mobility and nonphysical factors. *Journal of the American Geriatrics Society*, **42** (1994), 297–302.

80. J. Dichgans, K. H. Mauritz, J. H. J. Allum & T. Brandt, Postural sway in normals and atactic patients: analysis of the stabilising and destabilizing effects of vision. *Agressologie*, **17** (1976), 15–24.

81. K. H. Mauritz, J. Dichgans & A. Hufschmidt, Quantitative analysis of stance in late cortical cerebellar atrophy of the anterior lobe and other forms of cerebellar ataxia. *Brain*, **102** (1979), 461–82.

82. A. M. Bronstein, J. D. Hood, M. A. Gresty & C. Panagi, Visual control of balance in cerebellar and parkinsonian syndromes. *Brain*, **113** (1990), 767–79.

83. F. B. Horak & H. C. Diener, Cerebellar control of postural scaling and central set in stance. *Journal of Neurophysiology*, **72** (1994), 479–93.

84. H. C. Diener & J. G. Nutt, Vestibular and cerebellar disorders of equilibrium and gait. In *Gait Disorders of Aging: Falls and Therapeutic Strategies*, ed. J. C. Masdeu, L. Sudarsky & L. Wolfson (Philadelphia: Lippincott-Raven, 1997).

85. A. S. Robbins, L. Z. Rubenstein, K. R. Josephson *et al.*, Predictors of falls among elderly people – results of two population-based studies. *Archives of Internal Medicine*, **149** (1989), 1628–33.

86. G. M. Gehlsen & M. H. Whaley, Falls in the elderly. Part I. Gait. *Archives of Physical Medicine and Rehabilitation*, **71** (1990), 735–8.

87. S. M. Woolley, S. J. Czaja & C. G. Drury, An assessment of falls in elderly men and women. *Journal of Gerontology*, **52A** (1997), M80–7.

88. J. M. Hausdorff, H. K. Edelberg, S. L. Mitchell, A. L. Goldberger & J. Y. Wei, Increased gait unsteadiness in community-dwelling elderly fallers. *Archives of Physical Medicine and Rehabilitation*, **78** (1997), 278–83.

89. B. E. Maki, Gait changes in older adults: predictors of falls or indicators of fear? *Journal of the American Geriatrics Society*, **45** (1997), 313–20.

90. H. C. Hendrie, Epidemiology of dementia and Alzheimer's disease. *American Journal of Geriatric Psychiatry*, **6** (1998), S3–18.

91. D. M. Buchner & E. B. Larson, Falls and fractures in patients with Alzheimer-type dementia. *Journal of the American Medical Association*, **257** (1987), 1492–5.

92. J. C. Morris, E. H. Rubin, E. J. Morris & S. A. Mandel, Senile dementia of the Alzheimer's type: an important risk factor for serious falls. *Journal of Gerontology*, **42** (1987), 412–17.

93. D. M. Buchner & E. B. Larson, Transfer bias and the association of cognitive impairment with falls. *Journal of General Internal Medicine*, **3** (1988), 254–9.

94. Y. T. Gross, Y. Shimamoto, C. L. Rose & B. Frank, Why do they fall? Monitoring risk factors in nursing homes. *Journal of Gerontological Nursing*, **16** (1990), 20–5.

95. P. O. Jantti, V. I. Pyykko & A. L. Hervonen, Falls among elderly nursing home residents. *Public Health*, **107** (1993), 89–96.

96. T. Asada, T. Kariya, T. Kinoshita *et al.*, Predictors of fall-related injuries among community-dwelling elderly people with dementia. *Age and Ageing*, **25** (1996), 22–8.

97. C. Johansson & I. Skoog, A population-based study on the association between dementia and hip fractures in 85-year olds. *Aging – Clinical and Experimental Research*, **8** (1996), 189–96.

98. J. M. Mossey, Social and psychologic factors related to falls among the elderly. *Clinics in Geriatric Medicine*, **1** (1985), 541–53.

99. T. Nakamura, K. Meguro & H. Sasaki, Relationship between falls and stride length variability in senile dementia of the Alzheimer type. *Gerontology*, **42** (1996), 108–13.

100. E. M. Brody, M. H. Kleban, M. S. Moss & F. Kleban, Predictors of falls among institutionalized women with Alzheimer's disease. *Journal of the American Geriatrics Society*, **32** (1984), 877–82.

101. S. R. Lord, Predictors of nursing home placement and mortality in residents in intermediate care. *Age and Ageing*, **23** (1994), 499–504.

102. B. R. Baker, T. Duckworth & E. Wilkes, Mental state and other prognostic factors in femoral fractures of the elderly. *Journal of the Royal College of General Practitioners*, **28** (1978), 557–9.

103. D. Blazer & D. C. Hughes, The epidemiology of depression in an elderly community population. *The Gerontologist*, **27** (1987), 281–7.

104. M. E. Tinetti, M. Speechley & S. F. Ginter, Risk factors for falls among elderly persons living in the community. *New England Journal of Medicine*, **319** (1988), 1701–7.

105. A. H. Myers, S. P. Baker, M. L. Van Natta, H. Abbey & E. G. Robinson, Risk factors associated with falls and injuries among elderly institutionalized persons. *American Journal of Epidemiology*, **133** (1991), 1179–90.

106. N. G. Kutner, K. B. Schechtman, M. G. Ory & D. I. Baker, Older adults' perceptions of their health and functioning in relation to sleep disturbance, falling, and urinary incontinence. FICSIT Group. *Journal of the American Geriatrics Society*, **42** (1994), 757–62.

107. B. A. Liu, A. K. Topper, R. A. Reeves, C. Gryfe & B. E. Maki, Falls among older people: relationship to medication use and orthostatic hypotension. *Journal of the American Geriatrics Society*, **43** (1995), 1141–5.

108. M. A. Whooley, K. E. Kip, J. A. Cauley *et al.*, Depression, falls, and risk of fracture in older women. Study of Osteoporotic Fractures Research Group. *Archives of Internal Medicine*, **159** (1999), 484–90.

109. S. C. Samuels & I. B. Katz, Depression in the nursing home. *Psychiatry Annual*, **25** (1995), 419–24.

110. P. D. Sloane & J. Dallara, Clinical research and geriatric dizziness: the blind men and the elephant. *Journal of the American Geriatrics Society*, **47** (1999), 113–14.

111. W. S. Aronow, N. H. Lee, F. F. Sales & F. Etienne, Prevalence of postural hypotension in elderly patients in a long-term health care facility. *American Journal of Cardiology*, **62** (1988), 336.

112. V. Burke, L. J. Beilin, R. German *et al.*, Postural fall in blood pressure in the elderly in relation to drug treatment and other lifestyle factors. *Quarterly Journal of Medicine*, **84** (1992), 583–91.

113. F. I. Caird, G. R. Andrews & R. D. Kennedy, Effect of posture on blood pressure in the elderly. *British Heart Journal*, **35** (1973), 527–530.

114. R. H. Johnson, A. C. Smith & J. M. K. Spalding, Effect of posture on blood pressure in elderly patients. *The Lancet*, **1** (1965), 731–3.

115. I. M. Lennox & B. O. Williams, Postural hypotension in the elderly. *Clinical and Experimental Gerontology*, **2** (1980), 313–29.

116. K. H. Masaki, I. J. Schatz, C. M. Burchfiel *et al.*, Orthostatic hypotension predicts mortality in elderly men: the Honolulu Heart Program. *Circulation*, **98** (1998), 2290–5.

117. M. G. Myers, P. M. Kearns, D. S. Kennedy & R. H. Fisher, Postural hypotension and diuretic therapy in the elderly. *Canadian Medical Association Journal*, **119** (1978), 581–4.

118. I. Raiha, S. Luutonen, J. Piha *et al.*, Prevalence, predisposing factors, and prognostic importance of postural hypotension. *Archives of Internal Medicine*, **155** (1995), 930–5.

119. M. Rodstein & F. Zeman, Postural blood pressure changes in the elderly. *Journal of Chronic Diseases*, **6** (1957), 581–8.

120. R. S. Tilvis, S. M. Hakala, J. Valvanne & T. Erkinjuntti, Postural hypotension and dizziness in a general aged population: a four-year follow-up of the Helsinki Aging Study. *Journal of the American Geriatrics Society*, **44** (1996), 809–14.

121. K. T. Palmer, Studies into postural hypotension in elderly patients. *New Zealand Medical Journal*, **96** (1983), 43–5.

122. G. H. Rutan, B. Hermanson, D. E. Bild *et al.*, Orthostatic hypotension in older adults. The Cardiovascular Health Study. CHS Collaborative Research Group. *Hypertension*, **19** (1992), 508–19.

123. S. L. Mader, K. R. Josephson & L. Z. Rubenstein, Low prevalence of postural hypotension among community-dwelling elderly. *Journal of the American Medical Association*, **258** (1987), 1511–14.

124. T. F. Mets, Drug-induced orthostatic hypotension in older patients. *Drugs and Aging*, **6** (1995), 219–28.

125. S. Luutonen, P. Neuvonen, H. Ruskoaho *et al.*, The role of potassium in postural hypotension: electrolytes and neurohumoral factors in elderly hypertensive patients using diuretics. *Journal of Internal Medicine*, **237** (1995), 375–80.

126. M. E. Hillen, M. L. Wagner & J. I. Sage, "Subclinical" orthostatic hypotension is associated with dizziness in elderly patients with Parkinson disease. *Archives of Physical Medicine and Rehabilitation*, **77** (1996), 710–12.

127. P. A. Low, T. L. Opfer-Gehrking, B. R. McPhee *et al.*, Prospective evaluation of clinical characteristics of orthostatic hypotension. *Mayo Clinic Proceedings*, **70** (1995), 617–22.

128. C. J. Mathias, Orthostatic hypotension: causes, mechanisms, and influencing factors. *Neurology*, **45** (1995), S6–11.

129. J. H. Sheldon, On the natural history of falls in old age. *British Medical Journal*, **2** (1960), 1685–90.

130. A. J. Campbell, J. Reinken, B. C. Allan & G. S. Martinez, Falls in old age: a study of frequency and related clinical factors. *Age and Ageing*, **10** (1981), 264–70.

131. A. Gabell, M. A. Simons & U. S. Nayak, Falls in the healthy elderly: predisposing causes. *Ergonomics*, **28** (1985), 965–75.

132. P. V. Jonsson, L. A. Lipsitz, M. Kelley & J. Koestner, Hypotensive responses to common daily activities in institutionalized elderly. A potential risk for recurrent falls. *Archives of Internal Medicine*, **150** (1990), 1518–24.

133. L. Z. Rubenstein, A. S. Robbins, K. R. Josephson, B. L. Schulman & D. Osterweil, The value of assessing falls in an elderly population. A randomized clinical trial. *Annals of Internal Medicine*, **113** (1990), 308–16.

134. J. C. Brocklehurst, A. N. Exton-Smith, S. M. Lempert Barber, L. P. Hunt & M. K. Palmer, Fracture of the femur in old age: a two-centre study of associated clinical factors and the cause of the fall. *Age and Ageing*, **7** (1978), 2–15.

135. A. J. Kirshen, R. D. T. Cape, H. C. Hayes & J. D. Spencer, Postural sway and cardiovascular parameters associated with falls in the elderly. *Journal of Clinical Experimental Gerontology*, **6** (1984), 291–307.

136. S. R. Lord, K. J. Anstey, P. Williams & J. A. Ward, Psychoactive medication use, sensori-motor function and falls in older women. *British Journal of Clinical Pharmacology*, **39** (1995), 227–34.

137. L. A. Lipsitz, Abnormalities in blood pressure homeostasis that contribute to falls in the elderly. *Clinics in Geriatric Medicine*, **1** (1985), 637–48.

138. S. J. Peitzman & S. R. Berger, Postprandial blood pressure decrease in well elderly persons. *Archives of Internal Medicine*, **149** (1989), 286–8.

139. F. Puisieux, H. Bulckaen, A. L. Fauchais *et al.*, Ambulatory blood pressure monitoring and postprandial hypotension in elderly persons with falls or syncope. *Journal of Gerontology*, **55** (2000), M535–40.

140. E. Heitterachi, S. R. Lord, P. Meyerkort, I. McCloskey & R. Fitzpatrick, Blood pressure changes on upright tilting predict falls in older people. *Age and Ageing*, **31** (2002), 181.

141. K. E. Ensrud, M. C. Nevitt, C. Yunis *et al.*, Postural hypotension and postural dizziness in elderly women. The study of osteoporotic fractures. The Study of Osteoporotic Fractures Research Group. *Archives of Internal Medicine*, **152** (1992), 1058–64.

142. L. A. Lipsitz, The drop attack: a common geriatric symptom. *Journal of the American Geriatrics Society*, **31** (1983), 617–20.

143. I. Meissner, D. O. Wiebers, J. W. Swanson & W. M. O'Fallon, The natural history of drop attacks. *Neurology*, **36** (1986), 1029–34.

144. J. C. M. Brust, C. R. Plank & E. B. Healton, The pathology of drop attacks: a case report. *Neurology*, **29** (1979), 786–8.

145. M. Kameyama, Vertigo and drop attack. With special reference to cerebrovascular disorders and atherosclerosis of the vertebral-basilar system. *Geriatrics*, **20** (1965), 892–900.

146. M. J. Kubala & C. H. Millikan, Diagnosis, pathogenesis, and treatment of "drop attacks". *Archives of Neurology*, **11** (1964), 107–10.

147. S. Sheehan, R. B. Bauer & J. S. Meyer, Vertebral artery compression in cervical spondylosis: arteriographic demonstration during life of vertebral artery insufficiency due to rotation and extension of the neck. *Neurology*, **10** (1960), 968–72.

148. D. Williams & T. G. Wilson, The diagnosis of major and minor syndromes of basilar insufficiency. *Brain*, **85** (1962), 741–7.

149. M. Kremer, Sitting, standing and walking. *British Medical Journal*, **2** (1958), 121.

150. G. J. van Norel & W. I. Verhagen, Drop attacks and instability of the degenerate cervical spine. *Journal of Bone and Joint Surgery*, **78B** (1996), 495–6.

151. P. F. Walter, I. S. Crawley & E. R. Dorney, Carotid sinus hypersensitivity and syncope. *Neurology*, **27** (1978), 746–51.

152. A. L. Murphy, B. J. Rowbotham, R. S. Boyle *et al.*, Carotid sinus hypersensitivity in elderly nursing home patients. *Australian and New Zealand Journal of Medicine*, **16** (1986), 24–7.

153. R. A. Kenny & G. Traynor, Carotid sinus syndrome – clinical characteristics in elderly patients. *Age and Ageing*, **20** (1991), 449–54.

154. A. B. Dey, N. R. Stout & R. A. Kenny, Cardiovascular syncope is the most common cause of drop attacks in the elderly. *Pacing and Clinical Electrophysiology*, **20** (1997), 818–19.

155. L. M. Odkvist & J. Bergenius, Drop attacks in Meniere's disease. *Acta Otolaryngologica Supplementum*, **455** (1988), 82–5.

156. R. W. Baloh, K. Jacobson & T. Winder, Drop attacks with Meniere's syndrome. *Annals of Neurology*, **28** (1990), 384–7.

157. K. Fukushima, T. Fujiwara, K. Yagi & M. Seino, Drop attacks and epileptic syndromes. *Japanese Journal of Psychiatry and Neurology*, **47** (1993), 211–16.

158. P. Tinuper, A. Cerullo, C. Marini *et al.*, Epileptic drop attacks in partial epilepsy: clinical features, evolution, and prognosis. *Journal of Neurology, Neurosurgery and Psychiatry*, **64** (1998), 231–7.

159. A. N. Clark, Factors in fracture of the female femur. A clinical study of the environmental, physical, medical and preventive aspects of this injury. *Gerontologia Clinica*, **10** (1968), 257–70.

160. P. W. Overstall, A. N. Exton-Smith, F. J. Imms & A. L. Johnson, Falls in the elderly related to postural imbalance. *British Medical Journal*, **1** (1977), 261–4.

161. D. L. Stevens & W. B. Matthews, Cryptogenic drop attacks: an affliction of women. *British Medical Journal*, **1** (1973), 439–42.

162. A. J. Campbell, J. Reinken, B. C. Allan *et al.*, Falls in old age: a study of frequency and related clinical factors. *Age and Ageing*, **10** (1981), 262–70.

163. C. R. Ward, S. McIntosh & R. A. Kenny, Carotid sinus hypersensitivity – a modifiable risk factor for fractured neck of femur. *Age and Ageing*, **28** (1999), 127–33.

164. A. J. Davies & R. A. Kenny, Falls presenting to the accident and emergency department: types of presentation and risk factor profile. *Age and Ageing*, **25** (1996), 362–6.

165. D. O'Mahony & C. Foote, Prospective evaluation of unexplained syncope, dizziness, and falls among community-dwelling elderly adults. *Journals of Gerontology. Series A. Biological Sciences and Medical Sciences*, **53** (1998), M435–40.

166. J. Lawson, J. Fitzgerald, J. Birchall, C. P. Aldren & R. A. Kenny, Diagnosis of geriatric patients with severe dizziness. *Journal of the American Geriatrics Society*, **47** (1999), 12–17.

167. F. E. Shaw & R. A. Kenny, The overlap between syncope and falls in the elderly. *Postgraduate Medical Journal*, **73** (1997), 635–9.

168. L. A. Lipsitz, P. V. Jonsson, M. M. Kelley & J. S. Koestner, Causes and correlates of recurrent falls in ambulatory frail elderly. *Journal of Gerontology*, **46** (1991), M114–22.

169. L. M. March, A. J. Brnabic, J. C. Skinner & J. M. Schwarz, Musculoskeletal disability among elderly people in the community. *Medical Journal of Australia*, **168** (1998), 439–42.

170. J. Gibbs, S. Hughes, D. Dunlop, R. Singer & R. Chang, Predictors of change in walking velocity in older adults. *Journal of the American Geriatrics Society*, **44** (1996), 126–32.

171. M. V. Hurley, D. L. Scott, J. Rees & D. J. Newham, Sensorimotor changes and functional performance in patients with knee osteoarthritis. *Annals of the Rheumatic Diseases*, **56** (1997), 641–8.

172. L. Wegener, C. Kisner & D. Nichols, Static and dynamic balance responses in persons with bilateral knee osteoarthritis. *Journal of Orthopaedic and Sports Physical Therapy*, **25** (1997), 13–18.

173. B. Hassan, S. Mockett & M. Doherty, Static postural sway, proprioception, and maximal voluntary quadriceps contraction in patients with knee osteoarthritis and normal control subjects. *Annals of the Rheumatic Diseases*, **60** (2001), 612–18.

174. R. S. Hinman, K. L. Bennell, B. R. Metcalf & K. M. Crossley, Balance impairments in individuals with symptomatic knee osteoarthritis: a comparison with matched controls using clinical tests. *Rheumatology*, **41** (2002), 1388–94.

175. Y. C. Pai, W. Z. Rymer, R. W. Chang & L. Sharma, Effect of age and osteoarthritis on knee proprioception. *Arthritis and Rheumatism*, **40** (1997), 2260–5.

176. S. Studenski, P. W. Duncan & J. Chandler, Postural responses and effector factors in persons with unexplained falls: results and methodologic issues. *Journal of the American Geriatrics Society*, **39** (1991), 229–34.

177. R. Whipple, L. Wolfson, C. Derby, D. Singh & J. Tobin, Altered sensory function and balance in older persons. *Journal of Gerontology*, **48** (1993), 71–6.

178. A. Blake, K. Morgan, M. Bendall *et al.*, Falls by elderly people at home – prevalence and associated factors. *Age and Ageing*, **17** (1988), 365–72.

179. D. J. Torgerson, M. J. Garton & D. M. Reid, Falling and perimenopausal women. *Age and Ageing*, **22** (1993), 59–64.

180. A. Gabell, M. A. Simons & U. S. L. Nayak, Falls in the healthy elderly: predisposing causes. *Ergonomics*, **28** (1985), 965–75.

181. D. L. Sturnieks, A. Tiedemann, K. Chapman *et al.*, Physiological risk factors for falls in older people with lower limb arthritis. *Journal of Rheumatology*, **31** (2004), 2272–9.

182. R. Brain, D. Northfield & M. Wilkinson, Neurological manifestations of cervical spondylosis. *Brain*, **75** (1952), 187–225.

183. L. Sudarsky & M. Ronthal, Gait disorders among elderly patients. A survey study of 50 patients. *Archives of Neurology*, **40** (1983), 740–3.

184. J. Weitz, J. Byrne & P. Clagett, Diagnosis and treatment of chronic arterial insufficiency of the lower extremities: a critical review. *Circulation*, **94** (1996), 3026–49.

185. A. W. Gardner & P. S. Montgomery, Impaired balance and higher prevalence of falls in subjects with intermittent claudication. *Journal of Gerontology*, **56A** (2001), M454–8.

186. L. Halstead & C. Rossi, New problems in old polio patients: results of a survey of 539 polio survivors. *Orthopedics*, **8** (1985), 845–50.

187. J. Cosgrove, M. Alexander & E. Kitts, Late effects of poliomyelitis. *Archives of Physical Medicine and Rehabilitation*, **68** (1987), 4–7.

188. J. Silver & D. Aiello, Polio survivors: falls and subsequent injuries. *American Journal of Physical Medicine and Rehabilitation*, **81** (2002), 567–70.

189. J. Goerss, E. Atkinson & A. Windebank, Fractures in an aging population of poliomyelitis survivors: a community-based study in Olmsted County, Minnesota. *Mayo Clinic Proceedings*, **69** (1994), 333–9.

190. S. R. Lord, G. M. Allen, P. Williams & S. C. Gandevia, Risk of falling: predictors based on reduced strength in persons previously affected by polio. *Archives of Physical Medicine and Rehabilitation*, **83** (2002), 757–63.

191. K. J. Gorter, M. M. Kuyvenhoven & R. A. deMelker, Nontraumatic foot complaints in older people. A population-based survey of risk factors, mobility, and well-being. *Journal of the American Podiatric Medical Association*, **90** (2000), 397–402.

192. J. E. Dunn, C. L. Link, D. T. Felson *et al.*, Prevalence of foot and ankle conditions in a multiethnic community sample of older adults. *American Journal of Epidemiology*, **159** (2004), 491–8.

193. L. Greenberg, Foot care data from two recent nationwide surveys – a comparative analysis. *Journal of the American Podiatric Medical Association*, **84** (1994), 365–70.

194. I. Harvey, S. Frankel, R. Marks, D. Shalom & M. Morgan, Foot morbidity and exposure to chiropody: population based study. *British Medical Journal*, **315** (1997), 1054–5.

195. L. Hung, Y. Ho & P. Leung, Survey of foot deformities among 166 geriatric inpatients. *Foot and Ankle*, **5** (1985), 156–64.

196. A. E. Helfand, H. L. Cooke, M. D. Walinsky *et al.*, Foot problems associated with older patients – a focused podogeriatric study. *Journal of the American Podiatric Medical Association*, **88** (1998), 237–41.

197. A. A. Andervoort, B. M. Chesworth, D. A. Cunningham *et al.*, Age and sex effects on mobility of the human ankle. *Journal of Gerontology*, **47** (1992), M17–21.

198. F. Schiralid, Common dermatologic manifestations in the older patient. *Clinics in Podiatric Medicine and Surgery*, **10** (1993), 79–95.

199. G. A. Gorecki, Shoe related foot problems and public health. *Journal of the American Podiatry Association*, **4** (1978), 244–7.

200. S. Burns, G. Leese & M. McMurdo, Older people and ill-fitting shoes. *Postgraduate Medical Journal*, **78** (2002), 344–6.

201. C. Frey, F. Thompson, J. Smith, M. Sanders & H. Horstman, American Orthopedic Foot and Ankle Society women's shoe survey. *Foot and Ankle*, **14** (1993), 78–81.

202. H. B. Menz & M. E. Morris, Footwear characteristics and foot problems in older people. *Gerontology*, **51** (2005), 346–51.

203. J. Robbins & C. Austin, Common peripheral vascular diseases. *Clinics in Podiatric Medicine and Surgery*, **10** (1993), 205–19.

204. D. Green, Acute and chronic complications of diabetes mellitus in older patients. *American Journal of Medicine*, **80** (1986), 39–45.

205. A. Jacobs, Diabetes mellitus. *Clinics in Podiatric Medicine and Surgery*, **10** (1993), 231–48.

206. S. J. Benbow, A. Walsh & G. V. Gill, Diabetes in institutionalised elderly people: a forgotten population? *British Medical Journal*, **314** (1997), 1868.

207. J. D'Amico, The pathomechanics of adult rheumatoid arthritis affecting the foot. *Journal of the American Podiatry Association*, **66** (1976), 227–30.

208. J. R. Black, C. Cahalin & B. F. Germaine, Pedal morbidity in rheumatic disease. *Journal of the American Podiatry Association*, **72** (1982), 360–4.

209. M. J. Coughlin, Mallet toes, hammer toes, claw toes and corns. *Postgraduate Medicine*, **75** (1984), 191–8.

210. J. M. Guralnik, E. M. Simonsick, L. Ferrucci *et al.*, A short physical performance battery assessing lower extremity function: association with self-reported disability and prediction of mortality and nursing home admission. *Journal of Gerontology*, **49** (1994), M85–94.

211. F. Benvenuti, L. Ferrucci, J. M. Guralnik, S. Gangemi & A. Baroni, Foot pain and disability in older persons: an epidemiologic survey. *Journal of the American Geriatrics Society*, **43** (1995), 479–84.

212. D. DeLargy, Accidents in old people. *Medical Press*, **239** (1958), 117–20.

213. A. Helfand, Foot impairment – an etiologic factor in falls in the aged. *Journal of the American Podiatry Association*, **56** (1966), 326–30.

214. D. Wild, U. Nayak & B. Isaacs, Characteristics of old people who fell at home. *Journal of Clinical and Experimental Gerontology*, **2** (1980), 271–87.

215. H. B. Menz & S. R. Lord, The contribution of foot problems to mobility impairment and falls in older people. *Journal of the American Geriatrics Society*, **49** (2001), 1651–6.

216. H. B. Menz & S. R. Lord, Foot pain impairs balance and functional ability in community-dwelling older people. *Journal of the American Podiatric Medical Association*, **91** (2001), 222–9.

217. H. B. Menz, M. E. Morris & S. R. Lord, Foot and ankle characteristics associated with impaired balance and functional ability in older people. *Journal of Gerontology*, **60** (2005), 1546–52.

218. H. B. Menz, M. E. Morris & S. R. Lord, Foot and ankle risk factors for falls in older people – a prospective study. *Journal of Gerontology: Medical Sciences*, **61A** (2006), 866–70.

219. D. Thom, Variation in estimates of urinary incontinence prevalence in the community: effects of differences in definition, population characteristics, and study type. *Journal of the American Geriatrics Society*, **46** (1998), 473–80.

220. J. Gardner & D. Fonda, Urinary incontinence in the elderly. *Disability and Rehabilitation*, **16** (1994), 140–8.

221. J. Teno, D. P. Kiel & V. Mor, Multiple stumbles: a risk factor for falls in community-dwelling elderly. A prospective study. *Journal of the American Geriatrics Society*, **38** (1990), 1321–5.

222. S. Yasumura, H. Haga, H. Nagai *et al.*, Rate of falls and the correlates among elderly people living in an urban community in Japan. *Age and Ageing*, **23** (1994), 323–7.

223. H. Luukinen, K. Koski, S. L. Kivela & P. Laippala, Social status, life changes, housing conditions, health, functional abilities and life-style as risk factors for recurrent falls among the home-dwelling elderly. *Public Health*, **110** (1996), 115–18.

224. A. M. Tromp, J. H. Smit, D. J. Deeg, L. M. Bouter & P. Lips, Predictors for falls and fractures in the Longitudinal Aging Study Amsterdam. *Journal of Bone and Mineral Research*, **13** (1998), 1932–9.

225. T. Gluck, H. J. Wientjes & G. S. Rai, An evaluation of risk factors for in-patient falls in acute and rehabilitation elderly care wards. *Gerontology*, **42** (1996), 104–7.

226. B. Stevenson, E. M. Mills, L. Welin & K. G. Beal, Falls risk factors in an acute-care setting: a retrospective study. *Canadian Journal of Nursing Research*, **30** (1998), 97–111.

227. M. J. Ashley, C. I. Gryfe & A. Amies, A longitudinal study of falls in an elderly population. II. Some circumstances of falling. *Age and Ageing*, **6** (1977), 211–20.

228. M. E. Tinetti, J. Doucette, E. Claus & R. Marottoli, Risk factors for serious injury during falls by older persons in the community. *Journal of the American Geriatrics Society*, **43** (1995), 1214–21.

229. J. Brown, E. Vittinghoff, J. Wyman *et al.*, Urinary incontinence: does it increase risk for falls and fractures? *Journal of the American Geriatrics Society*, **48** (2000), 721–5.

7

Medications as risk factors for falls

Medications have long been implicated as an iatrogenic cause of falls and fractures, with a number of epidemiological and prospective cohort studies providing support for a link between medications and falls. This chapter will discuss the pharmacology of ageing and the potential physiological mechanisms by which medications may impact on postural stability. Specific drug classes will be highlighted where there is evidence to support a causal link between drug use and falls, and the concept of optimization of prescribing will be explored.

Drugs and ageing

Ageing is not a clearly defined single entity but more the result of a combination of anatomical, biochemical and physiological changes that occur with time. There are alterations to the physiological reserve capacity of the human body that can lead to marked haemodynamic and biochemical compromise even with the mildest of external stressor, e.g. a urinary tract infection.

The ageing process can be associated with an alteration of the body's ability to absorb, metabolize, distribute and excrete drugs (pharmacokinetics) as well as an alteration of the drug effect at its intended target site (pharmacodynamics). Changes with age are seen in body composition, with a reduction in total body water and lean body mass and a relative increase in body fat, which impact on the pharmacokinetics of a given drug. Advancing age can also be associated with an increase in the number of disease processes, which can impact on the body's ability to deal with and respond to drugs. Table 7.1 highlights the main pharmacokinetic changes that are associated with the ageing process, and the potential physiological and clinical mechanisms by which these changes may predispose an older person to fall. Pharmacodynamic changes with age are not well understood and in many instances the cause of the observed changes are unknown.

Table 7.1 Pharmacokinetic changes with ageing, and some of the potential physiological and clinical consequences in relation to risk of falling

	Effects of ageing	Examples of clinical consequences relating to falls and bone health
Drug absorption from gastrointestinal system	May be reduced.	Reduced absorption of calcium leading to deterioration in bone health. B_{12} deficiency leading to peripheral neuropathy and cognitive impairment.
First pass metabolism in liver and bioavailability	Decreased therefore increased toxicity for those drugs which undergo extensive first pass metabolism, e.g. propranolol and decreased effects from those drugs that are activated by first pass metabolism, e.g. perindopril.	Increased concentrations of beta blocker leading to bradycardias and hypotension. Decreased bioavailability of ACE inhibitor leading to poorly controlled blood pressure or heart failure.
Drug distribution (decreased total body water and relative increase in total body fat)	Smaller volume of distribution and therefore increased serum levels for water soluble drugs, e.g. digoxin and theophylline. Larger volume of distribution for lipid soluble drugs leading to prolonged half life of drug, e.g. benzodiazepines	Increased sensitivity to loading doses of both digoxin and theophylline, and possibility of toxicity and cardiac arrhythmias. Prolongation of half life of benzodiazepines causing day time drowsiness and impacting on postural stability.
Protein binding	Acidic compounds (e.g. diazepam and phenytoin) bind to albumin. Impaired nutritional states may lead to increased serum concentrations of such drugs.	Increased free serum concentrations of diazepam and phenytoin can have a direct effect on postural stability.

Table 7.1 (*cont.*)

	Effects of ageing	Examples of clinical consequences relating to falls and bone health
Drug clearance	*Liver* – reduction in blood flow and ability to extract drug. Therefore potential increased concentration of drugs which are predominantly cleared by the liver, e.g. chlormethiazole, codeine, morphine, propranolol and triazolam.	Increased toxicity from drugs which are largely metabolized by the liver – opiate analgesics, some beta blockers and benzodiazepines. All can be associated with falls.
	Renal – reduced renal function can affect rate of clearance of water soluble beta blockers, digoxin and lithium.	Increased toxicity from drugs with narrow therapeutic window, e.g. digoxin and lithium.

Physiological mechanisms by which drugs may alter performance

An understanding of the pharmacological properties, side-effect profile and effects of ageing can help explain how drugs can impair postural stability. Reduced mental alertness, slowed transmission within the central nervous system, sedation, blurred vision, confusion, neuromuscular incoordination, impaired balance and drug-induced parkinsonism are all potential mechanisms by which particular medications predispose older people to fall [1, 2].

Postural hypotension may also be a potential contributor to falls through a transient reduction in cerebral blood flow. This is a recognized side effect of anti-hypertensives, antidepressants, anti-psychotics and diuretics [3, 4]. In a large prospective study of community-dwelling women, we found a significant association between psychoactive medication use and postural hypotension [2]. Davie *et al.* [5] found that systolic hypotension contributed independently to dizziness and falls. However, other studies have not reported such a relationship [2, 6, 7].

Medications linked to falls

Despite the increase in the number of drugs available for diseases seen most commonly in older age, it has not been a feature of the pharmaceutical industry to record falls or any intermediate measures of postural stability as an outcome measure during drug development.

In the absence of good randomized controlled trial data, the majority of evidence linking drugs to falls comes from observational studies. Limitations observed in many of these studies include confounding by indication, small sample sizes, and questionable reliability and validity. Confounding by indication makes it difficult to ascertain whether the relationship between falls and medication is due to the actual drug, or the indications for its' use. Such confounders include physical disease, depression, anxiety and impaired cognitive status. While early studies failed to address possible confounding factors, more recent studies have taken this into account [8]. Due to small sample sizes, many studies have been unable to explore the effects of individual medications grouped within drug classes [9–11]. Retrospective studies have come under criticism for their lack of reliability and validity. Many involve the subjective recall of a fall event, which is questionable as up to one-third of older people forget about experiencing a fall three months to one year later [12]. Furthermore, drug use may change over time and a fall may lead to a change in the older person's medication [1, 10].

Prescription records may also be unreliable. In a study of hip fracture patients, Schwab *et al.* [13] reported that 18% had evidence of benzodiazepine use in their records, yet 41% tested positive for the drug in serum analyses. Even if prescription records are accurate, prospective falls risk factor studies that utilize a single baseline measurement of medication use for subsequent risk factor classification can be problematic. By studying the medication records of 2510 nursing home residents, Ray *et al.* [14] found high rates of misclassification at follow-ups, i.e. many patients had either stopped taking some of their medications or had commenced new medications. To avoid this, the authors suggest that studies of the acute effects of drugs or the effects of drugs taken intermittently may need to track exposure on a daily basis. However, the practical implementation of such an approach is challenging.

Despite these considerable impediments, many studies have now been undertaken in this area and patterns are emerging to indicate that some drug classes are indeed implicated in increasing falls risk in older people, whereas others are not.

Centrally acting medications

Elderly patients are more susceptible to the adverse effects from centrally acting (psychotropic) medications, including delirium, extrapyramidal symptoms,

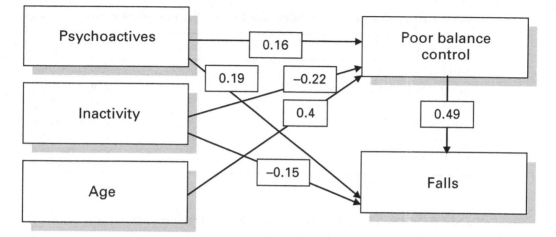

Fig. 7.1   A path analytic model for the relationship between psychoactive medication use and falls. The standardized relative strengths of the effects (similar to correlation coefficients) are indicated by the numerals near the path arrows. This model indicates that after adjusting for age and activity levels, approximately half of the association between psychoactive medication and falls is mediated via reduced stability. Notes: Psychoactives: nil, one or two. Activity: hours per week. Age: age in years. Poor balance control: a composite measure incorporating measures of tactile sensitivity, vibration sense, quadriceps strength, reaction time, sway and clinical stability. Falls: two or more falls versus nil or one. Postural hypotension was found to be a statistically insignificant variable in the development of the final model. Diagram adapted from Lord *et al.* [2].

arrhythmias and postural hypotension [15]. Advancing age is associated with increased sensitivity to the central nervous system effects of benzodiazepines [16], with sedation induced at lower doses and concentrations of diazepam [17, 18]. The exact mechanism responsible for the increased sensitivity to benzo-diazepines with ageing is unknown.

Many epidemiological studies have examined the association between the use of any centrally acting medication and falls in older people. These studies indicate that there is a two- to three-fold increased risk of falling when using any psychotropic medication [4, 19–25], and a two-fold increased risk of experiencing a hip fracture [26]. The use of multiple psychotropic agents has an additive effect on falls risk. For example, Weiner *et al.* [27] report that the odds ratio of experiencing a fall for community-dwelling older people taking one psychotropic medication was 1.5, whilst in those taking two or more of these drugs the odds ratio increased to 2.4.

In a prospective cohort study of factors associated with injurious falls, we have found associations between centrally acting medication use, quadriceps strength and measures of standing balance [28], which suggests that these medications impair balance both centrally and peripherally. Figure 7.1 shows a path analytic model for the relationship between centrally acting medication use

Table 7.2 Pooled odds ratios for falling associated with psychoactive medication classes

Drug Class	Number of Studies	Pooled Odds Ratio
Anti-psychotics	9	1.90 (1.35–2.67)
Any psychoactive medication	11	1.66 (1.40–1.97)
Antidepressants	11	1.62 (1.23–2.14)
Tricyclic antidepressants	8	1.40 (0.96–2.02)
Benzodiazepines	8	1.40 (1.11–1.76)
Sedatives/hypnotics	10	1.25 (0.98–1.60)

Adapted from Leipzig *et al.* [29]

and falls, derived from the Randwick Falls and Fractures Study [2]. This analysis reveals that after adjusting for other inter-related and confounding factors (increased age, postural hypotension and inactivity), the association between centrally acting medication use and falls is mediated, in part, through poor balance control (as measured by a composite measure of sensory, motor, speed and stability variables). The remaining direct effect is likely to be due to other postulated side effects of these medications such as increased sedation and reduced mental alertness.

In a published systematic review, Leipzig *et al.* included data from much of the literature in a meta-analysis to examine the relationship between centrally acting medications and falls in older people [29]. Significantly, only 40 studies were considered of a high enough quality to meet the author's inclusion criteria and none of these were randomized controlled trials. By pooling the odds ratios from the raw data of these studies, they found that psychotropic drugs were significantly associated with falls risk. These results are summarized in Table 7.2.

Sedative/hypnotics

The most consistent group of drugs found to be predictive of risk of falling have been the benzodiazepines, used primarily for sleep problems and less so for anxiety disorders and poorly controlled epilepsy. The benzodiazepines comprise the majority of drugs coming under the umbrella of sedative/hypnotics and have undergone the most extensive investigation with regard to an association with falls.

Prospective and cross-sectional studies have consistently reported that use of sedative/hypnotics (including benzodiazepines) increases the risk of falls two- to four-fold in both institutionalized and community-dwelling older people [8, 9, 24, 30–38]. The maximum risk from benzodiazepine use appears to be within the first two weeks of introduction of the drug, with two studies published in the literature to support this [37, 39].

The effect of sedative/hypnotic use on hip fracture risk is less clear, with some studies finding an increased risk [40,–42], and others not [43–45]. Herings *et al.* [36] reported that subjects taking more than the recommended dose of a benzodiazepine had double the risk of hip fracture regardless of the specific benzodiazepine prescribed.

Benzodiazepines have been found to impair reaction time and increase postural sway in older people [3, 18, 46–48], and an association has been reported between benzodiazepine use and decreased position sense in the toes [3].

The differential effects of short- and long-acting benzodiazepines remain unclear, and most studies fail to take into account the changing pharmacokinetic and dynamic profile of benzodiazepines in a heterogeneous population. Some studies have reported that long-acting benzodiazepines increase risk of falling [2, 8] and hip fracture [41] more than short-acting drugs, however, other studies have found no significant differences between the two [4, 21, 38]. In the largest study yet undertaken (8127 women), Ensrud *et al.* [49] found a marginally decreased risk associated with short-acting compared to long-acting benzodiazepines for single falls (OR 1.19 vs. 1.61) and frequent falls (OR 1.42 vs. 1.56). This half life distinction is perhaps academic. There is a considerably stronger rationale for not prescribing these drugs at all as they have consistently been linked to an increased risk of falls as well as having addictive properties when prescribed for a prolonged period of time.

Clinicians should therefore think critically about the necessity for the use of a benzodiazepine in an older population. A recent review regarding optimization of drug prescribing states clearly that benzodiazepines should rarely if ever be prescribed to older patients, specifically because of the increased risk of falls and nocturnal disorientation [50].

Antidepressants

Depression in itself has been shown to be a risk factor for falls in several studies [19, 51–55]. Ironically the pharmacological interventions available for the treatment of what can be a disabling mental health illness also appear to increase the propensity to fall.

Antidepressants include the drug groupings of selective serotonin re-uptake inhibitors (SSRIs), serotonin and noradrenaline re-uptake inhibitors (SNRIs), and tricyclics, tertracyclics and monamine oxidase inhibitors. Evidence for the association between antidepressant use and falls risk seems to be divided with some research supporting a direct link [2, 4, 19, 20, 30, 33, 34, 49, 56–59] and some not finding an association [8, 9, 60, 61]. These discrepant findings may be attributable, in part, to differing methodologies utilized. Overall, prospective designs have tended to report a significant association, whereas retrospective studies have not. The relationship between antidepressants and falls has been frequently observed even when controlling for variables such as medical conditions, dementia, functional status, age and body mass.

Specific classes of antidepressants and their effect on falls have also been investigated. Ray *et al.* [59] concluded that current users of tricyclic antidepressants had a significantly increased risk of hip fracture, while Ruthazer and Lipsitz [62] reported that falls risk was greatest among women using SSRIs and tricyclic antidepressants. However, both Tinetti *et al.* [51] and Ebly *et al.* [58] found that no individual drug class was specifically associated with falling. The small numbers of people taking these medications in the study samples limits the significance of trends observed between different classes of antidepressants.

Interestingly, the newer SSRIs do not appear to offer any significant benefit over the older tricyclic antidepressant medications in terms of falls risk [49] or hip fracture risk [42], despite the more favourable cardiovascular side-effect profile. Pacher and Ungvari [63] have speculated that this may be because the SSRIs may still have clinically significant cardiovascular effects such as syncope and orthostatic hypotension due to their inhibition of Ca^{2+} and Na^+ channels.

Antidepressant medication use may impair gait patterns. Draganich *et al.* [64] evaluated temporo-spatial and kinematic parameters of gait in older people walking on a level surface and when stepping over an obstacle, before and after they were administered a single dose of either a placebo, amitriptyline, desipramine or paroxetine. Compared to the placebo, amitriptyline reduced gait velocity, cadence and hip flexion when stepping over the obstacle, suggesting that older people taking this medication may be at greater risk of tripping. However, the underlying mechanisms by which the various antidepressants lead to an increased falls risk remain largely unanswered and is an area requiring further evaluation.

Anti-psychotics

Anti-psychotics encapsulate a broad range of drug classes used primarily to reduce the symptoms of psychosis such as anxiety, acute agitation, hallucinations, delusions and delirium. When prescribed in older people they are predominantly used to treat agitation and modify behaviour in those with dementia.

Yip and Cumming [4] found an association between falls and anti-psychotics among nursing home residents. After adjusting for potential confounders, they found that residents using anti-psychotic medications were four times more likely to fall than non-users. This risk was also linearly related to increasing dosage. Similarly, case-control studies of hospitalized older people [65, 66] and nursing home residents [11, 24] have reported that the use of anti-psychotic drugs is associated with a significantly increased risk of experiencing an injurious fall. As with the other centrally acting medications it is often difficult to determine whether it is the underlying disease or the treatment that is contributing to the reported increased falls risk. There has been one study which reported that the use of these drugs in patients with severe psychiatric illness actually decreases risk of falling [67].

In contrast to the general consensus that anti-psychotic drugs contribute to falls in long term care facilities, studies involving community or intermediate care samples have generally not found anti-psychotic drugs to be a risk factor for falls [2, 8, 61]. Possible reasons for this observation include disease severity, in that community dwellers are likely to represent a milder end of a spectrum of symptomatology. Community dwellers using anti-psychotic drugs may not comprise sufficient numbers to detect a significant relationship. Also the predisposing effects of anti-psychotics on falls may be more pronounced in long term care residents where the prevalence of frailty, cognitive impairment and immobility is higher.

Cardiovascular medications

Investigation of a relationship between cardiovascular medications and falls is meagre compared to studies exploring psychotropic medications and falls. Very few studies have specifically explored cardiovascular medications, choosing instead to view them concurrently with other medications. Furthermore, there are problems associated with the classification of drugs studied. In some studies, diuretics are classified as anti-hypertensives, while other studies choose to investigate them as a separate entity. Results from studies that group cardiovascular classes into 'cardiac drugs' have been inconsistent [10].

In the companion study to their work on centrally acting medications, Leipzig *et al.* conducted a systematic review and meta-analysis of the available research regarding cardiac and analgesic drugs [68], and falls in older people. As with the psychotropic review, only a minority of papers met the study's inclusion criteria and again none were randomized controlled trials. By pooling the odds ratios from the raw data of these studies, it was concluded that digoxin and type IA anti-arrhythmic drugs are only weakly associated with falls risk, while no significant association was found for other cardiac drugs or analgesics. The results of this meta-analysis are summarized in Table 7.3.

Digoxin

Digoxin is an anti-arrhythmic agent with positive inotropic properties used predominantly but not exclusively in the treatment of atrial fibrillation. Gales and Mernard [21] reported that digoxin use increased falls risk in older people by 90% in an acute hospital setting. A prospective study by Koski *et al.* [31] reported that the use of digoxin was associated with an increased risk of experiencing a fall-related minor injury for men, but not women. However, in

Table 7.3 Pooled odds ratios for falling associated with cardiac and analgesic medications

Drug class	Number of studies	Pooled odds ratio
Type 1A Anti-arrhythmics	10	1.59 (1.02–2.48)
Digoxin	17	1.22 (1.05–1.42)
ACE inhibitors	10	1.20 (0.92–1.58)
NSAIDs	13	1.16 (0.97–1.38)
Centrally acting anti-hypertensives	11	1.16 (0.87–1.55)
Nitrates	14	1.13 (0.95–1.36)
Aspirin	9	1.12 (0.80–1.57)
Non-narcotic analgesics	9	1.09 (0.88–1.34)
Thiazide diuretics	12	1.06 (0.97–1.16)
Any diuretic	9	1.05 (0.96–1.14)
Narcotic analgesics	13	0.97 (0.78–1.20)
Calcium channel blockers	13	0.94 (0.77–1.14)
Beta blockers	18	0.93 (0.77–1.11)
Loop diuretics	11	0.90 (0.73–1.12)

Leipzig *et al.* [68]

each of these studies it is possible that the use of digoxin is simply a marker of physical frailty and acute illness rather than a cause of falls.

Diuretics

Diuretics can be divided into three main groups – thiazides, loop diuretics and aldosterone antagonists. The thiazide diuretics (e.g. bendrofluazide) are predominantly used in the treatment of hypertension, whilst the loop diuretics (e.g. furosemide and bumetanide) and aldosterone antagonists (e.g. spironolactone) tend to play a greater role in the management of congestive cardiac failure. All have the capacity to cause volume depletion and postural hypotension via this mechanism.

There are few studies that report a significant relationship between the use of diuretics and falls. While a small number of studies have found that fallers are more likely to be users of diuretics than non-fallers [8, 69], most studies fail to report any significance of diuretic use in terms of falls risk [1, 8, 70, 71]. Interestingly, there is some evidence that thiazide diuretics, by decreasing excretion of calcium in the urine, may have positive effects on bone density, thereby decreasing the risk of hip fracture [72].

Other cardiovascular agents

ACE inhibitors, beta blockers, calcium channel blockers and vasodilators are commonly used drug classes in the treatment of hypertension and ischaemic heart disease. There have been mixed reports in the literature for an association between these drug classes and falls. While some studies have reported that the use of anti-hypertensives is associated with a moderately increased risk of falling [31, 61, 73], most studies have found a non-significant relationship for both older community-dwelling [2, 8, 30, 34, 60, 74–76] and long term care residents [9, 77, 78]. The only prospective, randomized controlled trial on hypertensive use found no difference in falls between subjects taking the medication and those taking a placebo [79].

Analgesic agents

Anti-inflammatories include corticosteroids and non-steroidal anti-inflammatory drugs (NSAIDs). These are often used to treat joint pain, stiffness, inflammation, gout and swelling associated with osteoarthritis in an older population. Most epidemiological studies of anti-inflammatory medications and falls have only been concerned with NSAIDs. Results have again been mixed, with one report suggesting a relationship between NSAID use and falls in institutionalized older people [80], and others reporting no relationship [2, 9]. Interestingly, Yip and Cumming [4] found that while NSAID use did not reach statistical significance for two or more falls, it was an independent risk factor for four or more falls. However, when the existence of arthritis is controlled for, odds ratios for falling are markedly reduced [8]. The mechanism by which a NSAID could increase the risk of falling is far from clear.

Narcotic analgesics (e.g. codeine and propoxyphene) have been found to produce psychomotor impairment and in one study were significantly associated with hip fracture [81]. However, no relationship has been reported between narcotic analgesics and falls [21, 49, 65].

Polypharmacy versus appropriate prescribing in older people

'Polypharmacy' is a term used to describe multiple medication prescribing (usually four or more medications). Multiple drug use has been shown to be a predictor of falls in several studies [8, 9, 19, 39, 57, 58, 61, 76, 82–85]. Cumming *et al.* [8] have reported that the relative risk of experiencing a fall when using one medication is 1.4, two medications 2.2, and three or more medications 2.4.

Multiple drug use may be partly a proxy measure for poor health. Lawlor *et al.* [32] undertook a cross-sectional study of 4050 women aged 60–79 in primary care and found that, after adjusting for underlying chronic disease, the number of prescribed medications was no longer an independent predictor of falls. Chronic obstructive pulmonary disease, circulatory disease, depression and arthritis were all associated with an increased risk of falling. Only two classes of drugs – hypnotics/anxiolytics and antidepressants – were independently associated with an increased risk of falling. However, there is other evidence that multiple medication use may lead to falls as a result of adverse reactions to one or more medication, detrimental drug interactions and/or incorrect use [10].

In an evolving world of evidence-based medicine there are an increasing number of pharmacological compounds emerging for the prevention and treatment of various diseases. Many of these new drugs are being developed for diseases related to the ageing process and older people are likely to be the primary users of these medications.

Within the UK, the proportion of the population aged 65 or over is currently 18%, yet this group accounts for 45% of the National Health Service drug dispensing [86]. Similar figures have been reported in the USA and other countries in Europe where it has been estimated that the aged population account for 25%–50% of expenditure on medications [87] with 85% of older subjects taking at least one medication and 48% taking three or more [8].

Optimization of prescribing medications for older people is a key priority and should reflect the expanding evidence-base, both in terms of potential benefits and harm of each medication as well as interactions with other co-prescribed medications. The RAND Corporation definition of appropriate prescribing is a widely accepted definition whereby 'the expected health benefit exceeds the expected negative consequences' [88]. Risk of falls and fractures should feature on the possible outcomes of poor prescribing practice.

Conclusions

Both the ageing process and disease affect an older person's ability to deal with and respond to drugs. A failure of clinicians to appreciate the pharmacology of ageing can lead to untoward and potentially avoidable events, including falls and fractures, in older people.

Certain classes of medication have been found to predispose older people to falls with the most convincing evidence for the centrally acting medications. Even after taking into account underlying disease, benzodiazepines, antipsychotics and antidepressants remain independent predictors of falling.

Methodological limitations and the multifactorial nature of falls aetiology have made it difficult to identify causal connections between medications and falls. Nevertheless, there is now evidence that changes in the central nervous system, postural hypotension, neuromuscular incoordination and impaired balance are physiological mechanisms that mediate the association between medication use and falls.

The prescription of multiple medications to older people will become increasingly more frequent in the context of evidence-based medicine, and the development of new medications for the prevention and treatment of age-related diseases. Clinicians need to 'optimize' prescribing, such that older people have access to, and can make informed choices about, the combination of medications from which they potentially stand to benefit. Further research is required to ascertain the mechanisms by which some drugs increase an individual's risk of falling. There is also a need to further investigate the risks and benefits of withdrawing medications known to increase an older person's propensity to fall.

REFERENCES

1. A. J. Campbell, Drug treatment as a cause of falls in old age. A review of the offending agents. *Drugs and Aging*, **1** (1991), 289–302.
2. S. R. Lord, K. J. Anstey, P. Williams & J. A. Ward, Psychoactive medication use, sensori-motor function and falls in older women. *British Journal of Clinical Pharmacology*, **39** (1995), 227–34.
3. G. S. Sorock & E. E. Shimkin, Benzodiazepine sedatives and the risk of falling in a community-dwelling elderly cohort. *Archives of Internal Medicine*, **148** (1988), 2441–4.
4. Y. B. Yip & R. G. Cumming, The association between medications and falls in Australian nursing-home residents. *Medical Journal of Australia*, **160** (1994), 14–18.
5. J. W. Davie, M. D. Blumenthal & S. Robinson-Hawkins, A model of risk of falling for psychogeriatric patients. *Archives of General Psychiatry*, **38** (1981), 463–7.
6. K. E. Ensrud, M. C. Nevitt, C. Yunis *et al.*, Postural hypotension and postural dizziness in elderly women. The study of osteoporotic fractures. The Study of Osteoporotic Fractures Research Group. *Archives of Internal Medicine*, **152** (1992), 1058–64.
7. B. A. Liu, A. K. Topper, R. A. Reeves, C. Gryfe & B. E. Maki, Falls among older people: relationship to medication use and orthostatic hypotension. *Journal of the American Geriatrics Society*, **43** (1995), 1141–5.
8. R. G. Cumming, J. P. Miller, J. L. Kelsey *et al.*, Medications and multiple falls in elderly people: the St Louis OASIS study. *Age and Ageing*, **20** (1991), 455–61.
9. M. Kerman & M. Mulvihill, The role of medication in falls among the elderly in a long-term care facility. *Mount Sinai Journal of Medicine*, **57** (1990), 343–7.
10. R. G. Cumming, Epidemiology of medication-related falls and fractures in the elderly. *Drugs and Aging*, **12** (1998), 43–53.
11. H. A. Nygaard, Falls and psychotropic drug consumption in long-term care residents: is there an obvious association? *Gerontology*, **44** (1998), 46–50.
12. S. R. Cummings, M. C. Nevitt & S. Kidd, Forgetting falls – the limited accuracy of recall of falls in the elderly. *Journal of the American Geriatrics Society*, **36** (1988), 613–16.
13. M. Schwab, F. Roder, T. Aleker *et al.*, Psychotropic drug use, falls and hip fracture in the elderly. *Aging – Clinical and Experimental Research*, **12** (2000), 234–9.

14. W. Ray, P. Thapa & P. Gideon, Misclassification of current benzodiazepine exposure by use of a single baseline measurement and its effects upon studies of injuries. *Pharmacoepidemiology and Drug Safety*, **11** (2002), 663–9.

15. C. Gregory & P. McKenna, Pharmacological management of schizophrenia in older people. *Drugs and Aging*, **5** (1994), 256–62.

16. W. H. Kruse, Problems and pitfalls in the use of benzodiazepines in the elderly. *Drug Safety*, **5** (1990), 328–34.

17. M. Reidenberg, M. Levy & H. Warner, Relationship between diazepam dose, plasma level, age, and central nervous system depression. *Clinical Pharmacology and Therapeutics*, **23** (1978), 371–4.

18. C. G. Swift, J. M. Ewen, P. Clarke & I. H. Stevenson, Responsiveness to oral diazepam in the elderly: relationship to total and free plasma concentrations. *British Journal of Clinical Pharmacology*, **20** (1985), 111–18.

19. A. J. Campbell, M. J. Borrie & G. F. Spears, Risk factors for falls in a community-based prospective study of people 70 years and older. *Journal of Gerontology*, **44** (1989), M112–17.

20. P. B. Thapa, P. Gideon, R. L. Fought & W. A. Ray, Psychotropic drugs and risk of recurrent falls in ambulatory nursing home residents. *American Journal of Epidemiology*, **142** (1995), 202–11.

21. B. J. Gales & S. M. Menard, Relationship between the administration of selected medications and falls in hospitalized elderly patients. *Annals of Pharmacotherapy*, **29** (1995), 354–8.

22. H. Luukinen, K. Koski, P. Laippala & S. L. Kivela, Predictors for recurrent falls among the home-dwelling elderly. *Scandinavian Journal of Primary Health Care*, **13** (1995), 294–9.

23. W. B. Mendelson, The use of sedative/hypnotic medication and its correlation with falling down in the hospital. *Sleep*, **19** (1996), 698–701.

24. C. A. Mustard & T. Mayer, Case-control study of exposure to medication and the risk of injurious falls requiring hospitalization among nursing home residents. *American Journal of Epidemiology*, **145** (1997), 738–45.

25. C. Neutel, S. Perry & C. Maxwell, Medication use and risk of falls. *Pharmacoepidemiology and Drug Safety*, **11** (2002), 97–104.

26. W. A. Ray, M. R. Griffin, W. Schaffner, D. K. Baugh & L. J. D. Melton, Psychotropic drug use and the risk of hip fracture. *New England Journal of Medicine*, **316** (1987), 363–9.

27. D. K. Weiner, J. T. Hanlon & S. A. Studenski, Effects of central nervous system polypharmacy on falls liability in community-dwelling elderly. *Gerontology*, **44** (1998), 217–21.

28. S. R. Lord, D. McLean & G. Stathers, Physiological factors associated with injurious falls in older people living in the community. *Gerontology*, **38** (1992), 338–46.

29. R. M. Leipzig, R. G. Cumming & M. E. Tinetti, Drugs and falls in older people: a systematic review and meta-analysis. I. Psychotropic drugs. *Journal of the American Geriatrics Society*, **47** (1999), 30–9.

30. A. Blake, K. Morgan, M. Bendall *et al.*, Falls by elderly people at home – prevalence and associated factors. *Age and Ageing*, **17** (1988), 365–72.

31. K. Koski, H. Luukinen, P. Laippala & S.-L. Kivela, Physiological factors and medications as predictors of injurious falls by elderly people: a prospective population-based study. *Age and Ageing*, **25** (1996), 29–38.

32. D. A. Lawlor, R. Patel & S. Ebrahim, Association between falls in elderly women and chronic diseases and drug use: cross sectional study. *British Medical Journal*, **327** (2003), 712–17.

33. E. Granek, S. P. Baker, H. Abbey *et al.*, Medications and diagnoses in relation to falls in a long-term care facility. *Journal of the American Geriatrics Society*, **35** (1987), 503–11.

34. M. E. Tinetti, M. Speechley & S. F. Ginter, Risk factors for falls among elderly persons living in the community. *New England Journal of Medicine*, **319** (1988), 1701–7.

35. O. P. Ryynanen, S. L. Kivela, R. Honkanen, P. Laippala & V. Saano, Medications and chronic diseases as risk factors for falling injuries in the elderly. *Scandinavian Journal of Social Medicine*, **21** (1993), 264–71.

36. R. M. Herings, B. H. Stricker, A. de Boer, A. Bakker & F. Sturmans, Benzodiazepines and the risk of falling leading to femur fractures. Dosage more important than elimination half-life. *Archives of Internal Medicine*, **155** (1995), 1801–7.

37. C. I. Neutel, J. P. Hirdes, C. J. Maxwell & S. B. Patten, New evidence on benzodiazepine use and falls: the time factor. *Age and Ageing*, **25** (1996), 273–8.

38. A. Passaro, S. Volpato, F. Romagnoni *et al.*, Benzodiazepines with different half-life and falling in a hospitalized population: the GIFA study. Gruppo Italiano di Farmacovigilanza nell'Anziano. *Journal of Clinical Epidemiology*, **53** (2000), 1222–9.

39. C. Neutal, S. Perry & C. Maxwell, Medication use and risk of falls. *Pharmacoepidemiology and Drug Safety*, **11** (2002), 97–104.

40. S. R. Cummings, M. C. Nevitt, W. S. Browner *et al.*, Risk factors for hip fracture in white women. Study of Osteoporotic Fractures Research Group. *New England Journal of Medicine*, **332** (1995), 767–73.

41. R. G. Cumming & R. J. Klineberg, Epidemiological study of the relation between arthritis of the hip and hip fractures. *Annals of the Rheumatic Diseases*, **52** (1993), 707–10.

42. W. A. Ray, M. R. Griffin & W. Downey, Benzodiazepines of long and short elimination half-life and the risk of hip fracture. *Journal of the American Medical Association*, **262** (1989), 3303–7.

43. M. Weintraub & B. M. Handy, Benzodiazepines and hip fracture: the New York State experience. *Clinical Pharmacology and Therapeutics*, **54** (1993), 252–6.

44. D. K. Wysowski, C. Baum, W. J. Ferguson *et al.*, Sedative-hypnotic drugs and the risk of hip fracture. *Journal of Clinical Epidemiology*, **49** (1996), 111–13.

45. C. Pierfitte, G. Macouillard, M. Thicoipe *et al.*, Benzodiazepines and hip fractures in elderly people: a case-control study. *British Medical Journal*, **322** (2001), 704–8.

46. C. G. Swift, M. R. Swift, S. I. Ankier, A. Pidgen, J. Robinson, Single dose pharmacokinetics and pharmacodynamics of oral loprazolam in the elderly. *British Journal of Clinical Pharmacology*, **20** (1985), 119–28.

47. D. W. Robin, S. S. Hasan, T. Edeki *et al.*, Increased baseline sway contributes to increased losses of balance in older people following triazolam. *Journal of the American Geriatrics Society*, **44** (1996), 300–4.

48. Y. J. Liu, G. Stagni, J. G. Walden, A. M. Shepherd & M. J. Lichtenstein, Thioridazine dose-related effects on biomechanical force platform measures of sway in young and old men. *Journal of the American Geriatrics Society*, **46** (1998), 431–7.

49. K. E. Ensrud, T. L. Blackwell, C. M. Mangione *et al.*, Central nervous system-active medications and risk for falls in older women. *Journal of the American Geriatrics Society*, **50** (2002), 1629–37.

50. S. H. D. Jackson, A. A. Mangoni & G. M. Batty, Optimization of drug prescribing. *British Journal of Clinical Pharmacology*, **57** (2004), 231–6.

51. M. E. Tinetti, T. F. Williams & R. Mayewski, Fall risk index for elderly patients based on number of chronic disabilities. *American Journal of Medicine*, **80** (1986), 429–34.

52. M. E. Tinetti, Factors associated with serious injury during falls by ambulatory nursing home residents. *Journal of the American Geriatrics Society*, **35** (1987), 644–8.

53. E. Granek, S. P. Baker, H. Abbey *et al.*, Medications and diagnoses in relation to falls in a long-term care facility. *Journal of the American Geriatrics Society*, **35** (1987), 503–11.

54. L. Z. Rubenstein, K. R. Josephson & A. S. Robbins, Falls in the nursing home. *Annals of Internal Medicine*, **121** (1994), 442–51.

55. M. A. Whooley, K. E. Kip, J. A. Cauley *et al.*, Depression, falls, and risk of fracture in older women. Study of Osteoporotic Fractures Research Group. *Archives of Internal Medicine*, **159** (1999), 484–90.

56. C. L. Arfken, H. W. Lach, S. J. Birge & J. P. Miller, The prevalence and correlates of fear of falling in elderly persons living in the community. *American Journal of Public Health*, **84** (1994), 565–70.

57. L. A. Lipsitz, P. V. Jonsson, M. M. Kelley & J. S. Koestner, Causes and correlates of recurrent falls in ambulatory frail elderly. *Journal of Gerontology*, **46** (1991), M114–22.

58. E. M. Ebly, D. B. Hogan & T. S. Fung, Potential adverse outcomes of psychotropic and narcotic drug use in Canadian seniors. *Journal of Clinical Epidemiology*, **50** (1997), 857–63.

59. W. A. Ray, M. R. Griffin & E. Malcolm, Cyclic antidepressants and the risk of hip fracture. *Archives of Internal Medicine*, **151** (1991), 754–6.

60. D. Prudham & J. G. Evans, Factors associated with falls in the elderly: a community study. *Age and Ageing*, **10** (1981), 141–6.

61. B. G. Wells, B. Middleton, G. Lawrence, D. Lillard & J. Safarik, Factors associated with the elderly falling in intermediate care facilities. *Drug Intelligence and Clinical Pharmacy*, **19** (1985), 142–5.

62. R. Ruthazer, L. A. Lipsitz, Antidepressants and falls among elderly people in long-term care. *American Journal of Public Health*, **83** (1993), 746–9.

63. P. Pacher & Z. Ungvari, Selective serotonin-reuptake inhibitor antidepressants increase the risk of falls and hip fractures in elderly people by inhibiting cardiovascular ion channels. *Medical Hypotheses*, **57** (2001), 469–71.

64. L. Draganich, J. Zacny, J. Klafta & T. Karrison, The effects of antidepressants on obstructed and unobstructed gait in healthy elderly people. *Journal of Gerontology*, **56A** (2001), M36–41.

65. G. S. Sorock, A case-control study of falling incidents among the hospitalized elderly. *Journal of Safety Research*, **14** (1983), 47–52.

66. L. C. Mion, S. Gregor, M. Buettner, D. Chwirchak, O. Lee & W. Paras, Falls in the rehabilitation setting: incidence and characteristics. *Rehabilitation Nursing*, **14** (1989), 17–22.

67. J. E. Spar, A. LaRue & C. Hewes, Multivariate prediction of falls in elderly inpatients. *International Journal of Geriatric Psychiatry*, **2** (1987), 185–8.

68. R. M. Leipzig, R. G. Cumming & M. E. Tinetti, Drugs and falls in older people: a systematic review and meta-analysis. II. Cardiac and analgesic drugs. *Journal of the American Geriatrics Society*, **47** (1999), 40–50.

69. K. G. Sobel & G. M. McCart, Drug use and accidental falls in an intermediate care facility. *Drug Intelligence and Clinical Pharmacology*, **17** (1983), 539–42.

70. D. K. Y. Chan & T. Gibian, Medications and falls in the elderly. *Australian Journal on Ageing*, **13** (1993), 22–6.

71. J. A. Cauley, S. R. Cummings, D. G. Seeley *et al.*, Effects of thiazide diuretic therapy on bone mass, fractures, and falls. The Study of Osteoporotic Fractures Research Group. *Annals of Internal Medicine*, **118** (1993), 666–73.

72. G. Jones, T. Nguyen, P. N. Sambrook & J. A. Eisman, Thiazide diuretics and fractures: can meta-analysis help? *Journal of Bone and Mineral Research*, **10** (1995), 106–111.

73. S. R. Lord, J. A. Ward, P. Williams & K. J. Anstey, Physiological factors associated with falls in older community-dwelling women. *Journal of the American Geriatrics Society*, **42** (1994), 1110–17.

74. B. C. Perry, Falls among the elderly living in high-rise apartments. *Journal of Family Practice*, **14** (1982), 1069–73.

75. J. L. O'Loughlin, Y. Robitaille, J. F. Boivin & S. Suissa, Incidence of and risk factors for falls and injurious falls among the community-dwelling elderly. *American Journal of Epidemiology*, **137** (1993), 342–54.

76. M. L. Svensson, A. Rundgren & S. Landahl, Falls in 84- to 85-year-old people living at home. *Accident Analysis and Prevention*, **24** (1992), 527–37.

77. M. R. Stegman, Falls among elderly hypertensives – are they iatrogenic? *Gerontology*, **29** (1983), 399–406.

78. B. E. Maki, P. J. Holliday & A. K. Topper, A prospective study of postural balance and risk of falling in an ambulatory and independent elderly population. *Journal of Gerontology*, **49** (1994), M72–84.

79. J. D. Curb, W. B. Applegate & T. M. Vogt, Antihypertensive therapy and falls and fractures in the Systolic Hypertension in the Elderly Program. *Journal of the American Geriatrics Society*, **41** (1993), SA15.

80. A. H. Myers, S. P. Baker, M. L. Van Natta, H. Abbey & E. G. Robinson, Risk factors associated with falls and injuries among elderly institutionalized persons. *American Journal of Epidemiology*, **133** (1991), 1179–90.

81. R. I. Schorr, M. R. Griffen & J. R. Daugherty, Opiod analgesics and the risk of hip fracture in the elderly: codeine and propoxyphene. *Journal of Gerontology*, **47** (1992), M111–15.

82. J. C. Close, R. Hooper, E. Glucksman, S. H. Jackson & C. G. Swift, Predictors of falls in a high risk population: results from the prevention of falls in the elderly trial (PROFET). *Emergency Medicine Journal*, **20** (2003), 421–5.

83. K. Lim, K. Ng, S. Ng & L. Ng, Falls amongst institutionalised psycho-geriatric patients. *Singapore Medical Journal*, **42** (2001), 466–72.

84. A. S. Robbins, L. Z. Rubenstein, K. R. Josephson *et al.*, Predictors of falls among elderly people – results of two population-based studies. *Archives of Internal Medicine*, **149** (1989), 1628–33.

85. H. Luukinen, K. Koski, P. Laippala & S.-L. Kivela, Risk factors for recurrent falls in the elderly in long-term institutional care. *Public Health*, **109** (1995), 57–65.

86. Department of Health, *Department of Health Statistics of prescriptions dispensed in the Family Health Service Authorities: England 1989–1999.* (Statistical Bulletin UK, 2000/2002).

87. D. Jones, Characteristics of elderly people taking psychotropic medication. *Drugs and Aging*, **2** (1992), 389–94.

88. M. Chassin R. Park & A. Fink, Indications for a selected medical and surgical procedure – a literature review and ratings appropriateness: coronary bypass graft surgery. 3204/2 (Santa Monica: RAND Corporation, 1986).

8

Environmental risk factors for falls

This chapter assesses the importance of a range of environmental factors that are predisposing to falls. This involves a discussion of aspects of indoor and outdoor environments which have been suggested to contribute to falls, the strength of the evidence for the role of these factors in falling, and the interaction between the environment and the older person's physical capabilities. Chapter 14 in the second part of this book examines the effectiveness of strategies to address potential environmental hazards as a falls prevention strategy.

Suggested environmental risk factors

Numerous environmental factors have been suggested to be associated with falls in older people and these are summarized in Table 8.1. These factors have been identified from reports by older people who have fallen and by structured observation of household environments [1–6]. In response to these observations and in an attempt to standardize home assessment procedures, a number of home hazard checklists have been developed [7–14]. These include the Home Environment Survey [7], the Westmead Home Safety Assessment [8, 9], the Home Assessment Profile [10], the Safety Assessment of Function and the Environment for Rehabilitation tool (SAFER) [11], the Home Falls and Accidents Screening Tool (HomeFAST) [12, 13], and the Home-Screen tool [14]. The content of these tools varies considerably with respect to the number of items (ranging from 10 to 73), the inclusion of footwear as an environmental risk factor, the inclusion of behavioural factors related to how the older person interacts with their environment and the level of training required to perform the assessment. Furthermore, most of these home hazard assessment tools have not been evaluated in relation to internal consistency and inter-rater reliability. These issues need to be considered when comparing the findings of different environmental risk factor studies.

Table 8.1 Posited environmental risk factors for falls

General
Slippery floor surfaces
Loose rugs
Upended carpet edges
Raised door sills
Obstructed walkways
Cord across walkways
Shelves or cupboards too high or too low
Spilt liquids
Pets

Furniture
Low chairs
Low or elevated bed height
Unstable furniture
Use of ladders and step ladders

Bathroom/toilet/laundry
Lack of grab rails shower/bathtub/toilet
Hob on shower recess
Low toilet seat
Outdoor toilet
Slippery surfaces
Use of bath oils

Stairs
No or inadequate handrails
Non-contrasting steps
Stairs too steep, tread too narrow
Distracting surroundings
Unmodifiable stairs or individual unable to manage stairs

Outdoors
Sloping, slippery, obstructed or uneven pathways, ramps and stairways
Rushing caused by inadequate time allowed for pedestrian crossings
Crowds
Certain weather conditions (leaves, snow, ice, rain)
Lack of places to rest
Unsafe garbage bin use

Evidence regarding environmental risk factors

Private residences

Most homes contain potential hazards that could increase the risk of falls. In fact, a recent survey found that the homes of all 570 older subjects had at least one environmental falls hazard [15]. It has been reported that many older people attribute their falls to trips or slips inside the home or immediate home surroundings [16]. However, what evidence is there that these hazards are either associated or causally linked to falls?

Six case-control studies have examined the association between environmental hazards and falls [17–22]. Two of these reported differences in the prevalence of household hazards between fallers and non-fallers. Isberner *et al.* [19] reported that the absence of handrails and the presence of uneven floors were more common in the households of 45 older people who had fallen compared to age- and sex-matched controls. Similarly, in a study involving 2304 older people, Fletcher and Hirdes [22] found that those who had one or more environmental hazards in their homes were more likely to have reported falling in the last three months. The remaining four studies, however, found no differences in home hazards between the faller and non-faller groups [17, 18, 20, 21].

Stronger evidence regarding the role of the environment is provided by prospective cohort studies, in which household hazards are assessed first and falls are monitored subsequently over a defined period. Of the five studies published [23–27], none found household hazards to be associated with falls in primary analyses (see Table 8.2).

Secondary analyses from two of these studies have highlighted important findings. Northridge *et al.* [28] re-evaluted the data from the Nevitt *et al.* study [24], classifying subjects as either vigorous or frail. Not surprisingly, they found that the frail group suffered more frequent falls. However, they also found that, while there was no effect of environmental hazards on fall rates among frail people, vigorous people living with more environmental hazards were more likely to fall. For this group, a four-point increase on a seven-point composite home hazard scale was associated with a three-fold increase in the odds of falling. Similarly, in a subsequent analysis of the Tinetti *et al.* study [23], Speechley and Tinetti [29] reported that environmental hazards were also more likely to contribute to falls in vigorous older people than in frail older people. However, in this study, these hazards were mostly outside the participants' homes.

Results from other studies have also reported that the mechanisms by which environmental hazards contribute to falls differ with varying health and

Table 8.2 Summary of prospective studies addressing environmental risk factors for falls in community-dwelling older people

Study	Participants	Risk factor assessment	Outcomes	Comments
Tinetti et al. [23]	■ n = 336 ■ aged 75+	Standard 30-point checklist administered by trained assessor	Number of hazards not associated with falls	■ Secondary analysis (Speechley and Tinetti [29]) found vigorous older people more likely to have a fall associated with an environmental hazard, many of which were outside the home
Nevitt et al. [24]	■ n = 325 ■ aged 60+	Self-administered questionnaire	No individual items or composite scores associated with falls	■ Participants who reported that environmental factors interfered with ADLs had a higher rate of multiple falls in the home (OR = 3.1, 95% CI = 1.4 to 6.2) ■ Secondary analysis (Northridge et al. [28]) found that hallway rugs and a composite home hazard scale were significantly associated with falls in vigorous older people
Campbell et al. [25]	■ n = 761 ■ aged 70+	OT assessment	Hazards not associated with falls	■ Majority of falls in the home occurred over normal household items
Teno et al. [26]	■ n = 586 ■ aged 65+	Telephone interviews regarding presence of loose rugs or non-slip strips in bath or shower	Neither factor associated with falls	■ Previous stumbles and falls, poor health status and hospitalization were identified as falls risk factors
Gill et al. [27]	■ n = 1088 ■ aged 72+	Standard assessment of 13 hazards by trained nurse assessor	No consistent associations between hazards and falls	■ Three year follow-up for falls ■ No consistent association after stratification according to vision, balance/gait or cognitive impairment

ADLs = activities of daily living, OT = Occupational Therapist, OR = odds ratio, CI = confidence interval mobility levels. In a study of over 1400 community-dwellers, Weinberg and Strain [30] found that those with better self-rated health and those falling outdoors were more likely to attribute a fall to the surroundings. Those with poorer self-rated health and those who reported having dexterity difficulties were more likely to attribute their falls to their own limitations.

Residential aged care facilities

Residents of aged care facilities (hostels and nursing homes) are generally frailer than those living in private homes. It is therefore likely that in these settings, the person's physical impairments will play a greater role in their risk of falling, i.e. these people may fall in the absence of any environmental hazard. In addition, these environments are often designed to minimize environmental hazards (e.g. absence of steps, wide corridors, presence of grab rails). Despite this, falls in residential care settings have also been found to involve environmental factors. Fleming and Pendergast [31] surveyed 294 fall incident reports for 95 residents of a residential care facility and found that 50% of the descriptions implicated an environmental factor, with pieces of furniture being the most common. A total of 57% of falls occurred in the residents' rooms. Similarly, Tinetti *et al.* [32] found that among recurrent fallers, at least one fall for 23 of the 25 residents involved an object (e.g. missing a chair while sitting down, falling while getting off the toilet). However, in each of these studies, the environmental factors identified were commonly used household items and the precipitant may well relate more to the individual's ability to function effectively in his/her environment than as a direct consequence of the object in question.

Public places

The issue of falls in public places is a vital one for public authorities. Over 10 000 claims for compensation for injuries sustained as a direct result of tripping over broken, uneven or loose paving stones are made against local authorities in England and Wales annually [33]. Despite this, the issue of environmental risk factors in public places has been given little attention in the literature.

Reports from fallers indicate that environmental factors may have a greater role to play in outdoor rather than indoor falls. Nevitt *et al.* [24] report that environmental factors (stairs or tripping and slipping hazards) were associated with 61% of falls that occurred away from home and 33% of those that occurred at home. Norton *et al.* [2] report similar results for those who have suffered a hip fracture: environmental factors were involved in 56% of falls occurring away from home. In a study of 237 Accident and Emergency patients who had fallen in public places, two-thirds fell on pavements, 11% when crossing the road and 9% in shops [34].

The STEPS project [35] was a participatory research project where people were encouraged to report falls in public places to a telephone hotline. Of the 533 callers, 35% had some type of physical disability. A total of 85% of incidents (falls and missteps) were in outdoor locations, and the majority were on the footpath (sidewalk), an uneven surface or on a concrete surface.

Environmental surfaces and fall injury

As might be expected, the surfaces onto which people fall are related to the risk of suffering an injury. Tinetti *et al.* [32] found that a fall on stairs within the home was associated with a two-fold increased risk of serious injury (defined as a fracture, joint dislocation or head injury) in 568 people during a 36-month follow-up period. Floor type may also play a role in fracture risk. A recent prospective study of 6641 falls in 34 residential care homes in the United Kingdom found that wooden carpeted floors were associated with a lower number of fractures compared to concrete floors, indicating that there may be some potential to reduce fractures by installing safer flooring materials [36]. In the outdoor environment, it is likely that the type of surface on which one falls also affects the chance of suffering an injury. In their prospective study, Nevitt *et al.* [37] report trends indicating an increased risk of injury with falls on hard surfaces, such as pavement or concrete. An earlier study [38] failed to find such an association. In a later case-control study, Nevitt and Cummings [39] found the risk of hip fracture to be significantly increased with falls on hard surfaces. However, two other case-control studies have not found such an association [40, 41].

The interaction between the individual and the environment

While it is evident from the studies outlined above that environmental factors are not the major cause of the majority of falls, the interaction between an environmental hazard (or extrinsic factor) and the person's physical abilities (intrinsic factors) seems to play an important role in falls. Lawton [42] describes a model of the interaction between an older person's competence and the demands of the environment. A person must have a high competence level to cope effectively in an environment with high demands, while a person with a low competence level will be able to cope with an environment with low demands. For example, if a more able person trips on a cracked footpath, they may have the ability to recover from this and avoid a fall, yet a person with impairments in proprioception, reaction time and/or muscle strength may not be able to recover in this way. This model is helpful in understanding why environmental factors have sometimes been reported to be more important contributors to falls in more vigorous older people [28, 29, 30].

In line with this concept, Chandler *et al.* [43] conducted a prospective study of 159 older men. Using a performance-based assessment tool, each subject's level of mobility was evaluated within their individual home environment. Thus, the performance score reflected the number of environmental hazards in each household and the degree to which the individual could negotiate these hazards. For example, using this tool, the absence of grab rails would not be considered a hazard if the subject has no difficulty with bathroom transfers. After six months of falls follow-up, and controlling for age, cognition and mobility, the performance score was found to be an independent predictor of falls, indicating that this approach may be addressing the interaction between the individual and his/her environment.

Non-linear factors may also be at play. Studenski *et al.* [10] used a mobility screen to classify 306 people aged 70 years and older into one of three categories: unable to sit or stand; having poor to fair mobility; and having fair to good mobility. Participants with poor to fair mobility experienced the highest rate of recurrent falls during a 6-month follow-up period and an elevated risk score on a standardized environmental home assessment scale. In this group, a ten-point increase in environmental risk score (out of a total 100) was associated with a 23% increase in falls risk. With regard to the other groups, it seems that those who could not sit or stand were not exposed to environmental hazards and those with good mobility were better able to withstand them.

Finally, a person's risk-taking behaviour is also an important part of the interaction between the person and their environment. It is possible that more vigorous people are more likely to undertake more challenging household activities, such as changing a light bulb or hanging curtains. Indeed, a person's attitude to risk (on a three-point scale) has been found to be associated with increased falls [10] and a 'type A behaviour pattern' has been shown to be associated with an increased risk of falling in men [44]. The development of valid tools to specifically assess these fall-related behavioural factors will provide further clarification of this relationship [45].

Conclusion

Environmental hazards are implicated as a contributory factor in a substantial proportion of falls in older people. However, the existence of home hazards alone is insufficient to cause falls. Rather, the interaction between an older person's physical abilities and their exposure to environmental stressors appears to be more important. Taking risks or impulsivity may further elevate falls risk.

Although fall rates are lower in vigorous older people than in their frailer counterparts, it has been reported that environmental hazards contribute to falls to a greater extent in older vigorous people than in older frail people. This appears to be due to increased exposure to risk and with an increase in the proportion of such falls occurring outside the home. There may also be a non-linear relationship between mobility and falls associated with hazards. House-hold environmental hazards may pose the greatest risk for older people with fair balance, whereas those with poor balance are less exposed to hazards and those with good mobility are more able to withstand them. Inappropriate environmental factors, such as bed and chair heights that are too high, may be at least as important as environmental 'hazards' in residential care. There is also some evidence that the type of surface on which an older person falls affects the likelihood of suffering an injury. The interaction between physical function, perception of risk and exposure to risk remains an area requiring further evaluation.

REFERENCES

1. R. W. Sattin, Falls among older persons: a public health perspective. *Annual Review of Public Health*, **13** (1992), 489–508.
2. R. Norton, A. J. Campbell, T. Lee-Joe, E. Robinson & M. Butler, Circumstances of falls resulting in hip fractures among older people. *Journal of the American Geriatrics Society*, **45** (1997), 1108–12.
3. J. C. Archea, Environmental factors associated with stair accidents by the elderly. *Clinics in Geriatric Medicine*, **1** (1985), 555–69.
4. H. Sjorgen & U. Bjornstig, Injuries among the elderly in the home environment: detailed analysis of mechanisms and consequences. *Journal of Aging and Health*, **3** (1991), 107–25.
5. B. R. Connell, Role of the environment in falls prevention. *Clinics in Geriatric Medicine*, **12** (1996), 859–80.
6. S. E. Kurrle, L. Day & I. D. Cameron, The perils of pet ownership: a new fall-injury risk factor. *Medical Journal of Australia*, **181** (2004), 682–3.
7. J. G. Rodriguez, A. L. Baughman, R. W. Sattin *et al.*, A standardized instrument to assess hazards for falls in the home of older people. *Accident Analysis and Prevention*, **27** (1995), 625–31.
8. L. Clemson, M. Roland & R. G. Cumming, Occupational therapy assessment of potential hazards in the homes of elderly people: an interrater reliability study. *Australian Occupational Therapy Journal*, **39** (1992), 23–6.
9. L. Clemson, M. H. Fitzgerald, R. Heard & R. G. Cumming, Inter-rater reliability of a home fall hazards assessment tool. *Occupational Therapy Journal of Research*, **19** (1999), 83–100.
10. S. Studenski, P. W. Duncan, J. Chandler *et al.*, Predicting falls: the role of mobility and nonphysical factors. *Journal of the American Geriatrics Society*, **42** (1994), 297–302.

11. L. Letts, S. Scott, J. Burtney, L. Marshall & M. McKean, The reliability and validity of the safety assessment of function and the environment for rehabilitation (SAFER Tool). *British Journal of Occupational Therapy*, **61** (1998), 127–32.

12. L. MacKenzie, J. Byles & N. Higginbotham, Designing the Home Falls and Accidents Screening Tool (HOME FAST): selecting the items. *British Journal of Occupational Therapy*, **63** (2000), 260–9.

13. L. MacKenzie, J. Byles & N. Higginbotham, Reliability of the Home Falls and Accidents Screening Tool (HOME FAST) for identifying older people at increased risk of falls. *Disability and Rehabilitation*, **24** (2002), 266–74.

14. M. Johnson, A. Cusick & S. Chang, Home-Screen: a short scale to measure fall risk in the home. *Public Health Nursing*, **18** (2001), 169–77.

15. M. Stevens, C. D. J. Holman & N. Bennett, Preventing falls in older people: impact of an intervention to reduce environmental hazards in the home. *Journal of the American Geriatrics Society*, **49** (2001), 1442–7.

16. B. R. Connell & S. L. Wolf, Environmental and behavioural circumstances associated with falls at home among healthy individuals. *Archives of Physical Medicine and Rehabilitation*, **78** (1997), 179–86.

17. D. McLean & S. R. Lord, Falling in older people at home: transfer limitations and environmental risk factors. *Australian Occupational Therapy Journal*, **43** (1996), 13–18.

18. L. Clemson, R. G. Cumming & M. Roland, Case-control study of hazards in the home and risk of falls and hip fractures. *Age and Ageing*, **25** (1996), 97–101.

19. F. Isberner, D. Ristzel, O. Sarvela, K. Brown, P. Hu & D. Newbolds, Falls in elderly rural home health clients. *Home Health Care Services Quarterly*, **17** (1998), 41–51.

20. R. W. Sattin, J. G. Rodriguez, C. A. DeVito & P. A. Wingo, Home environmental hazards and the risk of fall injury events among community-dwelling older persons. *Journal of the American Geriatrics Society*, **46** (1998), 669–76.

21. S. Kinn & D. Clawson, Health visitor risk assessment for preventing falls in elderly people. *British Journal of Nursing*, **11** (2002), 316–21.

22. P. C. Fletcher & J. P. Hirdes, Risk factors for falling among community-based seniors using home care services. *Journal of Gerontology*, **57A** (2002), M504–10.

23. M. E. Tinetti, M. Speechley & S. F. Ginter, Risk factors for falls among elderly persons living in the community. *New England Journal of Medicine*, **319** (1988), 1701–7.

24. M. Nevitt, S. Cummings, S. Kidd & D. Black, Risk factors for recurrent non-syncopal falls. *Journal of the American Medical Association*, **261** (1989), 2663–8.

25. A. J. Campbell, M. J. Borrie, G. F. Spears *et al.*, Circumstances and consequences of falls experienced by a community population 70 years and over during a prospective study. *Age and Ageing*, **19** (1990), 136–41.

26. J. Teno, D. P. Kiel & V. Mor, Multiple stumbles: a risk factor for falls in community-dwelling elderly. A prospective study. *Journal of the American Geriatrics Society*, **38** (1990), 1321–5.

27. T. M. Gill, C. S. Williams & M. E. Tinetti, Environmental hazards and the risk of non-syncopal falls in the homes of community-living older persons. *Medical Care*, **38** (2000), 1174–83.

28. M. E. Northridge, M. C. Nevitt, J. L. Kelsey & B. Link, Home hazards and falls in the elderly: the role of health and functional status. *American Journal of Public Health*, **85** (1995), 509–15.

29. M. Speechley & M. Tinetti, Falls and injuries in frail and vigorous community elderly persons. *Journal of the American Geriatrics Society*, **39** (1991), 46–52.

30. L. E. Weinberg & L. A. Strain, Community-dwelling older adults' attributions about falls. *Archives of Physical Medicine and Rehabilitation*, **76** (1995), 955–60.

31. B. E. Fleming & D. R. Pendergast, Physical condition, activity pattern, and environment as factors in falls by adult care facility residents. *Archives of Physical Medicine and Rehabilitation*, **74** (1993), 627–30.

32. M. E. Tinetti, J. T. Doucette & E. B. Claus, The contribution of predisposing and situational risk factors to serious fall injuries. *Journal of the American Geriatrics Society*, **43** (1995), 1207–13.

33. H. David & L. Freedman, Injuries caused by tripping over paving stones: an unappreciated problem. *British Medical Journal*, **300** (1990), 784–5.

34. J. Fothergill, D. O'Driscoll & K. Hashemi, The role of environmental factors in causing injury through falls in public places. *Ergonomics*, **38** (1995), 220–3.

35. E. M. Gallagher & V. J. Scott, The STEPS project: participatory action research to reduce falls in public places among seniors and persons with disabilities. *Canadian Journal of Public Health*, **88** (1997), 129–33.

36. A. H. R. W. Simpson, S. Lamb, P. J. Roberts, T. N. Gardner & J. G. Evans, Does the type of flooring affect the risk of hip fracture? *Age and Ageing*, **33** (2004), 242–6.

37. M. C. Nevitt, S. R. Cummings & E. S. Hudes, Risk factors for injurious falls: a prospective study. *Journal of Gerontology*, **46A** (1991), M164–70.

38. J. Waller, Falls among the elderly: human and environmental factors. *Accident Analysis and Prevention*, **10** (1978), 21–33.

39. M. C. Nevitt & S. R. Cummings, Type of fall and risk of hip and wrist fractures: the study of osteoporotic fractures. The Study of Osteoporotic Fractures Research Group. *Journal of the American Geriatrics Society*, **41** (1993), 1226–34.

40. J. A. Grisso, J. L. Kelsey & B. L. Strom, Risk factors for falls as a cause of hip fracture in women. *New England Journal of Medicine*, **324** (1991), 1326–31.

41. R. G. Cumming & R. J. Klineberg, Fall frequency and characteristics and the risk of hip fracture. *Journal of the American Geriatrics Society*, **42** (1994), 774–8.

42. M. Lawton, Environment and aging. In *Brooks/Cole Series in Social Gerontology*, ed. V. Bengison. (Monterey, California: Brooks/Cole, 1980).

43. J. M. Chandler, P. W. Duncan, D. K. Weiner & S. A. Studenski, The Home Assessment Profile – a reliable and valid assessment tool. *Topics in Geriatric Rehabilitation*, **16** (2001), 77–88.

44. J. G. Zhang, K. Ishikawa-Takata, H. Yamazaki & T. Ohta, Is type A behaviour pattern associated with falling among the community-dwelling elderly? *Archives of Gerontology and Geriatrics*, **38** (2004), 145–52.

45. L. Clemson, R. G. Cumming & R. Heard, The development of an assessment to evaluate behavioral factors associated with falling. *American Journal of Occupational Therapy*, **57** (2003), 380–8.

9

The relative importance of falls risk factors: an evidence-based summary

In this chapter, we have pooled the findings from published studies cited in Chapters 1 to 8 that have specifically addressed falls risk in older people. However, rather than simply listing the many and varied socio-demographic, physiological, psychological, health and environmental factors that have been posited as important falls risk factors, we have rated each factor according to the strength of the published evidence associating that factor with falls. To do this we have using the following four-level rating system:

- ***   strong evidence of association (consistently found in good studies)
- **   moderate evidence of association (usually but not always found)
- *   weak evidence of association (occasionally but not usually found)
- −   little or no evidence of association (not found in published studies despite research to examine the issue)

The factors have been classified into the following categories: socio-demographic factors; balance and mobility factors; sensory and neuromuscular factors; psychological factors; medical factors; medication factors; and environmental factors.

Socio-demographic factors

Table 9.1 shows a number of socio-demographic aspects that have been systematically studied as potential falls risk factors.

As falls are generally considered to be a marker of frailty and decreased mobility, it is not surprising that falls are associated with advanced age and impairments in activities of daily living. The finding that a history of falling is associated with future falls is also not surprising. Most studies undertaken in community settings have shown a higher incidence of falls in women. This may be due to reduced strength and increased visual field dependence in women [1]. In a recent study, our group has also found that older women are worse than older men at executing fast and accurate steps in a choice reaction stepping time

Table 9.1 Socio-demographic factors associated with falls

Factor	Strength of association
Advanced age	***
ADL/mobility limitations	***
History of falls	***
Female gender	**
Race	**
Living alone	**
Inactivity	**
Walking aid use	**
Alcohol consumption	–

ADL = activities of daily living

task that required whole body movement [2]. However, in hospitals and institutions, where the inpatient populations are subject to substantial selection biases (based on ill health, frailty and impaired mobility, etc.), the reported incidence of falling is similar for men and women. The finding that living alone is a risk factor for falls is most likely to be confounded by gender and age, in that older women comprise the majority of this group. The differences in fall rates among racial groups may reflect different lifestyle characteristics related to habitual physical activity rather than genetic differences.

As is described in Chapters 10 and 11, physical activity can improve strength, balance and functional abilities in older people [3], and can prevent falls [4]. However, being more physically active does not always prevent falls [5]. This is probably because the more physically active older person takes part in activities which increase exposure to falls risk situations. Clearly, this risk should be balanced against the benefits of increased physical functioning and independence that exercise brings.

The most surprising finding regarding associations between socio-demographic factors and falls is that alcohol consumption has not been shown to be a falls risk factor. Despite examining the issue, no significant associations have been found between alcohol use and falls in several large cohort studies [6–11]. In fact, most of these studies have found that those who are current drinkers have fewer falls than those who abstain [6–8, 10]. Campbell *et al.* [6] have suggested that this unexpected protective association may be due to alcohol use being lower in those with poor physical health or those taking psychoactive drugs; however, this was not the case in our community study [8]. It may also be the case that the lack of a positive association between alcohol use and falls is due to response and selection biases, in that heavy alcohol consumers may under-report their drinking levels or simply decline participation in research studies. However, despite the lack of an association between current alcohol use and falls, there is strong evidence that long term high alcohol intake can lead to multiple medical problems, including osteoporosis, cerebellar atrophy and peripheral neuropathy [12].

Postural instability

Table 9.2 summarizes the results of the many investigations that have been performed to evaluate whether various measures of balance and mobility are associated with an increased falls risk. Generally speaking, the more challenging the stability task, the stronger the evidence for it being a falls risk factor. For example, while impaired stability when standing and walking on level surfaces are moderate risk factors, measures of leaning balance, transfers and standing from a sitting position are consistently reported as strong risk factors in well-designed studies. On the other hand, the more global or non-specific measures provide less information with regard to the underlying mechanisms predisposing older people to falls.

Although many studies have been performed to evaluate age-related differences in responding to platform perturbations, performance on these tests is only weakly associated with falls. There are two possible reasons for this. Firstly, few large prospective studies have employed the mechanical perturbation model as it generally requires specialized equipment and is therefore restricted to testing of smaller numbers of subjects in a laboratory setting. Secondly, the artificial perturbations induced by platform tests are dissimilar to those that would lead to a fall in an older person's daily environment. Interestingly, a prospective study by Maki *et al.* [13] found that while standing sway in the medio-lateral direction predicted falls, performance on tests of medio-lateral and antero-posterior platform perturbation were not able to discriminate

Table 9.2 Balance and mobility factors associated with falls

Factor	Strength of association
Impaired sit-to-stand/transfer ability	***
Reduced gait velocity/cadence/step length	***
Impaired stability when standing	**
Impaired stability when leaning and reaching	**
Slow voluntary stepping	**
Increased step timing variability	**
Inadequate responses to external perturbations	*

between fallers and non-fallers. It appears that measures of postural stability will only predict falls if the tests used challenge balance in a realistic manner that represents the context of the specific task being performed.

Sensory and neuromuscular factors associated with falls

As outlined in Chapter 2, postural control is a complex process involving many body systems. Table 9.3 shows that reduced functioning in peripheral sensation, muscle strength and reaction time – major contributors to postural control – are strongly associated with falls. Impaired vision is also a strong falls risk factor and the fact that it is only moderately associated with falls in some studies appears to be due to the use of a sub-optimal test, i.e. Snellen letter charts. These charts measure discrimination of fine detail, whereas the ability to accurately perceive depth and detect larger visual stimuli under low contrast conditions are more pertinent visual measures for avoiding hazards and thus falls [14]. There is now emerging evidence that, if measured rigorously, vestibular impairments [15],

Table 9.3 Sensory and neuromuscular factors associated with falls

Factor	Strength of association
Vision	
Poor visual contrast sensitivity	***
Decreased depth perception	***
Poor visual acuity	**
Visual field loss	*
Increased visual field dependence	*
Poor hearing	–
Reduced vestibular function	*
Peripheral sensation	
Reduced vibration sense	***
Reduced tactile sensitivity	***
Reduced proprioception	**
Muscle strength	
Reduced muscle strength	***
Reduced muscle power	*
Reduced muscle endurance	*
Reaction time	
Poor simple reaction time	***
Poor choice reaction time	***

and reduced muscle power [16] and endurance [17] are also important falls risk factors in older people. Poor hearing is the only physiological risk factor found not to be a risk factor for falls, despite systematic study.

In our studies, we have found that measurements of vision, peripheral sensation, muscle strength, reaction time and balance, significantly and independently contribute to the discrimination between fallers and non-fallers in multivariate analyses [18, 19]. This suggests that poor functioning in any of these physiological domains predisposes older people to falls and that multiple impairments greatly increase falls risk. However, when the standardized weightings of each measure are compared, it is apparent that they do not contribute equally to the prediction of falls. Slow reaction time and increased sway (particularly when challenged by having subjects close their eyes or stand on a compliant surface) appear to be particularly strong physiological risk factors for falls [18, 19].

Psychological risk factors

Table 9.4 outlines the psychological factors that have been implicated in falls in older people. Several studies have shown that with increasing age, balance tasks become more attentionally demanding. Frail older people require even more attentional resources for postural control, to the extent that even simple tasks like answering a question may interfere with standing, stepping and walking [20]. In these situations, older people with attentional limitations are at an increased risk of falls [21].

Fear of falling is prevalent in older people. In many cases, this fear may be excessive, and lead to unnecessary restrictions in physical and social activity. Fear of falling is strongly associated with falls [22] but has not been shown to be a risk factor for falls after adjusting for physiological falls risk factors. Research is required to distinguish between rational and irrational levels of fear of falling as this distinction has implications for both falls risk assessment and interventions. There is only preliminary evidence that risk-taking behaviours increase falls risk in older people.

Table 9.4 Psychological factors associated with falls

Factor	Strength of association
Increased fear of falling	***
Impaired selective attention	**
Risk taking	*

Table 9.5 Medical factors associated with falls

Factor	Strength of association
Impaired cognition	***
Stroke	***
Parkinson's disease	***
Number of chronic conditions	***
Depression	**
Abnormal neurological signs	**
Incontinence	**
Acute illness	**
Arthritis	**
Foot problems	**
Dizziness	**
Orthostatic hypotension	*
Vestibular disorders	–

Medical factors

A number of researchers have now identified a range of medical factors that are associated with an increased risk of falls [6, 8–10, 23–25]. As illustrated in Table 9.5, these include the presence of stroke or Parkinson's disease, acute illness, arthritis, foot problems, depression, impaired cognition, incontinence and abnormal neurological signs. These conditions have been shown to be risk factors for falls in both community and institutional settings, although the importance of some of these, such as incontinence and impaired cognition, may be more important in institutions. The distinction between strong and moderate evidence for these factors relates to some extent to the difficulty in rigorously measuring some of these conditions. This has meant that fewer studies have addressed these factors or that crude measures (with resultant imprecision) have been used as substitutes. This is particularly the case for neurological conditions, arthritis and foot problems.

However, as also shown in Table 9.5, certain conditions commonly perceived to be strong risk factors for falls, such as vestibular disorders and orthostatic hypotension, have not been found to be important risk factors in research studies. The lack of reported associations between either vestibular disorders or dizziness and falls appears paradoxical, as such disorders have marked effects on balance. Three factors could account for the lack of association. Firstly, increased age results in a *loss* of vestibular functioning, not an increase in *aberrant* vestibular information, as is the case with vestibular disease. Older people with adequate peripheral sensation and/or vision may be able to compensate for reduced vestibular functioning. Secondly, vestibular disorders (as opposed to diminished vestibular function) do have a marked effect on balance in older people and this effect is patently clear to sufferers who as a result take steps to avoid falling – quite often by lying down. The final factor may relate to study limitations, in that assessment measures for accurately measuring vestibular functioning have not been carried out in large prospective studies on falls.

As indicated in Chapter 6, orthostatic hypotension, whether idiopathic or iatrogenic, has not been found to increase the risk of falling in older people. This indicates that in comparison with impairments of sensorimotor function, balance and gait, orthostatic hypotension is a relatively unimportant or rare cause of falls. As is the case with vestibular disorders, the lack of a demonstrated link between orthostatic hypotension and falls may be due to study limitations. Most studies have tested for orthostatic hypotension on a single occasion, usually when the older subject visits a clinic or laboratory. These subjects are then followed up in prospective studies to determine fall rates. It is possible that as orthostatic hypotension can be of an intermittent nature, subjects may test negatively on the baseline testing day, but suffer postural blood pressure drops and falls on one or more occasions in the follow-up period. Recent studies have also found that carotid sinus hypersensitivity, often cited as a cause of drop attacks and syncope, may be responsible for a proportion of unexplained falls [26].

Medication use

Table 9.6 outlines medications that have been implicated in falls in older people. Studies undertaken in both community and institutional settings have consistently reported significant associations between psychoactive medication use and falls. Many studies have examined anti-hypertensive use as a possible falls risk factor. Here the findings have been inconsistent, and a meta-analysis of the available published data by Leipzig et al. [27] concluded that there was little support for an association between anti-hypertensive use and falls. This meta-analysis also concluded that digoxin and type IA anti-arrhythmic drugs were weakly associated with falls, and that non-steroidal anti-inflammatory drugs do not appear to be an independent risk factor for falls once the confounding variable of arthritis is taken into account [27].

The use of multiple medications (usually four or more) has been shown to be a predictor of falls risk in several studies. However, multiple medication use may be primarily a marker for underlying chronic diseases. With the rising number of pharmacological treatments available from which older people have potential to benefit both in terms of morbidity and mortality, the priority is to ensure that

Table 9.6 Medication factors associated with falls

Factor	Strength of association
Use of multiple medications	***
Benzodiazepine use	***
Antidepressant use	***
Anti-psychotic use	***
Psychoactive medication use	***
Anti-arhythmics	*
Anti-hypertensive use	*
Analgesics	−
Anti-inflammatory drugs	−

Table 9.7 Environmental factors associated with falls

Factor	Strength of association
Poor footwear	*
Inappropriate spectacles	*
Home hazards	−
External hazards	−

older people are able to access treatments from which they stand to benefit while ensuring harmful drug interactions are avoided.

Environmental factors

In contrast to socio-demographic, medical and physiological factors, there is little evidence that environmental factors are strongly associated with falls risk (see Table 9.7). There is no conclusive data to indicate that the households of older people who fall are more 'hazardous' than those who do not fall. The lack of associations may reflect, at least in part, the difficulty of studying transient or intermittent risk factors. However, as many falls do involve environmental factors, it seems that the interaction between the older person's functional abilities and the environment is a crucial factor in determining whether a fall will occur. Further, as reported in Chapter 14, home hazard reduction is effective if targeted to older people with a history of falls and mobility limitations, and combined with strategies for improving transfer abilities and other behavioural changes.

There is now preliminary evidence that poor footwear [28] and inappropriate spectacles [29] are risk factors for falls. Both of these factors have also been found to affect important physiological falls risk factors. For example, high-heeled shoes impair balance [30], and bifocal and multifocal spectacles impair depth perception and contrast sensitivity at critical distances required for detecting obstacles in the environment [29].

Conclusion

Large epidemiological studies have identified many risk factors for falling in older people. Many socio-demographic factors, medical conditions, and impairments of sensorimotor function, balance and gait, have been shown to be strongly associated with falls. The lack of significant associations for other posited risk factors might indicate that these are relatively unimportant causes of falls or that these issues have not been subject to appropriate study. The risk factors that are of an intermittent nature have been especially difficult to study.

The above summaries have listed risk factors in isolation and have used a simple classification scheme. Many of the risk factors are inter-related as preliminary path analytic models have shown [31]. Furthermore, the intrinsic/extrinsic distinction is an oversimplification. A better understanding of falls is usually obtained when taking an ecological perspective, that is, examining the person in association with environmental factors [32]. Finally, the above summaries, by definition, are based on findings from population studies. Clearly, in clinical practice many medical conditions and disorders, in addition to those listed above as important risk factors, may well be the cause of falls in individual patients and require investigation.

REFERENCES

1. S. R. Lord, P. N. Sambrook, C. Gilbert *et al.*, Postural stability, falls and fractures in the elderly: results from the Dubbo Osteoporosis Epidemiology Study. *Medical Journal of Australia*, **160** (1994), 684–91.
2. S. R. Lord & R. C. Fitzpatrick, Choice stepping reaction time: a composite measure of falls risk in older people. *Journal of Gerontology*, **56A** (2001), M627–32.
3. D. M. Buchner, S. A. Beresford, E. B. Larson, A. Z. LaCroix & E. H. Wagner, Effects of physical activity on health status in older adults. II. Intervention studies. *Annual Review of Public Health*, **13** (1992), 469–88.
4. M. A. Province, E. C. Hadley, M. C. Hornbrook *et al.*, The effects of exercise on falls in elderly patients. A preplanned meta-analysis of the FICSIT Trials. Frailty and Injuries: Cooperative Studies of Intervention Techniques. *Journal of the American Medical Association*, **273** (1995), 1341–7.
5. S. Studenski, P. W. Duncan, J. Chandler *et al.*, Predicting falls: the role of mobility and nonphysical factors. *Journal of the American Geriatrics Society*, **42** (1994), 297–302.

6. A. J. Campbell, M. J. Borrie & G. F. Spears, Risk factors for falls in a community-based prospective study of people 70 years and older. *Journal of Gerontology*, **44** (1989), M112–17.

7. D. E. Nelson, R. W. Sattin, J. A. Langlois, C. A. DeVito & J. A. Stevens, Alcohol as a risk factor for fall injury events among elderly persons living in the community. *Journal of the American Geriatrics Society*, **40** (1992), 658–61.

8. S. R. Lord, J. A. Ward, P. Williams & K. J. Anstey, An epidemiological study of falls in older community-dwelling women: the Randwick Falls and Fractures Study. *Australian Journal of Public Health*, **17** (1993), 240–5.

9. S. L. Sheahan, S. J. Coons, C. A. Robbins *et al.*, Psychoactive medication, alcohol use, and falls among older adults. *Journal of Behavioral Medicine*, **18** (1995), 127–40.

10. M. E. Tinetti, M. Speechley & S. F. Ginter, Risk factors for falls among elderly persons living in the community. *New England Medical Journal*, **319** (1988), 1701–7.

11. M. C. Nevitt, S. R. Cummings, S. Kidd & D. Black, Risk factors for recurrent nonsyncopal falls. A prospective study. *Journal of the American Medical Association*, **261** (1989), 2663–8.

12. J. E. Carlson, Alcohol use and falls [letter]. *Journal of the American Geriatrics Society*, **41** (1993), 346.

13. B. E. Maki, P. J. Holliday & A. K. Topper, A prospective study of postural balance and risk of falling in an ambulatory and independent elderly population. *Journal of Gerontology*, **49** (1994), M72–84.

14. S. R. Lord, R. D. Clark & I. W. Webster, Visual acuity and contrast sensitivity in relation to falls in an elderly population. *Age and Ageing*, **20** (1991), 175–81.

15. R. P. Di Fabio, J. F. Greany, A. Emasithi & J. F. Wyman, Eye-head coordination during postural perturbation as a predictor of falls in community-dwelling elderly women. *Archives of Physical Medicine and Rehabilitation*, **83** (2002), 942–51.

16. D. A. Skelton, J. Kennedy & O. M. Rutherford, Explosive power and asymmetry in leg muscle function in frequent fallers and non-fallers aged over 65. *Age and Ageing*, **31** (2002), 119–25.

17. K. I. Schwender, A. E. Mikesky, W. S. Holt, M. Peacock & D. B. Burr, Differences in muscle endurance and recovery between fallers and nonfallers, and between young and older women. *Journal of Gerontology*, **52** (1997), M155–60.

18. S. R. Lord, R. D. Clark & I. W. Webster, Physiological factors associated with falls in an elderly population. *Journal of the American Geriatrics Society*, **39** (1991), 1194–200.

19. S. R. Lord, J. A. Ward, P. Williams & K. Anstey, Physiological factors associated with falls in older community-dwelling women. *Journal of the American Geriatrics Society*, **42** (1994), 1110–17.

20. M. Woollacott & A. Shumway-Cook, Attention and control of posture and gait: a review of an emerging area of research. *Gait and Posture*, **16** (2002), 1–14.

21. L. Lundin-Olsson, L. Nyberg & Y. Gustafson, "Stops walking when talking" as a predictor of falls in elderly people. *The Lancet*, **349** (1997), 617.

22. K. Letgers, Fear of falling. *Physical Therapy*, **82** (2002), 264–72.

23. A. J. Campbell, J. Reinken, B. C. Allan & G. S. Martinez, Falls in old age: a study of frequency and related clinical factors. *Age and Ageing*, **10** (1981), 264–70.

24. D. Prudham & J. Grimley Evans, Factors associated with falls in the elderly: a community study. *Age and Ageing,* **10** (1981), 141–6.

25. A. S. Robbins, L. Z. Rubenstein & K. R. Josephson, Predictors of falls among elderly people. Results of two population-based studies. *Archives of Internal Medicine,* **149** (1989), 1628–33.

26. S. W. Parry & R. A. Kenny, Drop attacks in older adults: systematic assessment has a high diagnostic yield. *Journal of the American Geriatrics Society,* **53** (2005), 74–8.

27. R. M. Leipzig, R. G. Cumming & M. E. Tinetti, Drugs and falls in older people: a systematic review and meta-analysis. II. Cardiac and analgesic drugs. *Journal of the American Geriatrics Society,* **47** (1999), 40–50.

28. A. F. Tencer, T. D. Koepsell, M. E. Wolf *et al.*, Biomechanical properties of shoes and risk of falls in older adults. *Journal of the American Geriatrics Society,* **52** (2004), 1840–6.

29. S. R. Lord, J. Dayhew & A. Howland, Multifocal glasses impair edge contrast sensitivity and depth perception and increase the risk of falls in older people. *Journal of the American Geriatrics Society,* **50** (2002), 1760–6.

30. S. R. Lord & G. M. Bashford, Shoe characteristics and balance in older women. *Journal of the American Geriatrics Society,* **44** (1996), 429–33.

31. S. R. Lord, K. Anstey, P. Williams & J. A. Ward, Psychoactive medication use, sensori-motor function and falls in older women. *British Journal of Clinical Pharmacology,* **39** (1995), 227–34.

32. C. C. Hogue, Falls and mobility in later life: an ecological model. *Journal of the American Geriatrics Society,* **32** (1984), 858–61.

Part II

Strategies for prevention

Falls prevention – an overview

The first section of this book provides detailed evidence on the physiological mechanisms integral to human balance and gait as well as describing in depth the factors that have been found to increase falls risk. While some of the identified risk factors are irreversible, there are many which are potentially modifiable or remediable with appropriate interventions. The irreversible factors are useful for identifying high-risk populations for targeted interventions, whilst the identification of modifiable risk factors provides a platform for focused interventions aimed at reducing falls risk. Heterogeneity is a major feature of the risk factor literature. This indicates that no single approach to prevention will adequately address the problem of falls and injury in older people.

Table 10.0 highlights the risk factors identified in Part I of this book that are most consistently associated with an increased falls risk, and suggests potential strategies for reducing or reversing such risks where possible.

This second part of the book concentrates on evidence-based assessments and interventions to prevent falls, and describes several different approaches applied to a range of at-risk populations. Exercise has been the most thoroughly investigated single intervention, and there is now a strong evidence base to support specific types of exercise for modifying falls risk factors and preventing falls. These findings are discussed in detail in Chapters 10 and 11. Chapter 12 appraises the efficacy of a range of medical interventions and Chapter 13 provides an overview of the role assistive devices can play in reducing falls risk. As outlined in Chapter 14, more evidence is emerging to support environmental assessment, in conjunction with safety advice and education, as a falls prevention strategy. Strategies for preventing falls in nursing home residents and hospital inpatients are discussed in Chapter 15. For these high-risk populations, multifactorial approaches have been shown to be the most beneficial. Chapter 16

Table 10.0 Falls risk factors: ability to be modified and possible intervention strategies

Risk factor	Able to be modified?	Intervention strategies
Advanced age	No	Can be used to identify high-risk populations.
Female	No	Can be used to identify high-risk populations.
Living alone	Possibly	Can be used to identify high-risk populations. Possible change of living arrangements.
History of falls	No	Can be used to identify high-risk populations. Probably the single best predictor of falls risk.
Inactivity	Yes	Exercise, education.
Limitations in activities of daily living	Yes	Exercise, motor training, use of aids, provision of assistance with ADL.
Medical factors	Possibly	Appropriate medical or surgical interventions. Ancillary treatment for osteoporosis as a mechanism for reducing fracture risk.
Medications	Possibly	Medication withdrawal if indicated, investigation of alternative strategies.
Poor vision	Possibly	Use of appropriate spectacles, medical/surgical interventions, environmental modifications.
Reduced peripheral sensation	No	Look for reversible cause. Discussion of increased risk and compensatory strategies.
Muscle weakness	Yes	Strength training.
Poor reaction time	Yes	Exercise/training of fast, coordinated responses, e.g. exercise to music.
Impaired balance	Yes	Exercise/training involving control of movements of centre of mass.
Impaired gait	Yes	Exercise, training targeting causes, consider use of aids and appliances.
Poor/inadequate assistive devices	Yes	Provision of appropriate spectacles, footwear, walking aids, hip protectors and other assistive devices.
Environmental hazards (home, hospital, residential care, public places)	Yes	Instillation of safety features, correction/removal of hazards and associated safety education.

ADL = activities of daily living

describes a physiological profile approach for assessing falls risk, tailoring a falls prevention programme and evaluating the effectiveness of interventions in both the research and clinical settings. Finally, Chapter 17 attempts to synthesize the existing successful approaches to intervention and discusses the opportunities and challenges to translating the evidence from the research arena into everyday clinical practice.

10

Exercise interventions to prevent falls

Written with Julie Whitney

Exercise has a major role to play in preventing falls among older people and is recommended in recent evidence-based guidelines for falls prevention [1–3]. As acknowledged in these guidelines, there are many different types of exercise, some of which are likely to result in greater reductions in falls than others. It is therefore incumbent upon health professionals to do better than merely suggest that older people should exercise. As Hadley [4] has stated 'telling an older person that 'exercise' can prevent falls is not much better than telling them that 'antibiotics' can cure an infection: although true, the advice would be much more useful if it were more specific'.

This chapter aims to assist the health professional to prescribe exercise for falls prevention. The first section reviews the findings of randomized controlled trials into exercise interventions for falls prevention. From this, a synthesis of the findings is undertaken in an effort to delineate the important components for successful exercise interventions.

Analysis of randomized controlled trials (RCTs) investigating exercise and falls

In revising and updating this chapter, a detailed analysis of the specific components of exercise was undertaken. A total of 44 RCTs of exercise interventions for falls prevention written in English were identified via searches of electronic databases (MEDLINE, CINAHL, EMBASE, PEDro), and reference lists of systematic reviews and clinical practice guidelines. An updated literature search, which has been undertaken for the next version of the Cochrane Collaboration systematic review of randomized controlled trials evaluating interventions for the prevention of falls in older people, and 'in press' articles, were obtained from colleagues. The terms 'tailored' and 'targeted' exercise have been used interchangeably in the literature. We have used the following definitions. *Tailored exercise* describes programmes where either the intensity and/or the type of exercise are specifically designed for individual participants. *Targeted* interventions describe programmes that are aimed at high-risk groups. We have not considered multifactorial interventions involving exercise in this chapter as it is not possible to differentiate the effects of exercise from those of the other interventions administered. We have used the term *transitional* to refer to those who either live in a low-support residential care setting (i.e. a hostel or congregate living facility but not a nursing home) or were recruited during a hospital admission.

Of the 44 studies, 16 were excluded from further analysis as they included fewer than 40 subjects per group and were therefore almost certainly underpowered to detect an effect on falls. Two further studies were excluded because they did not include a non-exercise or low-intensity exercise control group [5, 6], and one was excluded as the follow-up period was ten years after the intervention was prescribed [7]. Included and excluded trials are listed in Table 10.1.

Included trials were classified as preventing falls (12 trials) or not preventing falls (13 trials) on the basis of the intervention having a significant between-group effect on a falls outcome measure (number of fallers, fall rates or time delay to falling) during the trial period for the total sample. The use of intention to treat analysis was not considered when the studies were classified. Some studies reported statistically significant between-group differences for subgroups of subjects or for a part of the follow-up period only. These studies were grouped with the trials which did not prevent falls, but the positive findings are discussed. For one trial, a between-group analysis of fall rates was not reported but it was possible to calculate a relative risk from data provided in the paper. Features of the exercise programmes used in different studies are summarized in Tables 10.2 and 10.3. This was assessed from information given in publications about the studies rather than personal contact with authors.

Programmes which prevented falls

Exercise in groups – community dwellers

Barnett *et al.* [8] analysed the effect of a progressive programme of exercises carried out in a group with additional home exercise in 163 people at increased risk of falls with a mean age of 75 years. Exercises consisted of resistance training using graded resistance bands at individualized intensities, functional task training, endurance, flexibility, and gait and balance training. Exercise was not individually prescribed, but gait and balance training was carried out predominantly in standing positions, and aimed to progressively reduce the support provided by the upper limbs. The programme was designed by a

Table 10.1 List of trials included and excluded for review of effect of exercise on falls

Prevented falls	Didn't prevent falls	Low power (groups < 40)	Excluded
Barnett et al. 2003 [8]	Bunout et al. 2005 [23]	Alexander et al. 2003 [42]	No non-exercise control group
Buchner et al. 1997 [9]	Campbell et al. 1999 [32]	Buettner 2002 [43]	Means et al. 1996 [6]
Campbell et al. 1997 [17]	Campbell et al. 2005 [33]	Cerny et al. 1998 [44]	Steadman et al. 2003 [5]
Day et al. 2002 [10]	Carter et al. 2002 [24]	Fiatarone et al. 1997 [45]	
Li et al. 2005 [14]	Ebrahim et al. 1997 [22]*	Hauer et al. 2001 [46]	10-year follow-up period
Lord et al. 2003 [16]	Latham et al. 2003 [34]	Helbostad et al. 2004 [47]	Pereira et al. [7]
Means et al. 2005 [11]	Lord et al. 1995 [25]	Lui-Ambrose et al. 2004 [48]	
Robertson et al. 2001 [19]	McMurdo et al. 1997 [26]	MacRae et al. 1994 [49]	
Schnelle et al. 2003 [21]	Morgan et al. 2004 [27]	Nitz & Choy 2004 [50]	
Skelton et al. 2005 [12]	Mulrow et al. 1994 [35]	Nowalk 2001 [57]	
Wolf et al. 1996 [13]	Reinsch et al. 1992 [28]	Resnick 2002 [51]	
Voukelatos et al. [15]	Steinberg et al. 2000 [29]	Rubenstein et al. 2000 [52]	
	Wolf et al. 2003 [30]	Schoenfelder 2000 [53]	
		Sherrington et al. 2004 [54]	
		Shimada et al. 2004 [55]	
		Toulotte et al. 2003 [56]	
N = 12	N = 13	N = 16	N = 3

Studies classified as (a) preventing falls if at least one falls outcome measure showed a between-group difference, (b) not preventing falls if no between-group differences and more than 40 subjects per group, and (c) low power if less than 40 subjects per group.

*This study found an increased risk of falls in the intervention group.

physiotherapist and delivered to groups of 6–18 participants by a trained exercise instructor. Group sessions lasted one hour and took place once a week over four terms a year (37 sessions in total). A total of 34% of participants attended more than 30 classes, 91% exercised at home once a week and 13% reported exercising daily. Falls as measured for one year after the intervention were significantly reduced (incident rate ratio = 0.60, 95% CI = 0.36–0.99) and

Table 10.2 Description of exercise intervention programmes in random controlled trials *showing an effect* of the intervention on falls

| Study | Sample size | Effect size (follow-up period) | High-risk | Mean age | Time (mins) | Duration of exercise (months) | Freq. (per week) | Type of exercise | | | | | | Individualized | | Progressive | Most exercise in standing | Aim to reduce arm support |
								Resist.	Bal.	Funct.	End.	Walk.	Flex.	Type	Intensity			
Exercise in groups – community dwellers																		
Barnett et al. [8]	163	Incident rate ratio for rate of falls = 0.60, 95% CI 0.36–0.99 (1 year)	✓	75	60	12	1 (+ home ex.)	✓	✓	✓	✓	✗	✓	✗	✓	✓	✓	✓
Buchner et al. [9]	105	Relative risk for falls rate = 0.61, 95% CI 0.39–0.93 (median = 18 months)	✓	75	60	6	3	✓	✗	✗	✓	✗	✗	✗	✓	✓	✗	✗
Day et al. [10]	1090 (541)	Rate ratio for rate of falls = 0.82, 95% CI 0.70–0.97 (18 months)	✗	76	60	4	1 (+ home ex.)	✓	✓	✗	✗	✗	✓	✗	✓	✓	✓	✓
Li et al. [14]	256	Hazard ratio for multiple falls = 0.45, 95% CI 0.30–0.70 (1 year)	✗	77	60	6	3	✗	✓	✗	✗	✗	✓	✗	✗	✓	✓	✓
Lord et al.* [16]	551	Incident rate ratio for rate of falls = 0.78, 95% CI 0.62–0.99 (1 year)	✓	79	60	12	2 (+ home ex.)	✓	✓	✓	✓	✗	✓	✗	✓	✓	✓	✓
Means et al. [11]	205	Relative risk of being a faller = 0.40, 95% CI 0.25–0.63 (6 months) (calculated from data provided by paper)	✗	74	90	1.5	3	✓	✓	✓	✓	✓	✓	✗	✓	✓	✓	✓
Skelton et al. [12]	100	Incident rate ratio for rate of falls = 0.69, 95% CI 0.50–0.96 (mean = 86 weeks)	✓	73	60	9	1 (+ home ex.)	✓	✓	✓	✓	✗	✓	✓	✓	✓	✓	✓

Study	N	Outcome		Age															
Wolf et al. [13]	200	Risk ratio = 0.63, 95% CI 0.45–0.89 (13 months)	✗	76	45	4	2 (+ home ex.)	✗	✓	✗	✗	✗	✗	✗	✗	✓	✓	✓	✓
Voukelatos et al. [15]	702	Incident rate ratio for rate of falls = 0.65, 95% CI 0.47–0.89 (1 year)	✗	68	60	4	1	✗	✓	✗	✗	✗	✗	✗	✗	✓	✓	✓	✓
Sub-total			4/9	74	60#	6#	2#	6/9	8/9	4/9	3/9	1/9	5/9	5/9	1/9	7/9	9/9	8/9	8/9
Individual exercise – community dwellers																			
Campbell et al. [17]	233	Incident rate ratio for rate of falls = 0.47, 95% CI 0.04–0.90 (1 year)	✓	84	30	1	3	✓	✓	✓	✓	✓	✓	✗	✓	✓	✓	✓	✓
Robertson et al. [19]	240	Incident rate ratio for rate of falls = 0.54, 95% CI 0.32–0.90 (1 year)	✓	81	30	12	3	✓	✓	✓	✓	✓	✓	✗	✓	✓	✓	✓	✓
Sub-total			2/2	82.5	30	12	3	2/2	2/2	2/2	2/2	2/2	2/2	0/2	2/2	2/2	2/2	2/2	2/2
Individual exercise – institution dwellers																			
Schnelle et al. [21]	190	Relative risk of being a faller = 0.62, 95% CI (0.42–0.91) (8 months) (calculated from data provided by paper)	✓	88	20	8	20	✓	✓	✓	✗	✗	✗	✗	✗	✓	✓	✓	✗
Sub-total			1/1	88	20	17	20	1/1	1/1	1/1	0/1	0/1	0/1	0/1	0/1	1/1	1/1	1/1	0/1
Totals			7/12 (58%)	77	60#	7#	2.5#	9/12 (75%)	11/12 (92%)	7/12 (58%)	5/12 (50%)	3/12 (25%)	7/12 (58%)	5/12 (50%)	3/12 (25%)	10/12 (83%)	12/12 (100%)	11/12 (92%)	10/12 (83%)

Resist. = Resistance training, Bal. = balance training, Funct. = functional training, End. = endurance training, Walk. = walking programme, Flex. = flexibility

*retirement village and hostel residents

#Median

Table 10.3 Description of exercise intervention programmes in random controlled trials *not showing an effect* of the intervention on falls

Study	Sample size	Effect size (follow-up period)	High-risk	Mean age	Time (mins)	Duration of exercise (months)	Freq. (per week)	Resist.	Bal.	Funct.	End.	Walk.	Flex.	Type	Intensity	Progressive	Most exercise in standing	Aim to reduce arm support
									Type of exercise						Individualized			
Walking programmes – community dwellers																		
Ebrahim et al. [22]	165	Excess cumulative risk of falls = 15 per 100 person years, 95% CI 1.4–29 (2 years)	✓	67	40	24	3	✗	✗	✗	✗	✓	✗	✗	✓	✓	✓	✗
Sub-total			1/1	67	40	24	3	0/1	0/1	0/1	0/1	1/1	0/1	0/1	1/1	1/1	1/1	0/1
Exercise in groups – community dwellers																		
Bunout et al. [23]	294	24 falls in control group, 25 falls in exercise group (1 year)	✗	75	~60	12	2	✓	✗	✓	✗	✓	✗	✗	✓	✓	✓	✓
Carter et al. [24]	93	8 falls in control group, 7 falls in exercise group (20 weeks)	✗	69	40	5	2	✓	✓	✓	✗	✗	✓	✗	✓	✓	✗	✗
Lord et al. [25]	197	Relative risk of one or more falls = 0.99, 95% CI 0.65–1.5 (1 year)	✗	72	60	12	2	✓	✓	✗	✓	✗	✓	✗	✗	✗	✗	✗
McMurdo et al. [26]	118	31 falls in control group, 15 falls in exercise group (p=0.16) (2 years)	✗	65	45	24	3	✗	✓	✗	✓	✗	✓	✗	✗	✗	✓	✗
Morgan et al. [27]	294	Percentage who fell – 28.6 in exercise group and 30.9 in control group (1 year)	✓	81	45	2	3	✓	✓	✗	✗	✗	✓	✓	✓	✓	✓	✗
Reinsch et al. [28]	230	Percentage who fell – 25 in exercise group, 19 in CBT, 37 in combined group, 19 in discussion group (1 year).	✗	74	60	12	3	✗	✓	✓	✗	✗	✓	✗	✗	✗	✓	✗

Study	n	Outcome		Age	% female	Duration	Freq/wk										
Steinberg et al. [29]	252	Hazard ratio for time to first fall in the exercise vs. control group=0.67, 95% CI 0.42–1.07 (2 years)	✗	69	60	17	0.2	✓	✓	✗	✗	✓	✓	✓	✓	✓	✓
Wolf et al*. [30]	311	Risk ratio of falling = 0.75, 95% CI 0.52–1.08 (12 months)	✓	81	75	11	2	✗	✓	✗	✗	✓	✓	✓	✓	✓	✓
Sub-total			2/8	73	60#	12	2	5/8	7/8	3/8	2/8	2/8	6/8	2/8	5/8	6/8	4/8
Individual exercise – community dwellers																	
Campbell et al. [32]	93	Relative hazard ratio for exercise vs. no exercise = 0.87, 95% CI 0.36–2.09 (44 weeks)	✓	74	30	12	3	✓	✓	✗	✓	✓	✓	✓	✓	✓	✓
Campbell et al. [33]	391	Incident rate ratio for rate of falls = 1.15, 95% CI 0.82–1.61 (1 years)	✓	84	30	11	3	✓	✓	✓	✓	✓	✓	✓	✓	✓	✓
Latham et al. [34]	243	Relative risk of a fall = 0.96, 95% CI 0.67–1.36 (6 months)	✓	80	NK	2.5	3	✓	✗	✗	✗	✗	✗	✓	✓	✗	✗
Sub-total			3/3	80	30#	12	3	3/3	2/3	2/3	0/3	2/3	2/3	2/3	3/3	2/3	2/3
Individual exercise – institution dwellers																	
Mulrow et al. [35]	194	79 falls in exercise group and 60 falls among control subjects (?4 months).	✓	80	37	4	3	✓	✓	✓	✓	✓	✓	✓	✓	✓	✗
Sub-total			1/1	80	45#	4	3	1/1	1/1	1/1	1/1	0/1	1/1	1/1	1/1	1/1	0/1
Total			7/13 (53%)	75	45#	12#	3#	9/13 (69%)	10/13 (77%)	6/13 (45%)	3/13 (23%)	5/13 (38%)	7/13 (58%)	4/13 (31%)	8/13 (62%)	9/13 (69%)	7/13 (58%)	4/13 (31%)

Resist. = Resistance training, Bal. = balance training, Funct. = functional training, End. = endurance training, Walk. = walking program, Flex. = flexibility

*congregate living facility residents

#Median

CBT = cognitive behavioural therapy, NK = not known

there was also a trend indicating a reduction in fall injuries (incident rate ratio = 0.66, 95% CI = 0.38–1.15).

Buchner *et al.* [9] compared the effect of resistance training, endurance training and a combination of both to a control group. There were 105 community-dwelling participants with a mean age of 75 years. Participants attended a one-hour exercise group three times a week for the first 24–26 weeks of the study, and then chose whether to continue to exercise either with supervision in a group or at home without supervision. In the resistance, endurance and combination groups, exercises were individually prescribed in intensity but not type. The resistance training group carried out a series of lower limb strengthening exercises using resistance machines, performing the first set at 50–60% of one repetition maximum (1RM) and the second set at 75% 1RM. Endurance training was carried out on stationary cycles at 75% heart rate reserve (age-adjusted maximal heart rate minus resting heart rate). The combination group carried out endurance and resistance training. No specific exercises were aimed at functional task training, flexibility, or gait and balance training. After nine months, 58% of the 61 participants were exercising three times a week, 24% twice a week and 5% not at all. When the exercise groups were considered together, exercise resulted in significantly reduced fall rates (relative risk = 0.61, 95% CI = 0.39–0.93) and an increased time to first fall (Cox relative hazard = 0.53, 95% CI = 0.30–0.91).

Day *et al.* [10] used a factorial design to analyse the effect of a combination of exercise and/or reduced vision management and/or home hazard modification, compared to a control group, in 1090 community-dwelling participants with a mean age of 76 years. The exercise group consisted of individualized strength, gait, balance and flexibility exercises designed by a physiotherapist, and performed in a group setting for one hour once a week for 15 weeks. Additionally, participants were expected to exercise daily at home. Participants attended an average of ten exercise group sessions. In those randomized to exercise, the falls rate ratio of time to first fall was 0.82 (95% CI = 0.70–0.97). A larger risk reduction was seen when interventions aimed at improving vision and reducing home hazards were also undertaken (rate ratio = 0.67, 95% CI = 0.51–0.81).

Means *et al.* [11] compared an exercise programme involving six weeks of stretching, balance, endurance, coordination and strengthening exercises in groups of 6–8 people supervised by a physiotherapist, with an education seminar control programme. Training sessions 90 minutes long were held three times a week. Of the 181 people randomized to the intervention group, 169 attended exercise sessions but 19 ceased involvement for a range of reasons. Among the baseline fallers in the intervention group, 87% (compared with 34.5% for the controls) reported no falls in the subsequent six months. While no between-group comparison of fall rates was reported in the paper, we calculated the relative risk of falling in the six months after the intervention to be 0.40 (95% CI = 0.25–0.63) from the falls data given, i.e. 22 fallers among the exercise group (15%) and 36 fallers in the control group (38%).

Skelton *et al.* [12] tested the effect of group exercise with a supplementary home programme in 100 people with a mean age of 73 years. Subjects were at a high risk of falls, having fallen at least three times in the year prior to commencing the study. The exercise intervention consisted of progressive individualized resistance, gait, balance, functional activity, endurance and flexibility training, undertaken in a group of 6–8 people lasting one hour once a week for 36 weeks. Participants were also instructed to carry out exercise twice a week at home. Exercise was individually tailored in both type and intensity; most exercises were in weight-bearing positions and aimed to reduce upper limb support. Of those randomized to the exercise group, 17% refused and another 10% dropped out of the exercise sessions. The control group carried out a seated twice-weekly gentle exercise programme. There was a 31% reduction in the number of falls during the trial period for the exercise group compared with the control group (incident rate ratio = 0.69, 95% CI = 0.50–0.96). There was also a trend for a decrease in injurious falls (incident rate ratio = 0.60, 95% CI = 0.33–1.07).

Wolf *et al.* [13] compared Tai Chi, computerized balance training and an education control group in 200 community-dwelling participants with a mean age of 76 years. Participants who performed Tai Chi attended a group twice a week in which they received 45 minutes of individual attention. They were also expected to practise the Tai Chi exercises for 15 minutes twice every day. Computerized balance training was carried out once a week for 45 minutes and participants were given one-to-one supervision during the intervention. Both interventions lasted for 15 weeks and were progressive. Exercises were carried out in lower limb weight-bearing positions aiming to minimize the use of the arms for support. Most subjects completed the trial but ten exercise subjects ceased attendance at classes due to illness or carer responsibilities. Falls were measured between seven and 20 months after starting the intervention. Time to first fall was significantly increased after Tai Chi (risk ratio = 0.63, 95% CI = 0.45–0.89) (FISCIT fall definition of, unadjusted rate), but not after computerized balance training (risk ratio = 1.03, 95% CI = 0.74–1.41) compared to the education control group.

Li *et al.* [14] compared Tai Chi with a control stretching programme in 256 physically inactive community dwellers with a mean age of 77 years. Both groups attended a one-hour exercise class three times a week for six months.

The Tai Chi classes were taught by experienced Tai Chi instructors. They involved the Yang style, which is reported to focus on multidirectional weight shifting, awareness of body alignment and multi-segmental movement coordination, and synchronized breathing. The control programme focused on stretching for the trunk and upper body, in sitting and standing, and deep breathing. Median compliance was 61 sessions for both groups, and 80% of Tai Chi and 81% of stretching control participants attended 50 or more sessions. At the end of the six-month intervention period there were significantly fewer falls (n = 38 vs. 73, p = 0.007), lower proportions of fallers (28% vs. 46%, p = 0.01) and fewer injurious falls (7% vs. 18%, p = 0.03) in the Tai Chi group compared with the stretching control group. After adjusting for baseline covariates, the risk for multiple falls in the Tai Chi group was 55% lower than that of the stretching control group (risk ratio = 0.45, 95% CI = 0.30–0.70).

A recent, as yet, unpublished study [15] undertaken in Australia also evaluated Tai Chi as a strategy for preventing falls in a general population of older people with an average age of 68 years. This trial investigated the effectiveness of a one-hour Tai Chi class per week over 16 weeks for improving balance and reducing falls in 702 people aged 60 years or over. Within the intervention group, approximately 50% (173/322) of participants attended 13 out of 16 Tai Chi classes, with 75% (243/322) attending at least half of the classes. There was a 35% reduction in falls in the intervention group compared to the control group in the one-year follow-up period (incident rate ratio = 0.65, 95% CI = 0.47–0.89).

Exercise in groups – transitional

Our research group [16] studied the effect of a general exercise programme on 551 participants with a mean age of 79 years. Most of the participants were living in self-care apartments in retirement villages (78%) and the remainder were living in assisted-care hostels. Group exercise classes were held in common rooms at each retirement village randomized to receive the intervention, and consisted of resistance, gait, balance, flexibility and endurance exercise delivered by a trained exercise instructor. Exercise was tailored in intensity but not type and all exercise was progressive. Resistance training involved increasing the number of repetitions. Gait and balance training was undertaken mostly in standing with minimal use of the arms for support, and involved activity designed to improve coordination and reaction times such as stepping exercises to music. Endurance training consisted of 5–15 minutes of slow/moderate paced walking. Groups lasted for one hour and took place twice a week for 12 months. On average, 39 sessions (42% of available) were attended. The general exercise programme was compared to a non-exercise control and seated programme.

Falls measured after one year were significantly reduced for those in the exercise group (incident rate ratio = 0.78, 95% CI = 0.62–0.99). The effect was greater for previous fallers (incident rate ratio = 0.69, 95% CI = 0.48–0.99) and smaller in people without a history of falling (incident rate ratio = 0.79, 95% CI = 0.60–1.05).

Individual exercise – community dwellers

Campbell *et al.* [17] targeted a home exercise programme to a population at increased risk of falls; women aged over 80 years. The home exercise programme was taught to participants in their own homes by a physiotherapist and compared to social visits as a control in 233 women with a mean age of 84. Exercises were individually prescribed from a set number of warm up, muscle strength and balance training exercises. Each participant was provided with an exercise folder and advised to complete the programme three times each week. They were also encouraged to walk outdoors at their desired pace, building up to 30 minutes 2–3 times a week. The physiotherapist visited each intervention participant four times over the first two months. The first session took approximately one hour to establish the programme. Then three half-hour follow-up sessions took place at one, three and seven weeks after the first session to monitor and progress the exercises, and help to motivate participants to continue with the programme. Lower-limb strengthening exercise was carried out at moderate intensity and individually prescribed using ankle cuff weights. Balance and gait exercises were performed in standing and progressed by minimizing the use of the upper limbs for external support. After the fourth visit, the physiotherapist maintained regular contact with participants by telephone. After one year, 42% of the participants reported they were still exercising three times a week. In the 12-month trial period, the exercise group had a significantly lower rate of falls (between-group difference = 0.47, 95% CI = 0.04–0.90) and the relative hazard for the first four falls was 0.68 (95% CI = 0.52–0.90). The relative hazard for a first fall with injury was also significantly lower, i.e. 0.61(95% CI = 0.39–0.97).

Of the initial 233 trial participants, 213 completed the first year [18] of the study and were invited to continue for another year. Of this cohort, 71 women (69%) in the intervention group and 81 women (74%) in the control group agreed to continue. The physiotherapist did not visit the participants in this time, but remained in telephone contact. By the end of the two year period, 44% of the 71 intervention participants were still exercising three times a week. At the end of the two-year study period, the relative hazard for all falls and falls with moderate or severe injury remained significantly lower for the exercise group (0.69, 95% CI = 0.49–0.97 and 0.63, 95% CI = 0.42–0.95, respectively). Those who adhered to the exercise programme had significantly higher physical activity levels at baseline and one year, higher falls efficacy scores, and were more likely to report a fall before the intervention commenced.

This exercise intervention, now called the Otago Exercise Programme[1], was then investigated in a further randomized controlled trial of 240 community-dwelling participants with a mean age of 81 [19]. This time the exercise was delivered by a district nurse who had attended a week-long training course given by a research physiotherapist. The only change to the programme was that participants were given a fifth home visit six months after commencing the exercises. The research physiotherapist provided supervision and telephone support for the district nurses, who carried out the exercise programmes in addition to usual district nursing duties. A total of 43% of participants reported exercising more than three times a week after one year. Falls were reduced by 46% following exercise (incident rate ratio = 0.54, 95% CI = 0.32–0.90). The number of falls was reduced in subjects aged 80 and over (81 falls in the control group and 43 falls in the exercise group), but there was no difference in subjects aged 75–79 years.

The Otago Exercise Programme was then studied in routine healthcare settings [20] by allocating 32 general practices into three intervention centres and one control centre. The study included 450 people with a mean age of 84 years. District nurses were trained to deliver the exercise programme as described above. Falls in the exercise centres were reduced by 30% (incident rate ratio = 0.70, 95% CI = 0.59–0.84).

Individual exercise – institution dwellers

Schnelle *et al.* [21] recruited 190 nursing home residents with a mean age of 88 years and a history of incontinence, a risk factor for falls. Intervention participants were seen by a research assistant up to four times a day and given a continence prompt, a supervised walk, asked to sit-to-stand eight times and encouraged to take on fluids. Additional upper limb resistance training was provided at tailored intensity, walking distance was gradually increased if possible and sit-to-stand exercise encouraged with minimal use of upper limbs for support. These sessions took place five days a week for eight months and participants completed an average of 3.2 sessions a day. On logit analysis there was a significant difference between groups for the number of residents experiencing a fall (OR ± standard error = 0.46 ± 0.18). The control group had an increased incidence of falls from baseline to follow-up while the intervention group remained stable.

---

[1] http://www.acc.co.nz/wcm001/idcplg?IdcService=SS_GET_PAGE&nodeId=4003

Programmes which did not prevent falls

Walking programmes – community dwellers

Ebrahim *et al.* [22] investigated the effect of a brisk walking programme on 165 women with mean ages of 66–70 years. Participants were recruited if they had suffered a previous upper limb fracture. Exercise participants were visited by a research nurse every three months and encouraged to build up to walking for 40 minutes three times a week. The programme was progressive and tailored in intensity with the aim of participants walking 'briskly'. After two years, there was a 41% drop out rate and the cumulative risk of falling was actually higher in the walking group (excess risk of 15 per 100 person years, 95% CI = 1.4–29 per 100 person years, $p < 0.05$).

Exercise in groups – community dwellers

Bunout *et al.* [23] examined the effect of weight-bearing resistance training in 298 healthy community-dwelling older people with a mean age of 75 years. Participants randomized to the exercise intervention carried out progressive weight-bearing resistance exercises predominantly involving the lower limbs and performed in standing with the aim of reducing arm support. The programme also included 15 minutes walking before and after the resistance training. Exercise took place in supervised groups twice a week for one year. A total of 51 participants dropped out of the study before the follow-up was complete. The remaining participants attended 24% of scheduled sessions over the year. During the follow-up year there were 24 falls in the control group and 25 in the exercise group. It is possible that under-reporting of falls occurred, as subjects reported falls at monthly outpatient clinics and were considered dropouts if they failed to attend two or more times.

Carter *et al.* [24] recruited 93 people with a diagnosis of osteoporosis and an average age of 69 years. Intervention participants carried out resistance, gait, balance, functional activity practise and flexibility exercises in groups of 12, supervised by an exercise instructor. The exercise programme took 40 minutes to complete and participants were expected to attend twice a week for 20 weeks. Exercise was tailored and progressed in intensity but not type. Some balance exercise was carried out in standing but it was not clear if the aim of the exercise was to challenge postural stability by minimizing arm support. Completers participated in 89% of the exercise sessions. There were seven falls reported in the intervention compared to eight in the control group, indicating no significant difference in fall rates after 20 weeks of exercise.

Our research group [25] studied the effect of general exercise compared to a control group in 197 community-dwelling women not at increased risk of falls with a mean age of 72 years. Exercises included resistance, balance, gait, endurance and flexibility training. Balance exercises were carried out in weight-bearing positions but exercises were not tailored in intensity or type and nor were they progressive. Each exercise session lasted one hour and was held twice a week. The programme was delivered in four terms of 10–12 weeks over one year. Participants attended an average of 60 sessions. Falls were not significantly reduced after one year (relative risk of one or more falls = 0.99, 95% CI = 0.65–1.5) but there were fewer 'balance-related falls' (relative risk = 0.31, 95% CI = 0.11–0.91).

McMurdo et al. [26] recruited 118 women with a mean age of 65 years to take calcium supplements with or without exercise. Participants completed weight-bearing exercises in a group setting lasting 45 minutes and taking place three times a week for two years. The 78% of participants that completed the two-year programme attended 76% of classes. There was no overall between-group difference in fall rates (31 falls in the calcium only group and 15 falls in the calcium plus exercise group, $p = 0.158$). However, there was a significant reduction in falls between 12 and 18 months for the exercise group ($p = 0.011$).

Morgan et al. [27] compared resistance, gait and balance exercise to a control group in 294 older people at high risk of falls with a mean age of 81 years. Exercise participants carried out progressive resistance exercise using 2 lb ankle weights, and gait and balance training in groups of five. Group sessions were designed and delivered by a physiotherapist, lasted 45 minutes, and took place three times a week for eight weeks. Participants were then provided with a home exercise programme to continue when the group sessions were complete. Exercise was individualized in type and intensity but it is not clear how challenging the balance training was. Participants attended an average of 70% of sessions and 69% completed the study. When the intervention and control groups were compared, there was no significant difference in fall rates (28.6% of exercise group fell and 30.9% of the control group fell). However, among subjects with a low score on the physical function section of the SF36 health survey scale, the time to first fall was longer among exercise subjects than controls (Cox Hazard ratio = 0.51, $p \leq 0.03$). Conversely, among intervention subjects with a high score on the physical function section of the SF36, the time to first fall was actually longer among control subjects than intervention subjects (Cox Hazard ratio = 3.51, $p \leq 0.02$).

Reinsch et al. [28] randomized 230 people with a mean age of 74 years into four groups consisting of exercise alone, cognitive behavioural therapy (CBT), a combination of exercise and CBT, and a discussion group. In the exercise intervention, groups of 5–25 people carried out low-intensity resistance training, balance and gait training in weight-bearing positions, functional task training, and flexibility exercise. It was not clear whether exercises were progressive or tailored. Sessions lasted one hour and took place three times a week for 52 weeks. There was a 20% attrition rate over the year. The time to first fall was not significantly different between the groups, and the proportion of people in each group who fell one or more times was 25% for the exercise group, 19% for CBT, 37% for the combined group and 19% for the discussion group.

Steinberg et al. [29] used an 'add on' technique to analyse several interventions in 252 people aged over 50 years (70%–80% of participants were under 75 years). An education control group was compared with: (a) education and exercise; (b) education, exercise and home assessment; and (c) education, exercise, home and medical assessment. The exercise component consisted of exercise groups supplemented with a home exercise programme assisted by handouts and a video. Groups lasting one hour took place once a month for 17 months and participants were encouraged to exercise between classes. Exercises focused on strength, gait and balance but it was not clear whether exercise was progressive or tailored. When compared to the education control group, the hazard ratio for time to first fall in the exercise and education group was 0.67 (95% CI = 0.42–1.07).

Exercise in groups – transitional

Wolf et al. [30] evaluated the effect of Tai Chi compared to 'wellness' education in a cluster-randomized trial among 311 congregate living facility residents with a mean age of 81 years. Subjects were all 'transitionally frail' defined as neither frail nor vigorous on a set of criteria defined by Speechley and Tinetti [31]. Previous falls was an admission criterion for the study, making this a high-risk population. Tai Chi was taught to groups of up to 15 participants by a grand master or his student. The programme included progressively more challenging Tai Chi manoeuvres in weight-bearing positions with the aim of reducing the use of the arms for support. Groups took place in the participating centres twice a week, each session lasting 60–90 minutes and the programme ran for 48 weeks. Participants attended 76% of the sessions. The relative risk adjusted for each centre for the number of participants who fell at least once was 0.75 (95% CI = 0.52–1.08) reflecting a non-significant reduction in falls. However, the Tai Chi group had a significantly lower adjusted risk of falls in the final eight months of the trial (risk ratio = 0.54, 95% CI = 0.36–0.81).

Individual exercise – community dwellers

Campbell et al. [32] carried out a factorial trial on 93 community dwellers with group mean ages of between 73 and 76 years. The trial investigated the effect of: (a) the home exercise programme – the Otago Exercise Programme, described above [17]; (b) withdrawal of psychotropic medications; (c) both interventions; and (d) a control group. After 44 weeks, 63% of participants carried out the exercises three times a week and 72% walked more than twice a week. There was no significant difference in falls after exercise. The relative hazard ratio for exercise versus no exercise was 0.87 (95% CI = 0.36–2.09). While this study may have been under-powered to detect an effect of exercise on falls, it did find a reduction in falls following withdrawal of psychotropic medications.

The same research group have conducted a recent factorial trial among 391 older people with severe visual impairment [33]. Interventions comprised the Otago Exercise Programme plus vitamin D supplementation (n = 97), a home safety assessment and modification programme delivered by an occupational therapist (n = 100), both interventions (n = 98), or social visits (n = 96). Some 18% of the exercise participants completed the prescribed exercises three or more times a week for one year and 36% completed the exercises as least twice a week. Fewer falls occurred in the group randomized to the home safety programme but not in the exercise programme (incident rate ratio = 0.59, 95% CI = 0.42–0.83 and 1.15, 0.82–1.61, respectively). Among those allocated to the exercise intervention groups, the rate of falls was 77% lower in those who exercised at least three times a week compared with those exercising less than once a week.

Individual exercise – transitional

Latham *et al.* [34] compared vitamin D supplementation, resistance training, placebo control and attention control interventions in 243 people with a mean age of 80 years. Participants randomized to the resistance programme started the exercise while they were hospital inpatients, with the first two visits by the physiotherapist occurring during this time. A total of 90% of the participants were community dwellers, the remaining residing in care homes. Participants were categorized as frail on the basis of functional impairment, chronic diseases and falls. The resistance training programme consisted of a series of stretches and seated resisted knee extension exercises (three sets of eight repetitions). Participants were advised to exercise three times a week for ten weeks. The physiotherapist provided support once a week with alternating home visits and telephone calls. The authors aimed to increase the resistance used to 60%–80% 1RM but the actual mean resistance was 13% 1RM. Exercise participants completed 82% of the prescribed sessions. There was no significant reduction in fall rates for either vitamin D or resistance training compared to the controls (relative risk = 1.72, 95% CI = 0.79–1.37 and 0.96, 95% CI = 0.67–1.36, respectively) or time to first fall (hazard ratio = 1.14, 95% CI = 0.8–1.62 and 0.97, 95% CI = 0.68–1.37, respectively). However, there was a significantly higher rate of musculo-skeletal injury (that required medical attention or resulted in limitation in activities of daily living for at least two days) (relative risk = 3.6, 95% CI = 1.5–8.0) for the resistance training group.

Individual exercise – institution dwellers

Mulrow *et al.* [35] analysed the effect of one-to-one physiotherapy compared to controls in 194 people living in nursing homes who had a mean age of 80 years. The physiotherapists used an algorithm to choose from a standardized set of exercises. The programme consisted of resistance, balance, functional task training, endurance and flexibility exercises. The exercises were progressive, and tailored in both type and intensity. Resistance training was carried out with elastic bands and cuffs and increased if ten repetitions could be carried out easily. Some exercise was carried out in weight-bearing positions if deemed appropriate by the physiotherapist. Each session lasted 30–45 minutes and took place three times a week for four months. Participants attended 89% of the scheduled physiotherapy sessions. In the six months after the intervention commenced, 44 of the physiotherapy group fell 79 times and 38 of the control group fell 60 times. This difference was not statistically significant ($p = 0.11$). There were seven serious injuries in the physiotherapy group compared to two in the control group, again a non-significant difference ($p = 0.16$).

What do these studies tell us about exercise interventions for falls prevention?

Tables 10.2 and 10.3 summarize the features of the 12 intervention programmes which have been found to lead to a reduction in falls and the 13 which have not. This summary was collated from information given in the papers describing these studies. Direct contact with authors may have led to studies being differently described and was not undertaken for this chapter.

There does not appear to be a single factor that easily discriminates between programmes which have been found to prevent falls and those which have not. The success of exercise in reducing falls is probably a result of a combination of several key components acting together. Some studies that did not find an effect of exercise on falls were possibly under-powered to detect a difference between intervention and control groups, but this was not the case for all these studies. Features which are common to the programmes which prevented falls are summarized in box 10.1.

Box 10.1 Common features of effective exercise programmes for falls reduction.

(1) Type of exercise to include
   (a) balance exercises
   (b) exercises conducted in weight-bearing positions
   (c) exercises with the aim of reducing the amount of support provided by the arms
   (d) functional activity practise (i.e. stair climbing/sit-to-stand)
   (e) an additional component of endurance exercise to increase general fitness (but not a walking programme on its own)
   (f) an additional component of moderate-intensity resistance training

(2) Exercise prescription
   (a) progressive in intensity
   (b) individually prescribed intensity
   (c) exercises chosen to address the key risk factors of that individual or population group

(3) Nature of programme
   (a) sessions with a duration of 60 minutes (may need to build up to this level)
   (b) undertaken by participants at least three times a week
   (c) conducted for a minimum of six weeks (but long term exercise is probably required for sustained benefits)
   (d) either delivered in a group setting or on an individual basis
   (e) contain support mechanisms to motivate participants to maintain adherence (i.e. group camaraderie or telephone follow-up for home based programmes)

(4) Design and delivery
   (a) programmes designed by a trained professional (a physiotherapist in most cases)
   (b) exercises delivered by a trained instructor (to ensure exercises are challenging yet safe)

Type of exercise

Balance training

In all but one of the 12 exercise trials which prevented falls, balance training was undertaken. This supports the finding of the pre-planned meta-analysis [36] of the seven FICSIT (Frailty and Injuries: Cooperative Studies of Intervention Techniques) trials among a total of 2328 older people. The adjusted fall incidence ratio for the treatment arms including general exercise was 0.90 (95% CI = 0.81–0.99) and for those including balance training it was 0.83 (95% CI = 0.70–0.98). In other words, the incidence of falls was probably reduced by about 10% in those undertaking any exercise and by about 17% in those undertaking balance exercise.

Most successful balance training programmes are undertaken primarily in a weight-bearing position with an emphasis on reducing support from the upper limbs. These factors appear to be key discriminators between effective and ineffective interventions.

Tai Chi has now been found to be effective in preventing falls in three samples of community-dwelling participants [13–15]. We have classified Tai Chi as balance training but there may be additional benefits of Tai Chi over and above other types of balance training. This requires further investigation. In the study among frailer people, the reduction in falls was not quite significant [30] (risk ratio of falling $= 0.75$, 95% CI $= 0.52$–1.08). Perhaps in this study [30], the Tai Chi may have been too difficult for some subjects, thus they did not get as many benefits from the programme as they would have from an 'easier' programme that was still challenging for them. The authors did find a significant reduction in falls during the latter part of the study; this supports the idea that with practice, participants improved and were then able to obtain more benefits from Tai Chi.

Ten of the 13 randomized controlled trials that did not find an effect on falls from the interventions studied also involved balance training. Despite the lack of an effect on falls, several of these programmes led to some improvements in balance ability [24, 25]. The studies in which programmes including balance training did not affect falls were mostly conducted in relatively able populations. Perhaps the intervention was not challenging enough to balance to reduce falls in this group of people. Several of the studies involving balance training that did not affect falls, did not mention a specific aim of reducing arm support and several did not mention being primarily conducted in a standing position.

Functional training

Seven of the successful trials included functional task training in their programmes. This was often done in conjunction with balance or strength training. There is increasing evidence that both muscle strength and postural stability mechanisms are specific to a task [37], and that challenging, functionally relevant exercise is the optimal way to improve task-related balance function. Six of the randomized controlled trials that did not find an effect on falls from the interventions studied also involved functional task training, so, as for balance training, other aspects of exercise prescription are also important.

Endurance training/walking programmes

Five of the studies that found an effect of exercise on fall rates included endurance training. One study [9] found that endurance training either alone or combined with strength training led to increased aerobic capacity, but neither intervention led to improved balance or gait. Three trials not preventing falls also included endurance training. However, walking programmes when conducted as the only intervention have not been successful. The study conducted by Ebrahim *et al.* [22], in which participants (who had had a previous upper limb fracture) were encouraged to undertake brisk walking three times a week led to enhanced fitness but an increased frequency of falls. As subjects were only visited every three months it is possible that this programme was not closely supervised enough to encourage sufficient intensity or, alternatively, that these participants were put at increased risk by the advice to walk outdoors. Three studies showing an effect on falls included a walking programme as did five studies not finding an effect on falls.

Resistance training

Latham *et al.* [34] have conducted the only trial which has assessed the effect of seated resistance training alone on fall rates. This study involved progressive seated resistance training of the knee extension muscle groups and did not find an effect on falls (relative risk = 0.96, 95% CI = 0.67–1.36). The desired level of intensity, 60%–80% of 1RM, was found to be difficult to achieve in the home setting and this regime also increased the risk of musculo-skeletal injury. Moderate intensity strength training may take longer to achieve the desired increases in strength, but may minimize the risk of injury and optimize adherence [17].

As strength is a key risk factor for falls, there may be a role for strength training in isolation or as part of combined falls prevention exercise programmes. More research is needed to clarify the role of resistance training at various intensities and in various population groups. Nine of the studies finding an effect on falls included resistance training as did nine studies not finding an effect. As discussed in Chapter 11, the effect of resistance training on functional abilities is probably greatest in people whose muscle strength has fallen below a critical threshold associated with declining physical function, and when the training targets the lower-limb muscle groups involved in postural stability. There may also be a role for higher intensity strength training in early prevention programmes among 'fitter' people, to enable them to better withstand future age-related deterioration.

Flexibility training

No studies have evaluated the role of flexibility training alone in preventing falls. Elements of flexibility are included in most programmes (seven of the successful programmes and nine of the unsuccessful programmes). Flexibility exercise may play a direct role in improving the person's ability to withstand threats to their postural stability (i.e. increasing range of movement around the ankles) while others act as 'warm up' exercises or stretches which may prevent injury or discomfort as a result of other exercises. However, the optimal way to increase flexibility and the role of stretching in injury prevention remains unclear [38–40].

Combined training

Several types of exercise, which have not been shown to prevent falls in isolation, have been part of successful programmes. For example, resistance training was included in most of the effective trials. Endurance training to increase general fitness, exercise tolerance and reduce muscle fatigability is again probably an important supplement to balance exercise, as in everyday function balance must be maintained not just once, but continuously over sometimes protracted periods of time.

Prescription of exercise

Most trials involved progression of exercise (12/12 vs. 11/13 for studies finding or not finding an effect on falls respectively). While this did not distinguish greatly between successful and unsuccessful programmes, it is likely to be an important component of an exercise programme.

In trials finding an effect on falls, exercises were performed primarily in standing positions (11/12 vs. 9/13 for studies not finding an effect on falls) and challenged postural stability sufficiently to promote improved balance. One way of challenging postural stability is to gradually reduce reliance on the upper limbs for stability, retraining the use of lower-limb and trunk-balance mechanisms. Most successful programmes included a stated aim of reducing arm support during exercise (10/12 vs. 6/13 for studies not finding an effect on falls).

Successful programmes often involved individual prescription of the intensity of exercise (10/12) and some involved the individual prescription of type of exercise (3/12). However, these factors were just as common in the ineffective studies (10/13 and 5/13, respectively) so individual prescription in isolation does not appear to be an essential feature to prevent falls.

Time, duration and frequency of exercise

From the literature, it is difficult to determine the optimal exercise session frequency, exercise session time and programme duration for exercise to prevent falls. Effective sessions range from short interventions held 20 times a week in the residential aged care setting to 30–90 minute sessions conducted one to three times a week in a community setting. Several effective group community exercise programmes were held weekly in a group but also involved supplementary home exercise. Successful intervention programmes lasted for between six weeks and 12 months. It therefore seems that exercise frequency and programme duration are secondary in importance to exercise type and intensity.

It seems reasonable to conclude that exercise sessions should last for up to 60 minutes and take place at least three times a week. While it may be difficult for older people to attend a supervised exercise session more than once a week, home exercise programmes can be used in addition to group sessions [8, 10]. The minimum duration of exercise required to prevent falls was six weeks. However, if physical activity is not maintained in a meaningful way to preserve the gains in balance ability, muscle strength and fitness, the effect on falls is probably quickly lost. To maximize the effects of exercise, programmes should be ongoing.

Who provides the exercise?

All effective trials were designed and delivered by trained professionals, in most cases physiotherapists and exercise instructors. Training and experience in delivering exercise to older people seems necessary for several reasons. Firstly, the appropriate type of exercise should be built into programmes with opportunities for the intensity to be adjusted to appropriately challenging levels. Secondly, those delivering the exercise should have the confidence and experience to provide exercises that are sufficiently challenging, while minimizing the risk of falls and injury during exercise. As discussed in Chapter 11, strategies to enhance adherence should also be undertaken.

Group or individual (home based)

No studies with falls outcome measures have directly compared group and individual exercise. However, there appears to be little difference between individual and group settings in terms of adherence and effectiveness, providing attention is paid to other key elements such as type, intensity and progression of exercise. It is likely that some individuals will be more willing and able to exercise in a group setting and others in a home setting.

Target population

Seven of each group of trials (i.e. preventing falls and not preventing falls) were carried out among high-risk populations. Some studies have found exercise programmes to be more effective in people at higher risk. The Otago Exercise Programme was most effective for people aged over 80 years who had previously fallen [17] and was not effective with people in their 70s without a history of falls [41]. In our trial investigating group exercise among residents of retirement villages and hostels [16], we found people who had fallen previously had the greatest benefit in terms of falls reduction. Some studies have failed to demonstrate an effect because their participants were more vigorous and were not sufficiently challenged by the programme, and/or had low fall rates making between-group differences difficult to detect (e.g. [23–26]).

The ability of exercise alone to reduce falls probably also depends on the presence of other risk factors for falling among participating individuals. The Day *et al.* study [10] found a greater effect of a combined intervention programme than exercise alone, indicating that for some subjects the addition of other interventions was also necessary. The two factorial studies by Campbell *et al.* [32, 33] found greater effects of interventions targeted to particular needs for high-risk groups. The study of psychoactive medication reduction [32] among those taking these medications found that this strategy was more successful than exercise. Similarly, the study of exercise and home modification [33] among those with visual impairment found greater effects on falls from home modification. This finding may, in part, be due to the likely differences in exercise adoption and adherence levels among different populations. The recent study among older people with low visual acuity found that within the exercise group, better adherence to the exercise programme was associated with fewer falls ($p = 0.001$) [33].

Conclusion

Based on current evidence, effective exercise programmes for preventing falls comprise a combination of challenging and progressive balance exercises performed in weight-bearing positions that minimize the use of the upper limbs for support. Resistance, endurance and flexibility training may provide additional benefits if combined with the balance exercises. Exercise should be individualized in intensity, progressed over time, targeted to an appropriate population and conducted by trained personnel in a group or on an individual basis. As it is not the case that each form of exercise will reduce the risk of falling for every older person, careful consideration should be given to the type of exercise prescribed. As with other falls prevention interventions, exercise is likely to be more effective if targeted to the person's particular deficits and lifestyle.

REFERENCES

1. NICE, *Clinical Guideline 21. Falls: the Assessment and Prevention of Falls in Older People* (London: National Institute for Clinical Excellence, 2004).
2. J. Moreland, J. Richardson, D. H. Chan *et al.*, Evidence-based guidelines for the secondary prevention of falls in older adults. *Gerontology*, **49**(2) (2003), 93–16.
3. G. Feder, C. Cryer, S. Donovan & Y. Carter, Guidelines for the prevention of falls in people over 65. *British Medical Journal*, **321** (2000), 1007–11.
4. E. Hadley, The science of the art of geriatric medicine. *Journal of the American Medical Association*, **273** (1995), 1381–3.

5. J. Steadman, N. Donaldson & L. Kalra, A randomized controlled trial of an enhanced balance training program to improve mobility and reduce falls in elderly patients. *Journal of the American Geriatrics Society*, **51**(6) (2003), 847–52.

6. K. M. Means, D. E. Rodell, P. S. O'Sullivan & L. A. Cranford, Rehabilitation of elderly fallers: pilot study of a low to moderate intensity exercise program. *Archives of Physical Medicine and Rehabilitation*, **77** (1996), 1030–6.

7. M. A. Pereira, A. M. Kriska, R. D. Day *et al.*, A randomized walking trial in postmenopausal women: effects on physical activity and health 10 years later. *Archives of Internal Medicine*, **158**(15) (1998), 1695–701.

8. A. Barnett, B. Smith, S. R. Lord, M. Williams & A. Baumand, Community-based group exercise improves balance and reduces falls in at-risk older people: a randomised controlled trial. *Age and Ageing*, **32**(4) (2003), 407–14.

9. D. M. Buchner, M. E. Cress, B. J. de Lateur *et al.*, The effect of strength and endurance training on gait, balance, fall risk, and health services use in community-living older adults. *Journals of Gerontology. Series A, Biological Sciences and Medical Sciences*, **52**(4) (1997), M218–24.

10. L. Day, B. Fildes, I. Gordon *et al.*, A randomized factorial trial of falls prevention among older people living in their own homes. *British Medical Journal*, **325** (2002), 128–33.

11. K. M. Means, D. E. Rodell & P. S. O'Sullivan, Balance, mobility, and falls among community-dwelling elderly persons: effects of a rehabilitation exercise program. *American Journal of Physical Medicine and Rehabilitation*, **84**(4) (2005), 238–50.

12. D. Skelton, S. Dinan, M. Campbell & O. Rutherford, Tailored group exercise (FaME) reduces falls in community dwelling older frequent fallers (a RCT) (research letter). *Age and Ageing*, **34**(6) (2005), 636–9.

13. S. L. Wolf, H. X. Barnhart, N. G. Kutner *et al.*, Reducing frailty and falls in older persons: an investigation of Tai Chi and computerized balance training. Atlanta FICSIT Group. Frailty and injuries: cooperative studies of intervention techniques. *Journal of the American Geriatrics Society*, **44**(5) (1996), 489–97.

14. F. Li, P. Harmer, K. J. Fisher *et al.*, Tai Chi and fall reductions in older adults: a randomized controlled trial. *Journals of Gerontology. Series A, Biological Sciences and Medical Sciences*, **60**(2) (2005), 187–94.

15. A. Voukelatos, R. Cumming, S. Lord & C. Rissel, A randomised controlled trial of Tai Chi for prevention of falls: the Central Sydney Tai Chi trial. *Manuscript under review*.

16. S. R. Lord, S. Castell, J. Corcoran *et al.*, The effect of group exercise on physical functioning and falls in frail older people living in retirement villages: a randomized, controlled trial. *Journal of the American Geriatrics Society*, **51**(12) (2003), 1685–92.

17. A. J. Campbell, M. C. Robertson, M. M. Gardner *et al.*, Randomised controlled trial of a general practice programme of home based exercise to prevent falls in elderly women. *British Medical Journal*, **315**(7115) (1997), 1065–9.

18. A. J. Campbell, M. C. Robertson, M. M. Gardner, R. N. Norton & D. M. Buchner, Falls prevention over 2 years: a randomized controlled trial in women 80 years and older. *Age and Ageing*, **28**(6) (1999), 513–8.

19. M. C. Robertson, N. Devlin, M. M. Gardner & A. J. Campbell, Effectiveness and economic evaluation of a nurse delivered home exercise programme to prevent falls. 1. Randomised controlled trial. *British Medical Journal*, **322**(7288) (2001), 697–701.

20. M. C. Robertson, M. M. Gardner, N. Devlin, R. McGee & A. J. Campbell, Effectiveness and economic evaluation of a nurse delivered home exercise programme to prevent falls. 2. Controlled trial in multiple centres. *British Medical Journal*, **322**(7288) (2001), 701–4.

21. J. F. Schnelle, K. Kapur, C. Alessi *et al.*, Does an exercise and incontinence intervention save healthcare costs in a nursing home population? *Journal of the American Geriatrics Society*, **51**(2) (2003), 161–8.

22. S. Ebrahim, P. W. Thompson, V. Baskaran & K. Evans, Randomized placebo-controlled trial of brisk walking in the prevention of postmenopausal osteoporosis. *Age and Ageing*, **26**(4) (1997), 253–60.

23. D. Bunout, G. Barrera, M. Avendaño *et al.*, Results of a community-based weight-bearing resistance training programme for healthy Chilean elderly subjects.. *Age and Ageing*, **34**(1) (2005), 80–3.

24. N. D. Carter, K. M. Khan, H. A. McKay *et al.*, Community-based exercise program reduces risk factors for falls in 65- to 75-year-old women with osteoporosis: randomized controlled trial. *Canadian Medical Association Journal*, **167**(9) (2002), 997–1004.

25. S. Lord, J. Ward, P. Williams & M. Strudwick, The effect of a 12-month exercise trial on balance, strength, and falls in older women: a randomized controlled trial. *Archives of Physical Medicine and Rehabilitation*, **43** (1995), 1198–206.

26. M. E. McMurdo, P. A. Mole & C. R. Paterson, Controlled trial of weight bearing exercise in older women in relation to bone density and falls. *British Medical Journal*, **314**(7080) (1997), 569.

27. R. O. Morgan, B. A. Virnig, M. Duque, E. Abdel-Moty & C. A. DeVito, Low-intensity exercise and reduction of the risk for falls among at-risk elders. *Journals of Gerontology. Series A, Biological Sciences and Medical Sciences*, **59**(10) (2004), 1062–7.

28. S. Reinsch, P. MacRae, P. A. Lachenbruch & J. S. Tobis, Attempts to prevent falls and injury: a prospective community study. *Gerontologist*, **32**(4) (1992), 450–6.

29. M. Steinberg, C. Cartwright, N. Peel & G. Williams, A sustainable programme to prevent falls and near falls in community dwelling older people: results of a randomised trial. *Journal of Epidemiology and Community Health*, **54**(3) (2000), 227–32.

30. S. L. Wolf, R. W. Sattin, M. Kutner *et al.*, Intense tai chi exercise training and fall occurrences in older, transitionally frail adults: a randomized, controlled trial. *Journal of the American Geriatrics Society*, **51**(12) (2003), 1693–701.

31. M. Speechley & M. Tinetti, Falls and injuries in frail and vigorous community elderly persons. *Journal of the American Geriatrics Society*, **39** (1991), 46–52.

32. A. J. Campbell, M. C. Robertson, M. M. Gardner, R. N. Norton, D. M. Buchner, Psychotropic medication withdrawal and a home based exercise programme to prevent falls: results of a randomised controlled trial. *Journal of the American Geriatrics Society*, **47** (1999), 850–3.

33. A. Campbell, M. Robertson, S. La Grow *et al.*, Randomised controlled trial of prevention of falls in people aged 75 with severe visual impairment: the VIP trial. *British Medical Journal*, **331**(7520) (2005), 817–925.

34. N. K. Latham, C. S. Anderson, A. Lee *et al.*, A randomized, controlled trial of quadriceps resistance exercise and vitamin D in frail older people: the Frailty Interventions Trial in Elderly Subjects (FITNESS). *Journal of the American Geriatrics Society*, **51**(3) (2003), 291–9.

35. C. D. Mulrow, M. B. Gerety, D. Kanten *et al.*, A randomized trial of physical rehabilitation for very frail nursing home residents. *JAMA: Journal of the American Medical Association*, **271**(7) (1994), 519–24.

36. M. A. Province, E. C. Hadley, M. C. Hornbrook *et al.*, The effects of exercise on falls in elderly patients. A preplanned meta-analysis of the FICSIT trials. Frailty and injuries: cooperative studies of intervention techniques. *JAMA: the Journal of the American Medical Association*, **273**(17) (1995), 1341–7.

37. J. Carr & R. Shepherd, *Neurological Rehabilitation: Optimizing Motor Performance* (Oxford: Butterworth-Heinemann, 1998).

38. R. D. Herbert & M. Gabriel, Effects of stretching before and after exercising on muscle soreness and risk of injury: systematic review. *British Medical Journal*, **325**(7362) (2002), 468–71.

39. L. A. Harvey, A. J. Byak, M. Ostrovskaya, Randomised trial of the effects of four weeks of daily stretch on extensibility of hamstring muscles in people with spinal cord injuries. *Australian Journal of Physiotherapy*, **49**(3) (2003), 176–81.

40. A. M. Moseley, R. D. Herbert, E. J. Nightingale *et al.*, Passive stretching does not enhance outcomes in patients with plantarflexion contracture after cast immobilization for ankle fracture: a randomized controlled trial. *Archives of Physical Medicine and Rehabilitation*, **86** (6) (2005), 1118–26.

41. M. C. Robertson, A. J. Campbell, M. M. Gardner & N. Devlin, Preventing injuries in older people by preventing falls: a meta-analysis of individual-level data. *Journal of the American Geriatrics Society*, **50**(5) (2002), 905–11.

42. N. B. Alexander, N. Bentur, D. Strasburg & L. V. Nyquist, Fall risk reduction in Israeli day care centre attendees using exercise and behavior strategies [abstract]. *Journal of the American Geriatrics Society*, **51**(Suppl 4) (2003), S117.

43. L. L. Buettner, Focus on caregiving. Falls prevention in dementia populations: following a trial program of recreation therapy, falls were reduced by 164 percent. *Provider*, **28**(2) (2002), 41–3.

44. K. Cerny, R. Blanks, O. Mohamed *et al.*, The effect of a multidimensional exercise program on strength, range of motion, balance and gait in the well elderly [abstract]. *Gait and Posture*, **7**(2) (1998), 185–6.

45. M. Fiatarone, E. O'Neill, R. Doyle & K. Clements, *Efficacy of Home-Based Resistance Training in Frail Elders. Abstracts of the 16th Congress of the International Association of Gerontology.* (Bedford Park, South Australia, 1997).

46. K. Hauer, B. Rost, K. Rutschle *et al.*, Exercise training for rehabilitation and secondary prevention of falls in geriatric patients with a history of injurious falls. *Journal of the American Geriatrics Society*, **49** (2001), 10–20.

47. J. L. Helbostad, O. Sletvold & R. Moe-Nilssen, Effects of home exercises and group training on functional abilities in home-dwelling older persons with mobility and balance

problems. A randomized study. *Aging – Clinical and Experimental Research*, **16**(2) (2004), 113–21.

48. T. Liu-Ambrose, K. M. Khan, J. J. Eng *et al.*, Resistance and agility training reduce fall risk in women aged 75 to 85 with low bone mass: a 6-month randomized, controlled trial. *Journal of the American Geriatrics Society*, **52**(5) (2004), 657–65.

49. P. MacRae, M. Feltner & S. Reinsch, A 1-year exercise program for older women: Effects on falls, injuries and physical performance. *Journal of Aging and Physical Activity*, **2** (1994), 127–42.

50. J. C. Nitz & N. L. Choy, The efficacy of a specific balance-strategy training programme for preventing falls among older people: a pilot randomised controlled trial. *Age and Ageing*, **33**(1) (2004), 52–8.

51. B. Resnick, Testing the effect of the WALC intervention on exercise adherence in older adults. *Journal of Gerontological Nursing*, **28**(6) (2002), 40–9.

52. L. Rubenstein, K. Josephson, P. Trueblood *et al.*, Effects of a group exercise program on strength, mobility, and falls among fall-prone elderly men. *Journals of Gerontology. Series A, Biological Sciences and Medical Sciences*, **55A**(6) (2000), M317–21.

53. D. P. Schoenfelder, A fall prevention program for elderly individuals. Exercise in long-term care settings. *Journal of Gerontological Nursing*, **26**(3) (2000), 43–51.

54. C. Sherrington, S. R. Lord & R. D. Herbert, A randomized controlled trial of weight-bearing versus non-weight-bearing exercise for improving physical ability after usual care for hip fracture. *Archives of Physical Medical Rehabilitation*, **85**(2004), 710–6.

55. H. Shimada, S. Obuchi, T. Furuna & T. Suzuki, New intervention program for preventing falls among frail elderly people: the effects of perturbed walking exercise using a bilateral separated treadmill. *American Journal of Physical Medicine and Rehabilitation*, **83**(7) (2004), 493–9.

56. C. Toulotte, C. Fabre, B. Dangremont, G. Lensel & A. Thevenon, Effects of physical training on the physical capacity of frail, demented patients with a history of falling: a randomised controlled trial. *Age and Ageing*, **32**(1) (2003), 67–73.

57. M. P. Nowalk, J. M. Prendergast, C. M. Bayles, F. J. D'Amico & G. C. Colvin, A randomized trial of exercise programs among older Individuals living in two long-term care facilities: the Falls FREE program. *Journal of the American Geriatrics Society*, **49**(7) (2001), 859–65.

11

Exercise interventions to improve physical functioning

Written with Julie Whitney

As indicated in Chapter 10, exercise is a key intervention strategy for preventing falls in older people. Many diverse forms of exercise have been used in trials, ranging from highly prescribed resistance training regimes and laboratory-based balance training to unstructured general exercise programmes. In addition to studying the efficacy of exercise programmes on falls, many studies have also assessed the effectiveness of such programmes on a range of physical outcome measures, including strength, balance and gait. These studies elucidate the mechanisms by which exercise may prevent falls. Although falls are relatively common, most older individuals do not fall very frequently. Thus, large studies with long follow-up periods are required to detect the effects of exercise on fall rates. In contrast, the effects of exercise on risk factors for falls can be detected with smaller studies. Thus, complementary information can be gleaned from the analysis of studies with falls risk factors as outcome measures. Indeed, Liu-Ambrose and colleagues found that the risk of falling, as measured on the Physiological Profile Assessment tool (PPA, described in Chapter 16), could be reduced by around 50% by resistance or agility training [1].

This chapter describes the major forms of exercise that have been used in studies of older people, and summarizes the evidence for the effectiveness of each form on falls risk factors such as balance, strength and functional abilities. Additional considerations, including exercise setting selection, target population selection, and factors affecting adoption and adherence, are then explored.

Balance and functional task training

Background

As described in Chapter 2, balance or postural stability can be defined as the ability of an individual to maintain the position of the body, or more specifically, its centre of mass, within specific boundaries of space. Impaired balance is a clear risk factor for falls as is also discussed in Chapter 2. To maintain postural stability the person needs an awareness of where their body is in space and the ability to correct this by appropriately timed muscle contractions. These muscle contractions will be different for each task undertaken. To be able to safely carry out the variety of tasks necessary for daily living, the person needs to maintain balance in a range of situations, including standing still, reaching while standing, standing up from a chair, walking on different surfaces and responding to environmental challenges (e.g. stairs, slopes, obstacles, crowds). These everyday tasks can be considered to be motor skills.

As with any skilled activity, performance of functional tasks may be improved with motor training and practice. The motor learning model of rehabilitation [2, 3] emphasizes the role of practice, feedback and the environment in the performance of motor skills. This approach was originally developed for use after a stroke, but elements of it are relevant for motor task training in older people without neurological problems.

Among older people, performance of functional tasks may be hampered by a range of physical impairments. These limiting factors are likely to differ among individuals and differentially affect the range of functional tasks required for activities of daily living. It is likely that to maximize the functional effect of exercise, the physiotherapist or exercise leader needs to be able to assess what the major limitation is in performance of the task. An intervention programme tailored to these problems can then be developed and the effects of this intervention programme assessed using objective measures of motor performance (e.g. lowest height chair from which a person can stand up, timed walks). For some individuals, strength may be a limiting factor in the performance of a particular task and for others muscle shortening/joint stiffness may be more important. Different tasks also require different levels of skill. For example, the task of getting up from the floor is particularly difficult and seems likely to be amenable to motor training [4, 5]. As postural control is vital to safe performance of all daily tasks it is difficult to separate out balance training from functional motor task training.

Among older people without functional limitations, exercise programmes are also important to prevent age-related declines in strength and fitness which may lead to future functional impairments. A multi-component programme seems most sensible in this case.

Effects on balance

Many randomized controlled trials (RCTs) have now demonstrated that training can enhance balance abilities. Of the falls studies discussed in Chapter 10, seven of the exercise intervention programmes that prevented falls also led to improved balance [6–12]. Balance was also improved in three of the studies not finding an effect on falls [13–15]. Unfortunately a number of the falls studies did not measure balance [16–25]. Two of the RCTs that showed an effect on falls did not find an effect on balance [26, 27], but this may be due to the measurement tools chosen. Four of the studies that did not find an effect of their exercise programme on falls also did not find an effect on balance [28–31].

In a recent literature search, we identified 42 RCTs and five systematic reviews of training strategies primarily aimed to enhance balance in older people (we included only RCTs with between-group comparisons and more than 30 subjects; these trials are indexed on PEDro – the Physiotherapy Evidence Database[1]). These studies involved a mixture of group and individual training programmes. Of these studies 16 were published from 2003 onwards, indicating the recent growth of interest in this area. The majority of the RCTs identified (34 of the 42) found that balance training led to greater improvements in at least one measure of balance in the intervention group compared to a control group.

One exercise programme designed specifically to enhance balance and prevent falls is described by Lui-Ambrose et al. [1]. It involves a range of activities designed to challenge balance and coordination, including ball games, relay races, dance movements and obstacle courses. It reduced the risk of falls (on PPA assessment, see Chapter 16) by 48%.

One of the studies to show the effects of exercise on balance was conducted by Wolf et al. [32]. They found that among people aged 75 years and over with functional balance problems, an individualized balance training programme delivered in 12 sessions led to greater improvements in the Berg Balance Scale and Dynamic Gait Index than an attention control programme. Wolfson et al. [33] reported that balance training (involving various conditions with a computerized platform plus feedback, in standing, while sitting on a balance ball, and while walking on foam and a narrow beam) led to improved balance as measured by the sensory organization test, single stance time and voluntary limits of stability. Hansson et al. [34] trialled a group-based six-week balance and vestibular rehabilitation programme among people with dizziness of a central origin. They found greater improvements among the intervention group for the ability to stand on one leg with the eyes closed, but not for several other balance and gait tests, and a dizziness scale. Shimada et al. [35] have developed a bilateral separated treadmill system for training of perturbed walking. Among 32 long term care facility residents and outpatients, six months of this treadmill practice led to a significant improvement in balance and reaction time. However, gentle group-based programmes do not always enhance balance [36, 37].

---

[1] www.pedro.fhs.usyd.edu.au

In fact, all of the eight trials that did not find an effect on balance were group programmes.

A number of other studies investigating balance training programmes have not reported between-group differences (i.e. exercise vs. control), but found improved balance in the intervention group although not the control group. Examples of these programmes include: group exercise sessions for frail older people with an emphasis on balance and gait training [38]; group-based balance training for elderly people with non-peripheral vertigo and unsteadiness [39]; visual feedback-based balance training among frail care home residents [40]; and cobblestone mat walking [41]. Hiroyuki *et al.* [42] found that balance exercises improved 'static balance', and gait exercise improved 'dynamic balance' and gait.

Several studies have sought to distinguish between different types of balance training programmes. Nitz and Choy [43] found a specific balance strategy training programme delivered in a workstation format once a week for ten weeks was superior to a community-based general exercise class, in terms of the amount of improvement on functional measures. Other studies have not shown differences between two programmes but may not have been adequately powered to detect differences between fairly similar programmes [44–46].

Prescribing balance training programmes is particularly difficult as it is likely that to be effective a programme needs to be challenging, i.e. provide tasks that are difficult to do. To ensure that a programme remains difficult it needs to be monitored and progressed. The programme also needs to be able to be completed safely, so it does not cause falls or injury. Thus the prescription of effective balance training is particularly difficult where close supervision is not possible, i.e. at home and in a group setting. This may be why all of the trials of balance training we identified that were conducted in a group setting did not find an effect on balance. Several authors have developed programmes that can be safely and successfully conducted in these settings [6, 8, 47].

Effects on functional abilities

It is now clear from a number of RCTs that well-prescribed training can enhance a range of functional abilities. Seven of the falls exercise intervention studies found enhanced functional abilities among exercise subjects [7, 9–11, 22, 31, 48]. In five of these studies, falls were also prevented [7, 9–11, 22].

Many of the exercise programmes that aim to enhance functional task performance have included multiple components. Several studies have been conducted among community dwellers with functional limitations. Gill *et al.* [49, 50] evaluated a six-month home based physiotherapy 'prehabilitation' programme 'that focused primarily on improving underlying impairments in physical abilities, including balance, muscle strength, ability to transfer from one position to another and mobility', among 188 persons 75 years of age or older who were physically frail and living at home. They found that participants in the intervention group had less functional decline over time as indicated by their disability scores [49]. Intervention subjects also had improved functional scores and gains in mobility and physical performance at seven and 12 months [50]. The programme was more effective in those with moderate rather than severe frailty.

Worm *et al.* [51] evaluated a multi-component exercise programme among 46 community-dwelling frail older people above 74 years of age not able to leave their home without mobility aids. They found the intervention group had a significant improvement in balance, muscle strength, walking function and self-assessed functional ability compared with the control group. Similarly, the multi-component programme described by DeVito *et al.* [13] and Morgan *et al.* [52] (which included low-intensity resistance training, flexibility and postural exercise as well as balance and gait training in small groups for 24 sessions, followed by a home exercise programme) led to significantly greater improvements in functional abilities (as well as strength, balance and gait tests) among exercise subjects than control subjects. Subjects were all assessed as being at a high risk of falls due to recent hospitalization or bed rest. Timonen *et al.* [53] found benefits on strength, balance and gait speed from a programme of strength training and functional exercise among frail older women soon after hospital stays. Hauer *et al.* [54] found that, among people soon after hospital discharge with a history of injurious falls, intensive (three sessions a week for three months) training with a focus on strength, functional performance and balance improved physical performance significantly, and that between-group differences were maintained two years later [55].

Functional training has also been investigated among fitter people. Thompson and Osness [56] found that an eight-week programme of strength and flexibility training led to improved strength, range of motion and golf performance (measured via golf-club head speed). Nelson *et al.* [57] compared a home based progressive strength, balance and general physical activity intervention with an attention control programme among community dwellers. There was a between-group difference for the tandem walk test but not for measures of strength, gait speed or endurance. Hofmeyer *et al.* [5] found that it is possible to train older adults to get off the floor more easily using a strategy focusing on key intermediate body positions.

It seems that greater functional effects are likely with more functionally relevant exercises. To test this hypothesis, we compared weight-bearing exercise programmes with traditional non-weight-bearing programmes in 120 community-dwelling older people who had suffered a hip fracture. We found greater improvements in balance and functional ability with a home exercise programme of weight-bearing exercises (sit-to-stand, stepping up, stepping in different directions) than a bed exercise programme (hip flexion, hip abduction, knee flexion, knee extension, ankle dorsiflexion, ankle plantar flexion) [58].

Resistance training

Background

Muscle weakness is an important risk factor for falls [59]. Resistance training aims to increase the ability of a muscle or group of muscles to generate force. It is based on the overload principle first described by Roux and Lange in the early twentieth century, who suggested that performance of work of an intensity beyond its accustomed load would cause a muscle to grow in size and strength [60]. Progressive resistance training regimes for a range of patient groups were initially described by DeLorme and Watkins in the 1940s and 1950s [61]. Patients performed three sets of ten repetitions at increasing proportions of a weight that could only be lifted ten times (ten repetition maximum or 10RM). The 10RM was assessed weekly so that as the person became stronger, the load lifted was increased.

A large number of controlled trials have found resistance training can improve strength and power among older adults [62]. While it remains unclear whether resistance training alone can prevent falls in older people, resistance training has formed part of many successful falls prevention programmes and can also decrease risk of falling as measured on the PPA [1]. While the popular perception of resistance training continues largely to involve muscle-bound young men, several books aimed at older people outline practical aspects of strength training programmes for this age group [63, 64].

The American College of Sports Medicine (ACSM) [65] recommends that healthy sedentary adults undertake a strength training programme involving one set of 8–12RM of 8–10 different exercises twice weekly. It also recommends that older adults and people with cardiac disease carry out similar programmes at a slightly lower intensity (10–15RM) to decrease the risk of musculo-skeletal injury and cardiac complications [66, 67]. While few studies have compared strength training at different intensities for older people, there is some evidence for a greater relative effectiveness of lower-intensity programmes compared with higher-intensity programmes than in younger people [68, 69]. While there is evidence that high-intensity resistance training is more beneficial in terms of increasing muscle strength [70], this type of exercise has been associated with a greater risk of muscle soreness, injury and consequently non-adherence to a programme [30]. To decrease the risk of injury, it is common for strength training programmes for older people to include a warm-up set at a lower intensity [71].

Older people with various medical conditions may still be able to benefit from a strength training programme. For example, resistance training has been shown to reduce physical disability and pain among older people with osteoarthritis [72, 73], and high-intensity strength training (80% of 1RM) has been found to be safe and effective among aerobically trained cardiac patients [74]. Ades *et al.* [75] also found that among disabled older female cardiac patients, resistance training led to greater improvements in ability to perform a range of household physical activities than a light yoga and breathing exercise programme.

However, the risk of a cardiovascular event occurring during exercise is substantially increased among those with cardiac disease. Guidelines published by the American College of Sports Medicine and the American Heart Association (AHA) [76] suggest that cardiovascular screening be undertaken before a person of any age commences a moderate to high intensity exercise programme. Two screening tools are suggested, the revised *physical activity readiness questionnaire* (PAR-Q) and the AHA/ACSM *health/fitness facility pre-participation screening questionnaire*. If potential risk is identified on these brief questionnaires, the person is advised to contact their doctor for possible further investigation. These people should also exercise in a setting where medical or professional supervision is available.

Effects on strength

Epidemiological studies have shown that muscle strength decreases with increased age [77] and that reduced muscle strength is one of the major risk factors for falling [59, 78, 79]. Exercise interventions aimed at improving muscle strength have been widely identified as a key strategy for reducing frailty [80] and maintaining function [67] in old age. However, the role of strength training in the prevention of falls remains unclear.

It is now clear from a number of RCTs that resistance training can substantially increase muscle strength among community-dwelling older people [33, 81–85]. The recent Cochrane review [62] pooled the results of 41 studies using progressive resistance training in 1955 people aged over 65 and found significant improvements in muscle strength (standardized mean difference 0.68 95% CI = 0.52–0.84). On further examination high-intensity resistance training for longer than 12 weeks duration was most effective compared to moderate-to-low intensity training carried out for less than 12 weeks. A typical programme would involve the person lifting a weight of 50%–80% of their 1RM (the weight they are able to lift only once) using an exercise machine, two or three times weekly.

Resistance training can be carried out at home if well set up. For example, Jette *et al.* [86] trialled a six-month programme of exercise resisted with elastic sheeting among 215 older people with disability. They also used a motivational video and a range of behavioural strategies which included rewards for mailing completed exercise logs. This programme led to improved strength and balance, and decreased disability, but did not improve gait. In an earlier study among non-disabled community dwellers [87], a similar programme over 12–15 weeks led to improved strength among the younger subjects and psychological benefits among the male participants. However, there is also evidence that it is difficult to increase strength among frailer people with a home programme [30]. Some groups of people may require more supervision of resistance training to maximize benefits.

Resistance-training programmes are also possible among people living in supported accommodation. In a RCT of a ten-week resistance exercise programme among 100 frail nursing home residents, Fiatarone *et al.* [88] demonstrated significant increases in muscle strength, gait velocity, stair-climbing power and level of spontaneous physical activity in the exercisers compared with the controls. Hruda *et al.* [89] found positive effects on muscle power and functional abilities from power training. Several other non-controlled studies have also demonstrated the feasibility of this type of approach among nursing home residents [90, 91].

Effects on functional abilities

There is some controversy in the literature about the effect of strength training on functional abilities [67, 92]. Pooled results from the Cochrane review of RCTs on strength training found equivocal results of progressive resistance training on functional abilities. Resistance training in older people resulted in a significant improvement in gait speed (weighted mean difference 0.07 m/s, 95% CI = 0.04–0.09) and timed chair rise (standard mean difference −0.67, 95% CI = 1.31–0.02). However, there were no significant improvements in aerobic capacity, balance, Timed Up and Go, activities of daily living, physical function, health related quality of life and pain. Unfortunately, many strength training studies do not measure functional abilities and so do not offer additional information on this question. Keysor and Jette [93] reviewed 21 studies of aerobic and resistance training. They found that only half the studies included a measure of disability and of those that did most found no beneficial effect on this measure.

It has been found that a non-linear relationship exists between strength and function among older people. Buchner *et al.* [94] reported that among weaker people, leg strength and gait speed were associated, whereas among stronger people there was no relationship between the variables. It appears that stronger people were able to generate sufficient levels of muscle tension to successfully carry out the task, while the weaker people's lack of strength impaired performance of the task [94]. The level of strength required for a particular task has been referred to as the threshold value [95]. Threshold values have been identified for various tasks [96–101] but a minority of studies have found a more linear relationship between strength and function [102].

It seems likely that for people below a critical level of strength, strength training will lead to improved functional abilities [103]. Indeed, the studies which have shown functional improvements from non-weight-bearing strength training programmes have tended to be on weaker or less active people. The RCT which has shown some of the most substantial functional effects of strength training [88] took place among frail nursing home residents. Similarly, in a RCT [104] among people with knee osteoarthritis, decreased pain and improved function was found among the exercise group after six months of daily lower-limb strengthening exercise. Other studies finding effects on functional abilities have also been among the functionally impaired [95], and older people with osteoarthritis [105] and physical disability [72].

Among stronger people (who already have sufficient strength for functional tasks), an increase in strength will not improve functional performance of daily tasks but may be evident when more difficult tasks are assessed. For example, studies have shown improved abilities after strength training on backward tandem walk [106], stair-climbing endurance [107] and obstacle negotiation [108].

Several studies have shown that muscle power is more closely related to functional ability than muscle strength [109, 110] and recent studies have focused more on power training than strength training [89], with some conflicting findings on whether it leads to greater functional effects [111, 112].

It seems that task-related resistance training could have a greater effect on functional abilities than the more traditional non-weight-bearing resistance training. Studies among younger people have shown that the greatest improvements in muscle strength occur for the muscle action which has been trained and that carry-over to other muscle actions is limited [60, 113]. This principle of specificity of training has been shown to apply to the task trained [114], the velocity of contractions [115] and the angle of isometric contractions [116]. This means that strength training for isolated muscle groups in positions and velocities not relevant to everyday tasks may not be the most effective way to increase functional ability. For example, seated resistance training may improve the ability to lift a weight using the quadriceps muscle in sitting, but may not be the best way to improve stair-climbing ability. As Rutherford [117] suggests 'rather than using conventional exercises to strengthen individual muscle groups it may be more advantageous to identify particular functional deficits and then repeatedly practise these with or without added resistance'.

In recent years, a number of authors have reported using this approach [118–120]. For example, Rooks *et al.* [121] had subjects carry out weighted stair-climbing and resisted plantarflexion exercises in addition to seated knee extension exercise. This led to increased strength as well as improved performance on a number of weight-bearing tasks (stair-climbing, single leg balance and ability to reach down to the floor in standing). Similarly, Shaw and Snow [122] had subjects carry out weight-bearing exercises with weight vests to provide resistance. This led to significant increases in lower-limb strength and subjective reports of enhanced functional abilities among the intervention group. After an initial study [123] showing that weighted stair-climbing led to greater increases in muscle power than a walking programme, Bean *et al.* [124] compared two 12-week exercise programmes among community dwellers. They found greater improvements in leg power and chair stand time in a group who did resisted exercises, designed to be specific to mobility tasks, at the fastest possible velocity (called Increased Velocity Exercise Specific to Task – InVEST) than in a group who carried out slow-velocity, low-resistance exercise. In a RCT among 161 disabled older adults, Alexander *et al.* [125] found a 12-week task-specific resistance-training intervention (training in bed- and chair-rise subtasks with the addition of weights) enhanced overall ability and decreased bed- and chair-rise time compared to a control flexibility intervention.

Functional benefits have also been demonstrated when strength training is undertaken in combination with other types of training. As discussed previously, strength training has been a component of many studies that have enhanced functional abilities and prevented falls. However, the relative benefits of the different interventions could not be assessed in these studies. One such study, of both strength and endurance training [126], was conducted in a nursing home setting, where participants are likely to have had low initial levels of both strength and endurance. Work by Judge *et al.* showed that a programme of strength training, combined with endurance and balance training, improved balance [127] and gait velocity [128] among community dwellers. Binder *et al.* found that a six-months outpatient rehabilitation programme, which included resistance training, improved physical function and quality of life, and reduced disability, compared with low-intensity home exercise among frail older people [129] and among those after hip fracture [130].

The data reviewed above suggest that weaker older people can show improved functional abilities following traditional non-weight-bearing strength training programmes. However, older people with greater initial muscle strength do not always show such a carry-over. These individuals may have the capacity to improve functional ability with strength training in weight-bearing or skill training. Thus, the principles of specificity of training may be most important among stronger older adults. However, older people with less muscle strength may also derive greater benefit from training programmes designed around these principles, than from non-weight-bearing resistance training. This issue requires further investigation.

Endurance training

Background

Endurance training is not commonly discussed as a falls prevention strategy. However, increased age is associated with a loss of aerobic capacity [67] and difficulty performing activities of daily living. Difficulties in walking and transferring (e.g. from bed to chair) have been consistently associated with an increased risk of falling.

Even seemingly simple physical activities such as walking across a room, getting dressed or climbing stairs have energy requirements associated with them. Therefore, a certain level of cardiovascular fitness is required to successfully undertake such activities. Morey *et al.* have found that individuals with a peak oxygen uptake of less that 18 ml/kg per minute report significantly more difficulties performing daily tasks [131]. If a person's cardiovascular system is unable to meet the energy requirements of these simple tasks, functional ability and independence will be severely impaired. Such a person is then likely to become increasingly less active. This lack of activity associated with such low levels of functional ability will in turn contribute to greater losses in cardiovascular fitness and muscle strength.

Other older people may be able to carry out daily activities successfully, yet they may have a reduced physiological reserve and be operating close to their maximum aerobic capacity [80]. When faced with a task with higher demands (e.g. a flight of stairs) they are unable to meet these energy needs and their poor fitness becomes apparent. Reduced reserve may also become apparent if the person suffers an acute illness followed by a further loss of fitness.

The American College of Sports Medicine position on exercise for older adults [67] recommends that older adults with sufficient strength and balance should undertake an aerobic exercise programme. Such a programme should first target frequency (at least three days per week), then duration (at least 20 minutes) and finally appropriate intensity (40%–60% of heart rate reserve or 11–13 on the Borg scale of perceived exertion [132]).

A range of endurance training strategies are available for older people. These include: group exercise classes; walking programmes; pedometer-based walking; treadmill walking or running; stationary cycling; step test; and arm cranking [133–135]. Strategies need to be appropriate for individuals and depend in part on the level of fitness and skill. Intermittent exercise could be considered for high-risk individuals. Morris et al. have shown that when exercising at the same percentage of VO_{2max} and with the total amount of work fixed, intermittent exercise results in significantly lower physiological responses [136] yet similar fitness adaptations [137] compared to continuous exercise in older men.

Studies have now established the feasibility of endurance training among community-dwelling older people [138–140], those requiring institutional care [141], and among people with peripheral vascular disease [142–144], stroke [145, 146], coronary artery disease [147], arthritis [72, 148–150], chronic airflow limitation [151] and following lower limb amputation [152]. One study found that ten years after a RCT of an intervention to encourage walking, people in the walking group still reported more frequent walking for exercise [21].

Endurance training is contraindicated in some individuals. As for strength training, it is important that proper screening takes place before aerobic exercise programmes are undertaken [67, 153, 154]. While it has been found that health problems can arise during strength or endurance training despite medical screening [155], it seems that generally the risk associated with a lack of exercise is greater [67]. In a recent editorial, Buchner [156] reminds us that sudden death is actually more common among sedentary adults.

Effects on endurance

It has now been shown that older people can benefit from fitness training [67, 138]. From a review of 22 studies investigating the effects of aerobic training among older adults, Buchner et al. [103] concluded that 3–12 months of exercise improves aerobic capacity by between 5% and 20%. From a meta-analysis of 29 studies of endurance training among older people, Green and Crouse [157] found an average increase in maximum oxygen consumption of around 23%. These improvements may be enough to lead to improved functional abilities and therefore decrease the person's risk of falling.

The optimal intensity at which older people should undertake endurance training requires further investigation. While moderate-to high-intensity exercise is recommended to increase fitness [67], light-to moderate-intensity physical activity has been associated with a range of other health benefits [158, 159, 160]. There is also some evidence that fitness benefits can be obtained among older people from lower-intensity endurance training (i.e. 30%–45% heart rate reserve) [161] or 60% to 73% of peak treadmill heart rate [162].

Effects on functional abilities

Although endurance training has the potential to lead to improvements in functional abilities, most studies of aerobic training have not measured these abilities. As with muscle strength, it is likely that there is a non-linear relationship between fitness and functional ability, and that threshold levels of fitness are required for particular tasks. It would be reasonable to expect aerobic training to have a greater effect on the functional abilities of deconditioned people, than on those who had sufficient aerobic fitness to complete the task in question prior to the intervention.

In one of the few studies designed to address this question, Ettinger *et al.* [72] compared both aerobic (group exercise 50%–70% of heart rate reserve) and resistance training (10RM) with health education, among 439 older people with osteoarthritic knees causing pain and disability. The participants attended three months of group exercise then completed a 15-month home programme. When compared with health education, both aerobic and resistance training led to decreased pain and disability, and improved six-minute walk distance, stair-climbing ability, performance of a lift-and-carry task and time taken to get out of a car. Only aerobic training led to an increased aerobic capacity and neither intervention increased strength. Both interventions prevented the development of activity of daily living disability in those without disability at baseline and the lowest activity of daily living disability risks were found for participants with the highest compliance to exercise [163].

General exercise

Background

General exercise programmes do not always involve the intensity of stimulus which seems necessary to improve strength, balance or endurance. Some general exercise programmes are conducted primarily in seated positions. This is appealing for the safe conduct of exercise in a large-group setting and means that minimal training is required for exercise leaders. However, as discussed above, this may limit the usefulness of the programme in terms of improved balance and functional abilities.

Effects on function

Group exercise conducted in weight-bearing positions can enhance functional abilities. While some of these programmes are not targeting balance or functional ability as specifically as those described above, it is likely they are challenging these abilities sufficiently by providing exercise in functionally relevant positions. These programmes may have an important role in preventing decline in people who do not yet have substantial functional limitations, but such long term benefits have yet to be assessed in research studies.

Our group has designed a group exercise programme which is effective in improving performance on a number of measures of falls risk [15, 164, 165]. In a 12-month RCT of this exercise programme in 197 women, improvements were evident in lower-limb strength (ankle dorsiflexion, knee flexion and extension, and hip flexion and extension), reaction time, neuromuscular control, postural sway, maximal balance range and coordinated stability in the exercise group. The exercise subjects also showed significantly increased walking speed, cadence, stride length and decreased stride times. The intervention involved twice-weekly one-hour group exercise classes. These included a warm-up, conditioning (aerobic exercises, strengthening exercises, and activities for balance, flexibility, endurance and coordination), stretching and relaxation components.

A number of other RCTs have investigated group exercise programmes among relatively healthy older people. Programmes found to be effective in falls risk factor modification generally involve exercise carried out in weight-bearing positions which require controlled body movements (i.e. weight transference). Improvements among exercise subjects have been shown in strength [166], balance [167, 168], gait velocity [168], range of movement [169, 170], life satisfaction [169], psychological well-being [171], maximum physical exertion level [169] and perceived health status [169].

However, general exercise programmes do not always enhance balance, strength and function. In particular, seated flexibility exercise programmes have been used as a control programme in several studies and have generally failed to be associated with improved physical abilities [81]. General group-based programmes do not always enhance balance in community dwellers [36, 37] so need to be carefully designed.

Among institutional dwellers there may be more of a role for seated exercise. For example, McMurdo and Rennie [172, 173] compared the effects of a seated exercise class (involving isometric gravity-resisted exercises) with those of a reminiscence group, and found greater improvements in quadriceps strength [173], grip strength, spinal flexion, chair-to-stand time, activities of daily living and self-rating of depression [172] among the exercise group. Although this intervention was of a relatively low intensity and conducted in a seated position, it appears to have been intense enough to improve functional performance among this group.

Home exercise programmes also need to be well prescribed as several RCTs have failed to find improvements in falls risk factors with home based gentle exercise programmes [174]. Similarly, a 'lifestyle' home exercise programme, which involved stretching, theraband strength training and walking, improved quality of life but not physical variables in older women following vertebral fracture [175]. The programme was prescribed in a one-hour information session and followed up in monthly visits from an exercise therapist. It seems that the intervention was not sufficiently tailored or intensive to affect balance and gait.

Thus, it seems that if not sufficiently challenging, general exercise programmes are unlikely to affect functional abilities. However, a more challenging general exercise programme can enhance performance on a range of falls risk measures.

Vestibular rehabilitation

Background

The vestibular system contributes to the maintenance of postural stability by providing information on the head's position in relation to gravity as well as linear and rotational accelerations. This information is used in conjunction with somatosensory and visual inputs. The vestibulo-ocular reflex (VOR) stabilizes vision while the head is moving to maintain visual acuity during movement such as walking. Vestibular dysfunction can result from a wide variety of causes, including benign paroxysmal positional vertigo, Meniere's disease, acoustic neuroma and ototoxic medication. Vestibular impairment can be bilateral or unilateral, complete or incomplete. Impairment of one or both labyrinthine organs can result in loss of gaze stability (oscillopsia), vertigo, nausea and postural instability.

Although there is limited evidence to date that vestibular dysfunction contributes to falls risk in the general community, vertiginous symptoms or dizziness may be a factor in some falls for those with particular pathologies. In a recent study, Pothula *et al.* [176] found that 80% of unexplained fallers attending an accident and emergency department over a six month period had symptoms of dizziness on the vertigo symptom scale. A total of 40% of these cases were classified as true vertigo.

Vestibular rehabilitation (VR) aims to improve symptoms through a combination of habituation to the sensation of dizziness, sensory substitution by using the somatosensory or visual systems, and/or adaptation by re-balancing of tonic inputs in the brain stem and vestibular nuclei. The stimulus for improvements in symptoms is retinal slip. This can be elicited by repeated practice of movements and activities known to provoke moderate dizziness and visual disturbance. The following section is intended as a brief overview of VR. For further information please refer to Herdman [177] and Herdman *et al.* [178].

Effects on dizziness/falls risk factors and functional abilities

To date there have been no prospective RCTs analysing the effect of VR on falls. However, there have been several studies investigating the effect of VR on symptoms of dizziness, balance control and quality of life. Hall et al. [179] used the dynamic gait index (DGI) as an indication of falls risk, defining people with a DGI of ≤ 19 as 'at risk' of falls. Using this classification, in a retrospective before/after study, they found a significant reduction in risk of falling after a 4–6 week VR programme consisting of gaze stability and balance exercise. Although further investigation with controlled trials is required, these initial results are promising.

Several studies have analysed the effect of VR on balance and symptoms of dizziness (RCTs [34, 180–186], before after study designs [187–190] and a matched control design [191]). Tailored programmes of VR have resulted in significant improvements on computerized dynamic posturography and sensory organization tests [185, 189, 191], clinical balance measures [34, 185], gait velocity [180, 183, 186], stability during a stepping task [190], and subjective reports of vertigo [182, 184, 185, 187–189, 191]. These studies described VR as: progressive, frequent and repetitive practise of head or body movements that provoke a sensation of moderate dizziness; exercises to challenge gaze stability, such as head movements while focusing on a visual reference; and balance exercise. Recent studies have suggested that other interventions may also be of benefit in reducing dizziness. Corna et al. [192] compared five days of treatment using instrumental rehabilitation (standing on a sinusoidally moving platform) to more traditional VR (Cawthorne-Cooksey exercise), and found significantly more improvement in sway scores and the dizziness handicap inventory after the instrumental rehabilitation. Pavlou et al. [193] reported significantly better outcomes with the addition of optokinetic stimulation (five different simulator-based visual and self-motion stimulation experiences) compared to a conventional customized programme of VR. Viirre and Sitarz [194] carried out a small RCT using interactive computer displays, where they set the screen magnification controlling image motion at 5% higher than the participant's VOR gain for the intervention and did not alter the image motion for controls. After ten 30 minute sessions over five days the intervention participants significantly improved VOR gain (if the movement of the eyes matches the speed and amplitude of the head movement, the VOR gain is one).

In one of the largest RCTs investigating the effect of VR, Yardley et al. [195] recruited 170 people with chronic dizziness from general practices in the UK and provided one 30–60 minute session delivered by a trained nurse. Exercises to be carried out daily consisted of simple head turning and gaze stability exercise, tailored to be performed at a level that provoked moderate symptoms of dizziness. Additional balance exercises were provided if deemed necessary. Participants in the intervention group were given a support booklet with information on how to continue and progress the exercise programme, and what to expect. After three months there were significant improvements in postural stability with the eyes open and closed, self-reported dizziness, and dizziness-related quality of life. These improvements were maintained for six months after the intervention. The intervention group overall had a significant improvement in clinical symptoms.

Some studies have investigated factors affecting the outcome of VR. Whitney *et al.* [196] found that VR was equally effective in a group of participants aged 20–40 compared with those aged 60–80, when there was no significant difference between the two groups in vestibular diagnosis, duration of symptoms and vestibular function tests. Cohen and Kimball [182] also found that age did not significantly affect the outcome of VR. Bamiou *et al.* [197] studied people with unilateral vestibular hypofunction, and found that non-performance of the exercises, late initiation of rehabilitation and late presentation to the balance unit were predictors of a poor outcome following VR. Cohen and Kimball [181] investigated whether the speed of head movements during the exercise affected outcome. Both fast and slow head movements were equally effective in improving symptoms of vertigo.

Additional considerations for exercise prescription

To optimize the prescription of exercise, the health professional can assess the person's performance on key physical measures of falls risk. The most appropriate form of exercise to address individual deficits found can then be determined. Possible exercise settings should then be discussed with the client. A range of other factors may also need to be considered when deciding on the most appropriate exercise for an individual. Among these are financial status, carer responsibilities, availability of transport and personal preferences.

Factors affecting adoption and adherence

Most of those who participate in an exercise programme for six months will continue to do so in the longer term [198]. Therefore, it is important that the healthcare professional is aware of factors that may influence both adoption and adherence to interventions. The motivators and barriers to exercise in older people are diverse. Motivation to take up exercise after the age of 65 depends on previous exercise experience, general health, knowledge about exercise and psychological factors [199]. The populations at the highest risk of falls and therefore most likely to benefit from interventions, are likely to have poorer general health and reduced physical function – a commonly cited barrier to exercise in older people [199–201]. This makes it all the more crucial that efforts are made to reduce barriers and increase motivation to exercise in this population.

In order to promote the uptake of exercise it is important to provide adequate information to allow older people to decide whether to commence a programme. Exercise interventions require active participation. Therefore, motivation to perform these exercises is paramount to adherence and consequently the efficacy of the exercise. Feedback relating to improved performance in assessments of muscle strength, gait or balance may provide additional incentives for continued participation. There is some evidence to suggest that not all older people view falls prevention as the most important problem they face, therefore additional benefits of exercise such as improvements in strength, balance and function should be discussed. Finally, it is important that participants know what to expect when they start an exercise programme. Muscle soreness after exercise could easily be interpreted as harmful if a person is not informed that this is not unusual or harmful.

The theory of planned behaviour explains to some degree why older people take up exercise interventions [202]. This theory states that intention is formed by a weighted appraisal of attitude towards a behaviour and the subjective norms of this behaviour. Attitude depends on beliefs both that the behaviour will lead to a certain outcome and the desirability of that outcome. In older people, the attitudes to behaviour appear to be more important than the reference to social norms [199]. Therefore in order to increase uptake of interventions, it may be important to understand each individual's desirable outcome and provide information as to the possibility of achieving it.

Self-efficacy is thought to be an important determinant of adherence to exercise. It has been defined as 'an individual's belief in their ability to successfully perform a behaviour' [201] (p. 1059). McAuley *et al.* [203] found that the frequency of exercise, associated social support from the exercise group and the effects of the exercise, were the most important components of self-efficacy contributing to adherence six and 18 months after starting a walking or stretching programme in people with a mean age of 66 years. This suggests that social support is an important mediator of adherence and since effects of exercise are not always immediately apparent, social support is especially important at the beginning of a programme. Support can be provided either within an exercise group or from an exercise instructor (either face to face or by telephone [204]), and by involving family, friends and the person's general practitioner.

Several studies have now sought to evaluate the use of these interventions to enhance exercise programmes. Williams *et al.* [205] compared a low-to-moderate intensity balance programme for older adults, emphasizing self-efficacy information, to an exercise only control intervention. While adherence was higher among self-efficacy programme subjects, balance and mobility did not show greater improvements for this group. The 'Stepping On' multi-faceted falls prevention programme includes self-efficacy as a key component and reduced falls by 31% [206].

Setting

The different types of exercise described above can be conducted in various settings. The preferred setting for an individual will depend on lifestyle, other responsibilities and the person's ability to maintain motivation. Exercise can be conducted individually or in a group, can have various levels of supervision, and can be conducted within a healthcare centre, in a community setting or within the person's home. Several systematic reviews have failed to find overall benefits of one setting over another although direct comparisons in trials are lacking [207, 208].

Advantages of exercise within a group setting include support and assistance from an instructor, the structure provided by having a regular period of time allocated to exercise, the mutual encouragement and socialization provided by a group, and the enjoyable use of music. A recent study among physically frail older people compared home training (of functional balance and strength exercises) with and without additional group training. Few differences were found in physical outcome measures [209], but there were greater effects on mental health of group training, which lasted six months after the end of the study [210]. Classes may be necessary to maintain improvements in older persons attending centre-based exercise. King *et al.* [211] found that compared with a home control, centre-based exercise improved gait, chair-rise time and balance over one year. Improvements were not sustained with the transition to home exercise from months 13 to 18. General exercise is often carried out in a group setting and resistance training has also been shown to be effective in this setting [26, 212].

However, some individuals may not enjoy group environments and may prefer to exercise alone or with one other person [213]. For some older people it may be difficult to physically access venues where exercise classes are held (e.g. due to frailty and/or dependence on others for transport) or to find time to attend a regular class (e.g. due to responsibilities of caring for a partner or grandchildren, or social engagements). There is evidence that strength training can be successfully undertaken at home either alone [214] or supervised [95]. Endurance training can be as effective at home as in a group setting [162]. In fact, in a RCT [162], King *et al.* found that 12-month adherence rates were higher in home based groups.

Equipment requirements may also limit venues where exercise can be undertaken. Resistance training can involve expensive non-portable equipment used under supervision in a healthcare facility. However, after full assessment, community-dwelling older people could be taught to use exercise machines in a local gymnasium. In addition, several authors have shown increased strength among older people with the application of the principles of resistance training to more readily available tools, such as free weights, body weight and elastic sheeting [95, 121, 214]. Gait and balance training requires sufficient space and usually the presence of a firm surface to use for support if required. This could consist of parallel bars in a healthcare setting, firm chairs in a community setting and a bench or chair in the home.

Different types of exercise intervention require differing levels of supervision. For example, functional task training requires ongoing input from a physiotherapist in training sessions at a healthcare facility or within the person's home [215]. However, the ongoing practice/exercise undertaken by the client after input from the physiotherapist is also crucial. Exercise diaries or practice records may assist in this. Some examples of exercise cards for task-related practice are shown in Figure 11.1. Others can be obtained from the website: www.physiotherapyexercises.com. If exercises are to be performed without supervision, adequate information should be provided to ensure the exercises are carried out effectively and safely. This is usually in the form of exercise sheets or folders containing a written description of the exercises along with a diagram of the exercise in question – as in the Otago Exercise Programme [47]. A recent study involved a video being taken of the home exercise instruction session with the physiotherapist. The subjects were then given the video and advised to watch it in conjunction with their exercise sessions. This study showed marked improvements in the functional reach test performance from the home exercise programme [216].

Older people with varying levels of physical function may require differing levels of supervision. Frailer individuals, and those with mild cognitive impairment, poor motivation and/or reduced self-efficacy, may require a greater level of supervision both in order to exercise safely and to boost adherence. There is evidence that ongoing supervision and support is important in maintaining adherence to exercise [217–219], and the efficacy of this exercise. Kerschan *et al.* [220] found that while 5–10 year compliance with an unvarying home exercise programme was reasonable (36%), the resulting intensity was not enough to reduce fracture risk. Although ongoing supervision of exercise programmes may appear expensive, this may be outweighed by the potential savings from falls prevented by a successful programme.

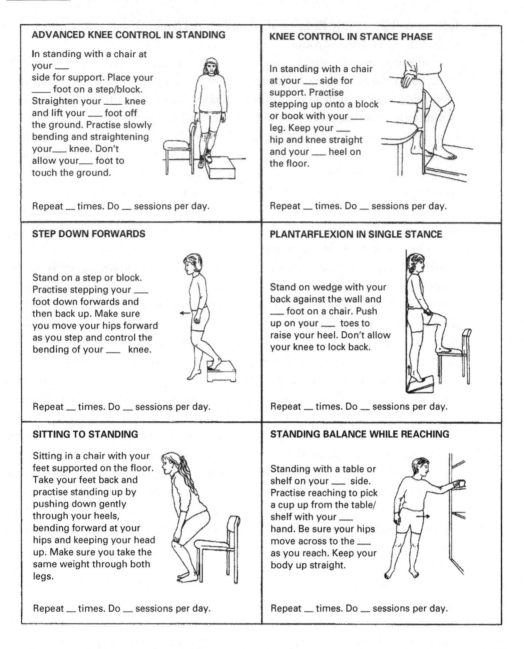

ADVANCED KNEE CONTROL IN STANDING

In standing with a chair at your ___
side for support. Place your ___ foot on a step/block. Straighten your ___ knee and lift your ___ foot off the ground. Practise slowly bending and straightening your___ knee. Don't allow your___ foot to touch the ground.

Repeat __ times. Do __ sessions per day.

KNEE CONTROL IN STANCE PHASE

In standing with a chair at your ___ side for support. Practise stepping up onto a block or book with your ___ leg. Keep your ___ hip and knee straight and your ___ heel on the floor.

Repeat __ times. Do __ sessions per day.

STEP DOWN FORWARDS

Stand on a step or block. Practise stepping your ___ foot down forwards and then back up. Make sure you move your hips forward as you step and control the bending of your ___ knee.

Repeat __ times. Do __ sessions per day.

PLANTARFLEXION IN SINGLE STANCE

Stand on wedge with your back against the wall and ___ foot on a chair. Push up on your ___ toes to raise your heel. Don't allow your knee to lock back.

Repeat __ times. Do __ sessions per day.

SITTING TO STANDING

Sitting in a chair with your feet supported on the floor. Take your feet back and practise standing up by pushing down gently through your heels, bending forward at your hips and keeping your head up. Make sure you take the same weight through both legs.

Repeat __ times. Do __ sessions per day.

STANDING BALANCE WHILE REACHING

Standing with a table or shelf on your ___ side. Practise reaching to pick a cup up from the table/shelf with your ___ hand. Be sure your hips move across to the ___ as you reach. Keep your body up straight.

Repeat __ times. Do __ sessions per day.

Fig. 11.1   Examples of exercise cards. Reproduced with permission from St Joseph's Hospital Physiotherapy Department, Sydney, Australia.

The ideal exercise setting therefore depends on the nature of the exercise, the purpose of this exercise (i.e. whether it aims to address particular deficits), and the preferences and social situation of the older person.

Conclusion

It is clear that well-prescribed exercise can improve physical abilities that are risk factors for falls. As we require balance for all tasks of daily life, it is often difficult to separate out the measurement and training of postural control from the measurement and training of functional task performance. It is clear that various aspects of postural control can be improved by well-designed training programmes. A group programme which does not allow individual prescription and safe performance of sufficiently challenging tasks does not appear to enhance balance. Functional abilities can be improved with training and practice of relevant tasks, and have often been trained with multi-component programmes. This approach is also likely to have a role in the prevention of age-related decline and the maintenance of functional ability.

Strength can be improved by strength training, fitness training can improve endurance and VR can lead to reduced dizziness. Functional ability may also be improved by strength training – particularly among frailer older people. Recent work has indicated the potential of task-related strength training to have greater functional benefits. Endurance training may also have greater effects on functional ability in frailer people but can offer health benefits to all older people.

General exercise can enhance functional ability if well-prescribed, and needs to be intensive and conducted in a weight-bearing position in more vigorous older people. There may be a role for seated programmes among frailer people, yet the greatest benefits are likely to be obtained from programmes which offer a greater challenge to postural control. In healthy older people, general exercise programmes should be undertaken to prevent age-related declines.

In summary, exercise programmes for older people need to be carefully designed after consideration of their aims and their target population. As with other falls prevention interventions, exercise will be more effective if targeted to the person's particular deficits and lifestyle. While adequate attention must be given to safety issues [76], there is certainly much scope to increase levels of exercise participation among older people. This will be enhanced if exercise providers take into account the factors which have been found to influence adoption of and adherence to exercise programmes. As well as assisting in the improvement of physical ability and the prevention of falls, this will provide a range of additional health benefits [160, 213].

REFERENCES

1. T. Liu-Ambrose, K. M. Khan, J. J. Eng et al., Resistance and agility training reduce fall risk in women aged 75 to 85 with low bone mass: a 6-month randomized, controlled trial. *Journal of the American Geriatrics Society*, **52**(5) (2004), 657–65.

2. J. Carr, & R. Shepherd, *Neurological Rehabilitation: Optimizing Motor Performance*, (Oxford: Butterworth-Heinemann, 1998).

3. J. Gordon, Assumptions underlying physical therapy intervention: theoretical and historical perspectives. In *Movement Science: Foundations for Physical Therapy in Rehabilitation*, ed. J. Carr, R. Shepherd, J. Gordon et al. (Maryland: Aspen, 1987).

4. A. C. Reece & J. M. Simpson, Preparing older people to cope after a fall. *Physiotherapy*, **82** (4) (1996), 227–35.

5. M. R. Hofmeyer, N. B. Alexander, L. V. Nyquist, J. V. Medell & A. Koreishi, Floor-rise strategy training in older adults. *Journal of the American Geriatrics Society*, **50**(10) (2002), 1702–6.

6. A. Barnett, B. Smith, S. R. Lord, M. Williams & A. Baumand, Community-based group exercise improves balance and reduces falls in at-risk older people: a randomised controlled trial. *Age and Ageing*, **32**(4) (2003), 407–14.

7. A. J. Campbell, M. C. Robertson, M. N. Gardner et al., Randomised controlled trial of a general practice programme of home based exercise to prevent falls in elderly women. *British Medical Journal*, **315**(7115) (1997), 1065–9.

8. L. Day, B. Fildes, I. Gordon, M. Fitzharris, H. Flamer & S. Lord, A randomized factorial trial of falls prevention among older people living in their own homes. *British Medical Journal*, **325** (2002), 128–33.

9. F. Li, P. Harmer, K. J. Fisher et al., Tai Chi and fall reductions in older adults: a randomized controlled trial. *Journals of Gerontology. Series A, Biological Sciences and Medical Sciences*, **60**(2) (2005), 187–94.

10. K. M. Means, D. E. Rodell, & P. S. O'Sullivan, Balance, mobility, and falls among community-dwelling elderly persons: effects of a rehabilitation exercise program. *American Journal of Physical Medicine and Rehabilitation*, **84**(4) (2005), 238–50.

11. M. C. Robertson, N. Devlin, M. M. Gardner & A. J. Campbell, Effectiveness and economic evaluation of a nurse delivered home exercise programme to prevent falls. 1. Randomised controlled trial. *British Medical Journal*, **322**(7288) (2001), 697–701.

12. A. Voukelatos, R. Cumming, S. Lord & Rissel, A randomised controlled trial of Tai Chi for prevention of falls: the Central Sydney Tai Chi trial. Unpublished findings.

13. C. A. DeVito, R. O. Morgan, M. Duque, E. Abdel-Moty & B. A. Virnig, Physical performance effects of low-intensity exercise among clinically defined high-risk elders. *Gerontology*, **49**(3) (2003), 146–54.

14. N. D. Carter, K. M. Khan, H. A. McKay et al., Community-based exercise program reduces risk factors for falls in 65- to 75-year-old women with osteoporosis: randomized controlled trial. *Canadian Medical Association Journal*, **167**(9) (2002), 997–1004.

15. S. Lord, J. Ward, P. Williams & M. Strudwick, The effect of a 12-month exercise trial on balance, strength, and falls in older women: a randomized controlled trial. *Archives of Physical Medicine and Rehabilitation*, **43** (1995), 1198–206.

16. D. Bunout, G. Barrera, M. Avendaño *et al.*, Results of a community-based weight-bearing resistance training programme for healthy Chilean elderly subjects. *Age and Ageing*, **34**(1) (2005), 80–3.

17. A. J. Campbell, M. C. Robertson, M. M. Gardner, R. N. Norton & D. M. Buchner, Psychotropic medication withdrawal and a home based exercise programme to prevent falls: results of a randomised controlled trial. *Journal of the American Geriatrics Society*, **47** (1999), 850–3.

18. A. Campbell, M. Robertson, S. La Grow *et al.*, Randomised controlled trial of prevention of falls in people aged 75 with severe visual impairment: the VIP trial. *British Medical Journal*, **331**(7520) (2005), 817–925.

19. S. Ebrahim, P. W. Thompson, V. Baskaran & K. Evans, Randomized placebo-controlled trial of brisk walking in the prevention of postmenopausal osteoporosis. *Age and Ageing*, **26**(4) (1997), 253–60.

20. M. E. McMurdo, P. A. Mole & C. R. Paterson, Controlled trial of weight bearing exercise in older women in relation to bone density and falls. *British Medical Journal*, **314**(7080) (1997), 569.

21. M. A. Pereira, A. M. Kriska, R. D. Day *et al.*, A randomized walking trial in postmenopausal women: effects on physical activity and health 10 years later. *Archives of Internal Medicine*, **158** (15) (1998), 1695–701.

22. J. F. Schnelle, K. Kapur, C. Alessi *et al.*, Does an exercise and incontinence intervention save healthcare costs in a nursing home population? *Journal of the American Geriatrics Society*, **51**(2) (2003), 161–8.

23. M. Steinberg, C. Cartwright, N. Peel & G. Williams, A sustainable programme to prevent falls and near falls in community dwelling older people: results of a randomised trial. *Journal of Epidemiology and Community Health*, **54**(3) (2000), 227–32.

24. D. Skelton, S. Dinan, M. Campbell & O. Rutherford, Tailored Group Exercise (FaME) reduces falls in community dwelling older frequent fallers (an RCT) (research letter). *Age and Ageing*, **34**(6) (2005), 636–9.

25. S. L. Wolf, H. X. Barnhart, N. G. Kutner *et al.*, Reducing frailty and falls in older persons: an investigation of Tai Chi and computerized balance training. Atlanta FICSIT Group. Frailty and injuries: cooperative studies of intervention techniques. *Journal of the American Geriatrics Society*, **44**(5) (1996), 489–97.

26. D. M. Buchner, M. E. Cress, B. J. de Lateur *et al.*, The effect of strength and endurance training on gait, balance, fall risk, and health services use in community-living older adults. *Journals of Gerontology. Series A, Biological Sciences and Medical Sciences*, **52**(4) (1997), M218–24.

27. S. R. Lord, S. Castell, J. Corcoran *et al.*, The effect of group exercise on physical functioning and falls in frail older people living in retirement villages: a randomized, controlled trial. *Journal of the American Geriatrics Society*, **51**(12) (2003), 1685–92.

28. S. Reinsch, P. MacRae, P. A. Lachenbruch & J. S. Tobis, Attempts to prevent falls and injury: a prospective community study. *Gerontologist*, **32**(4) (1992), 450–6.

29. S. L. Wolf, R. W. Sattin, M. Kutner *et al.*, Intense tai chi exercise training and fall occurrences in older, transitionally frail adults: a randomized, controlled trial. *Journal of the American Geriatrics Society*, **51**(12) (2003), 1693–701.

30. N. K. Latham, C. S. Anderson, A. Lee et al., A randomized, controlled trial of quadriceps resistance exercise and vitamin D in frail older people: the Frailty Interventions Trial in Elderly Subjects (FITNESS). *Journal of the American Geriatrics Society,* **51**(3) (2003), 291–9.

31. C. D. Mulrow, M. B. Gerety, D. Kanten et al., A randomized trial of physical rehabilitation for very frail nursing home residents. *JAMA: the Journal of the American Medical Association,* **271**(7) (1994), 519–24.

32. B. Wolf, H. Feys, W. De Weerdt et al., Effect of a physical therapeutic intervention for balance problems in the elderly: a single-blind, randomized, controlled multicentre trial. *Clinical Rehabilitation,* **15**(6) 2001, 624.

33. L. Wolfson, R. Whipple, C. Derby et al., Balance and strength training in older adults: intervention gains and Tai Chi maintenance. *Journal of the American Geriatrics Society,* **44** (5) (1996), 498–506.

34. E. E. Hansson, N. Mansson & A. Hakansson, Effects of specific rehabilitation for dizziness among patients in primary health care. A randomized controlled trial. *Clinical Rehabilitation,* **18**(5) (2004), 558–65.

35. H. Shimada, S. Obuchi, T. Furuna & T. Suzuki, New intervention program for preventing falls among frail elderly people: the effects of perturbed walking exercise using a bilateral separated treadmill. *American Journal of Physical Medicine and Rehabilitation,* **83**(7) (2004), 493–9.

36. R. G. Crilly, D. A. Willems, K. J. Trenholm, K. C. Hayes & L. F. Delaquerriere-Richardson, Effect of exercise on postural sway in the elderly. *Gerontology,* **35**(2–3) 1989, 137–43.

37. M. J. Lichtenstein, S. L. Shields, R. G. Shiavi & M. C. Burger, Exercise and balance in aged women: a pilot controlled clinical trial. *Archives of Physical Medicine and Rehabilitation,* **70**(2) (1989), 138–43.

38. H. Shimada, Y. Uchiyama & S. Kakurai, Specific effects of balance and gait exercises on physical function among the frail elderly. *Clinical Rehabilitation,* **17**(5) (2003), 472–9.

39. A. C. Kammerlind, J. K. Hakansson & M. C. Skogsberg, Effects of balance training in elderly people with nonperipheral vertigo and unsteadiness. *Clinical Rehabilitation,* **15**(5) (2001), 463–70.

40. S. E. Sihvonen, S. Sipila & P. A. Era, Changes in postural balance in frail elderly women during a 4-week visual feedback training: a randomized controlled trial. *Gerontology,* **50**(2) (2004), 87–95.

41. F. Li, P. Harmer, N. L. Wilson & K. J. Fisher, Health benefits of cobblestone-mat walking: preliminary findings. *Journal of Aging and Physical Activity,* **11**(4) (2003), 487–501.

42. S. Hiroyuki, Y. Uchiyama & S. Kakurai, Specific effects of balance and gait exercises on physical function among the frail elderly. *Clinical Rehabilitation,* **17**(5) (2003), 472–9.

43. J. C. Nitz & N. L. Choy, The efficacy of a specific balance-strategy training programme for preventing falls among older people: a pilot randomised controlled trial. *Age and Ageing,* **33**(1) (2004), 52–8.

44. M. R. Hinman, Comparison of two short-term balance training programs for community-dwelling older adults. *Journal of Geriatric Physical Therapy,* **25**(3) (2002), 10–5.

45. J. Steadman, N. Donaldson & L. Kalra, A randomized controlled trial of an enhanced balance training program to improve mobility and reduce falls in elderly patients. *Journal of the American Geriatrics Society,* **51**(6) (2003), 847–52.

46. K. M. Means, D. E. Rodell, P. S. O'Sullivan & L. A. Cranford, Rehabilitation of elderly fallers: pilot study of a low to moderate intensity exercise program. *Archives of Physical Medicine and Rehabilitation*, **77** (1996), 1030–6.

47. M. C. Robertson, A. J. Campbell, M. M. Gardner & N. Devlin, Preventing injuries in older people by preventing falls: a meta-analysis of individual-level data. *Journal of the American Geriatrics Society*, **50**(5) (2002), 905–11.

48. C. A. DeVito, R. O. Morgan, M. Duque, E. Abdel-Moty & B. A. Virnig, Physical performance effects of low-intensity exercise among clinically defined high-risk elders. *Gerontology*, **49**(3) (2003), 146–54.

49. T. M. Gill, D. I. Baker, M. Gottschalk *et al.*, A program to prevent functional decline in physicaly frail, elderly persons who live at home. *New England Journal of Medicine*, **347** (14) (2002), 1068–74.

50. T. M. Gill, D. I. Baker, M. Gottschalk *et al.*, A prehabilitation program for the prevention of functional decline: effect on higher-level physical function. *Archives of Physical Medicine and Rehabilitation*, **85**(7) (2004), 1043–9.

51. C. H. Worm, E. Vad, L. Puggaard *et al.*, Effects of a multicomponent exercise program on functional ability in community-dwelling, frail older adults. *Journal of Aging and Physical Activity*, **9**(4) (2001), 414–24.

52. R. O. Morgan, B. A. Virnig, M. Duque, E. Abdel-Moty & C. A. DeVito, Low-intensity exercise and reduction of the risk for falls among at-risk elders. *Journals of Gerontology. Series A, Biological Sciences and Medical Sciences*, **59**(10) (2004), 1062–7.

53. L. Timonen, T. Rantanen, O. P. Ryynanen *et al.*, A randomized controlled trial of rehabilitation after hospitalization in frail older women: effects on strength, balance and mobility. *Scandinavian Journal of Medicine and Science in Sports*, **12**(3) (2002), 186–92.

54. K. Hauer, N. Specht, M. Schuler, P. Bartsch & P. Oster, Intensive physical training in geriatric patients after severe falls and hip surgery. *Age and Ageing*, **31**(1) (2002), 49–57.

55. K. Hauer, M. Pfisterer, M. Schuler, P. Bartsch & P. Oster, Two years later: a prospective long-term follow-up of a training intervention in geriatric patients with a history of severe falls. *Archives of Physical Medicine and Rehabilitation*, **84**(10) (2003), 1426–32.

56. C. J. Thompson & W. H. Osness, Effects of an 8-week multimodal exercise program on strength, flexibility, and golf performance in 55- to 79-year-old men. *Journal of Aging and Physical Activity*, **12**(2) (2004), 144–56.

57. M. E. Nelson, J. E. Layne, M. J. Bernstein *et al.*, The effects of multidimensional home-based exercise on functional performance in elderly people. *Journals of Gerontology. Series A, Biological Sciences and Medical Sciences*, **59**(2) (2004), 154–60.

58. C. Sherrington, S. R. Lord & R. D. Herbert, A randomized controlled trial of weight-bearing versus non-weight-bearing exercise for improving physical ability after usual care for hip fracture. *Archives of Physical Medical Rehabilitation*, **85** (2004), 710–6.

59. J. D. Moreland, J. A. Richardson, C. H. Goldsmith & C. M. Clase, Muscle weakness and falls in older adults: a systematic review and meta-analysis. *Journal of the American Geriatrics Society*, **52** (2004), 1121–9.

60. D. Jones, O. Rutherford & D. Parker, Physiological changes in skeletal muscle as a result of strength training. *Quarterly Journal of Experimental Physiology*, **74** (1989), 233–56.

61. T. DeLorme & A. Watkins, *Progressive Resistance Exercise: Technical and Medical Application*, (New York: Appleton-Century-Crofts, 1951).

62. N. Latham, C. Anderson, D. Bennett & C. Stretton, Progressive resistance strength training for physical disability in older people. *The Cochrane Database of Systematic Reviews*, (2) (2003).

63. M. Nelson & S. Wernick, *Strong Women Stay Young (Revised Edition)*, (New York: Bantam Books, 2000).

64. M. Nelson, K. Baker, R. Roubenoff, L. Linder & K. Baker, *Strong Women and Men Beat Arthritis*, (New York: G. P. Putnam's Sons, 2002).

65. ACSM: American College of Sports Medicine Position Stand, The recommended quantity and quality of exercise for developing and maintaining cardiorespiratory and muscular fitness, and flexibility in healthy adults. *Medicine and Science in Sports and Exercise*, **30**(6) 1998, 975–91.

66. M. S. Feigenbaum & M. L. Pollock, Prescription of resistance training for health and disease. *Medicine and Science in Sports and Exercise*, **31**(1) (1999), 38–45.

67. ACSM: American College of Sports Medicine Position Stand, Exercise and physical activity for older adults. *Medicine and Science in Sports and Exercise*, **30**(6) 1998, 992–1008.

68. T. Hunter, Relative training intensity and increases in strength in older women. *Journal of Strength and Conditioning Research*, **9** (1995), 188–91.

69. D. R. Taaffe, L. Pruitt, G. Pyka, D. Guido & R. Marcus, Comparative effects of high- and low-intensity resistance training on thigh muscle strength, fiber area, and tissue composition in elderly women. *Clinical Physiology*, **16**(4) (1996), 381–92.

70. O. Seynnes, M. A. F. Singh, O. Hue *et al.*, Physiological and functional responses to low-moderate versus high-intensity progressive resistance training in frail elders. *Journals of Gerontology. Series A, Biological Sciences and Medical Sciences*, **59**(5) (2004), 503–9.

71. S. Fleck & W. Kraemer, *Designing Resistance Training Programs*, 2nd edn (Champaign: Human Kinetics, 1997).

72. W. H. Ettinger, Jr., R. Burns, S. P. Messier *et al.*, A randomized trial comparing aerobic exercise and resistance exercise with a health education program in older adults with knee osteoarthritis. The Fitness Arthritis and Seniors Trial (FAST). *JAMA: Journal of the American Medical Association*, **277**(1) (1997), 25–31.

73. K. R. Baker, M. E. Nelson, D. T. Felson *et al.*, The efficacy of home based progressive strength training in older adults with knee osteoarthritis: a randomized controlled trial. *Journal of Rheumatology*, **28**(7) (2001), 1655–65.

74. L. C. Ghilarducci, R. Holly & E. Amsterdam, Effects of high resistance training in coronary artery disease. *The American Journal of Cardiology* **64** (1989), 866–70.

75. P. A. Ades, P. D. Savage, M. E. Cress *et al.*, Resistance training on physical performance in disabled older female cardiac patients. *Medicine and Science in Sports and Exercise*, **35**(8) (2003), 1265–70.

76. ACSM: American College of Sports Medicine and American Heart Association Joint Position Statement. Recommendations for cardiovascular screening, staffing, and emergency policies at health/fitness facilities. *Medicine and Science in Sports and Exercise*, **30**(6) (1998), 1009–18.

77. B. F. Hurley, Age, gender, and muscular strength. *Journals of Gerontology. Series A, Biological Sciences and Medical Sciences*, **50**(Spec No) (1995), 41–4.

78. A. J. Campbell, M. J. Borrie & G. F. Spears, Risk factors for falls in a community-based prospective study of people 70 years and older. *Journal of Gerontology*, **44**(4) (1989), M112–7.

79. S. R. Lord, J. A. Ward, P. Williams & K. J. Anstey, Physiological factors associated with falls in older community-dwelling women. *Journal of the American Geriatrics Society*, **42**(10) (1994), 1110–7.

80. D. M. Buchner & E. H. Wagner, Preventing frail health. *Clinics in Geriatric Medicine*, **8**(1) (1992), 1–17.

81. J. O. Judge, M. Underwood & T. Gennosa, Exercise to improve gait velocity in older persons. *Archives of Physical Medicine and Rehabilitation*, **74**(8) (1993), 837–9.

82. J. F. Nichols, D. K. Omizo, K. K. Peterson & K. P. Nelson, Efficacy of heavy-resistance training for active women over sixty: muscular strength, body composition, and program adherence. *Journal of the American Geriatrics Society*, **41**(3) (1993), 205–10.

83. G. Pyka, E. Lindenberger, S. Charette & R. Marcus, Muscle strength and fiber adaptations to a year-long resistance training program in elderly men and women. *Journal of Gerontology*, **49**(1) (1994), M22–7.

84. N. McCartney, A. L. Hicks, J. Martin & C. E. Webber, Long-term resistance training in the elderly: effects on dynamic strength, exercise capacity, muscle, and bone. *Journals of Gerontology. Series A, Biological Sciences and Medical Sciences*, **50**(2) (1995), B97–104.

85. C. Morganti, M. Nelson, M. Fiatarone *et al.*, Strength improvements with 1 year of progressive resistance training in older women. *Medicine and Science in Sports and Exercise*, **27**(6) (1995), 906–12.

86. A. M. Jette, M. Lachman, M. M. Giorgetti *et al.*, Exercise – it's never too late: the strong-for-life program. *American Journal of Public Health*, **89**(1) (1999), 66–72.

87. A. M. Jette, B. A. Harris, L. Sleeper *et al.*, A home-based exercise program for nondisabled older adults. *Journal of the American Geriatrics Society*, **44**(6) (1996), 644–9.

88. M. A. Fiatarone, E. F. O'Neill, N. D. Ryan *et al.*, Exercise training and nutritional supplementation for physical frailty in very elderly people. *New England Journal of Medicine*, **330**(25) (1994), 1769–75.

89. K. V. Hruda, A. L. Hicks & N. McCartney, Training for muscle power in older adults: effects on functional abilities. *Canadian Journal of Applied Physiology*, **28**(2) (2003), 178–89.

90. M. A. Fiatarone, E. C. Marks, N. D. Ryan *et al.*, High-intensity strength training in nonagenarians. Effects on skeletal muscle. *JAMA: Journal of the American Medical Association*, **263**(22) (1990), 3029–34.

91. N. M. Fisher, D. R. Pendergast & E. Calkins, Muscle rehabilitation in impaired elderly nursing home residents. *Archives of Physical Medicine and Rehabilitation*, **72**(3) (1991), 181–5.

92. B. K. Barry & R. G. Carson, The consequences of resistance training for movement control in older adults. *Journals of Gerontology. Series A, Biological Sciences and Medical Sciences*, **59**(7) (2004), 730–54.

93. J. J. Keysor & A. M. Jette, Have we oversold the benefit of late-life exercise? *Journals of Gerontology. Series A, Biological Sciences and Medical Sciences*, **56**(7) (2001), M412–23.

94. D. M. Buchner, E. B. Larson, E. H. Wagner, T. D. Koepsell & B. J. DeLateur, Evidence for a non-linear relationship between leg strength and gait speed. *Age and Ageing*, **25** (1996), 386–91.

95. J. M. Chandler, P. W. Duncan, G. Kochersberger & S. Studenski, Is lower extremity strength gain associated with improvement in physical performance and disability in frail, community-dwelling elders? *Archives of Physical Medicine and Rehabilitation*, **79**(1) (1998), 24–30.

96. D. Skelton & A. Young, Are the national fitness survey strength and power thresholds for performance of everyday tasks too high? *Journal of Physiology*, **473** (1993), 84P.

97. M. Brown, D. R. Sinacore & H. H. Host, The relationship of strength to function in the older adult. *Journals of Gerontology. Series A, Biological Sciences and Medical Sciences*, **50** (Spec No) 1995, 55–9.

98. T. Rantanen, P. Era & E. Heikkinen, Maximal isometric knee extension strength and stair-mounting ability in 75- and 80-year-old men and women. *Scandinavian Journal of Rehabilitation Medicine*, **28**(2) (1996), 89–93.

99. T. Rantanen, J. M. Guralnik, G. Izmirlian *et al.*, Association of muscle strength with maximum walking speed in disabled older women. *American Journal of Physical Medicine and Rehabilitation*, **77**(4) (1998), 299–305.

100. I. S. Kwon, S. Oldaker, M. Schrager *et al.*, Relationship between muscle strength and the time taken to complete a standardized walk-turn-walk test. *Journals of Gerontology. Series A, Biological Sciences and Medical Sciences*, **56**(9) (2001), B398–404.

101. L. L. Ploutz-Snyder, T. Manini, R. J. Ploutz-Snyder & D. A. Wolf, Functionally relevant thresholds of quadriceps femoris strength. *Journals of Gerontology. Series A, Biological Sciences and Medical Sciences*, **57**(4) (2002), B144–52.

102. Y. Ostchega, C. F. Dillon, R. Lindle, M. Carroll & B. F. Hurley, Isokinetic leg muscle strength in older Americans and its relationship to a standardized walk test: data from the National Health and Nutrition Examination Survey 1999–2000. *Journal of the American Geriatrics Society*, **52**(6) (2004), 977–82.

103. D. M. Buchner, S. A. Beresford, E. B. Larson, A. Z. LaCroix & E. H. Wagner, Effects of physical activity on health status in older adults. II. Intervention studies. *Annual Review of Public Health*, **13** (1992), 469–88.

104. S. O'Reilly, K. Muir & M. Doherty, Effectiveness of home exercise on pain and disability from osteoarthritis of the knee: a randomised controlled trial. *Annals of the Rheumatic Diseases*, **58** (1999), 15–19.

105. S. P. Messier, T. D. Royer, T. E. Craven *et al.*, Long-term exercise and its effect on balance in older, osteoarthritic adults: results from the Fitness Arthritis and Seniors Trial (FAST). *Journal of the American Geriatrics Society*, **48**(2) (2000), 131–8.

106. M. E. Nelson, M. A. Fiatarone, C. M. Morganti *et al.*, Effects of high-intensity strength training on multiple risk factors for osteoporotic fractures: a randomized controlled trial. *JAMA: Journal of the American Medical Association*, **272**(24) (1994), 1909–14.

107. N. McCartney, A. L. Hicks, J. Martin & C. E. Webber, A longitudinal trial of weight training in the elderly: continued improvements in year 2. *Journals of Gerontology. Series A, Biological Sciences and Medical Sciences*, **51**(6) (1996), B425–33.

108. E. Lamoureux, W. A. Sparrow, A. Murphy & R. U. Newton, The effects of improved strength on obstacle negotiation in community-living older adults. *Gait and Posture*, **17** (3) (2003), 273–83.

109. J. F. Bean, D. K. Kiely, S. Herman *et al.*, The relationship between leg power and physical performance in mobility-limited older people. *Journal of the American Geriatrics Society*, **50**(3) (2002), 461–7.

110. J. F. Bean, S. G. Leveille, D. K. Kiely *et al.*, A comparison of leg power and leg strength within the InCHIANTI study: which influences mobility more? *Journals of Gerontology. Series A, Biological Sciences and Medical Sciences*, **58**(8) (2003), 728–33.

111. T. A. Miszko, M. E. Cress, J. M. Slade *et al.*, Effect of strength and power training on physical function in community-dwelling older adults. *Journals of Gerontology. Series A, Biological Sciences and Medical Sciences*, **58**(2) (2003), 171–5.

112. S. P. Sayers, J. Bean, A. Cuoco *et al.*, Changes in function and disability after resistance training: does velocity matter? A pilot study. *American Journal of Physical Medicine and Rehabilitation*, **82**(8) (2003), 605–13.

113. D. Sale & D. MacDougall, Specificity in strength training: a review for the coach and athlete. *Canadian Journal of Applied Sports Sciences*, **6** (1981), 87–92.

114. G. Wilson, A. Murphy & A. Walshe, The specificity of strength training: the effect of posture. *European Journal of Applied Physiology*, **73** (1996), 346–52.

115. H. Kanehisa & M. Miyashita, Specificity of velocity in strength training. *European Journal of Applied Physiology*, **52** (1983), 104–6.

116. M. Lindh, Increase of muscle strength from isometric quadriceps exercises at different knee angles. *Scandanavian Journal of Rehabilitation Medicine*, **11** (1979), 33–6.

117. O. Rutherford, Muscular coordination and strength training. Implications for injury rehabilitation. *Sports Medicine*, **5** (1988), 196–202.

118. J. V. Jessup, C. Horne, R. K. Vishen & D. Wheeler, Effects of exercise on bone density, balance, and self-efficacy in older women. *Biological Research for Nursing*, **4**(3) (2003), 171–80.

119. N. Lindelof, H. Littbrand, B. Lindstrom & L. Nyberg, Weighted belt exercise for frail older women following hip fracture – a single subject design. *Advances in Physiotherapy*, **4** (2) (2002), 54–64.

120. C. Barrett & P. Smerdely, A comparison of community-based resistance exercise and flexibility exercise for seniors. *Australian Journal of Physiotherapy*, **48**(3) (2002), 215–9.

121. D. S. Rooks, D. P. Kiel, C. Parsons & W. C. Hayes, Self-paced resistance training and walking exercise in community-dwelling older adults: effects on neuromotor performance. *Journals of Gerontology. Series A, Biological Sciences and Medical Sciences*, **52** (3) (1997), M161–8.

122. J. M. Shaw & C. M. Snow, Weighted vest exercise improves indices of fall risk in older women. *Journals of Gerontology. Series A, Biological Sciences and Medical Sciences*, **53**(1) (1998), M53–8.

123. J. Bean, S. Herman, D. K. Kiely *et al.*, Weighted stair climbing in mobility-limited older people: a pilot study. *Journal of the American Geriatrics Society*, **50**(4) (2002), 663–70.

124. J. F. Bean, S. Herman, D. K. Kiely *et al.*, Increased Velocity Exercise Specific to Task (InVEST) training: a pilot study exploring effects on leg power, balance, and mobility in community-dwelling older women. *Journal of the American Geriatrics Society*, **52**(5) (2004), 799–804.

125. N. B. Alexander, A. T. Galecki, M. L. Grenier *et al.*, Task-specific resistance training to improve the ability of activities of daily living-impaired older adults to rise from a bed and from a chair. *Journal of the American Geriatrics Society*, **49**(11) (2001), 1418–27.

126. L. R. Sauvage, Jr., B. M. Myklebust, J. Crow-Pan *et al.*, A clinical trial of strengthening and aerobic exercise to improve gait and balance in elderly male nursing home residents. *American Journal of Physical Medicine and Rehabilitation*, **71**(6) (1992), 333–42.

127. J. O. Judge, C. Lindsey, M. Underwood & D. Winsemius, Balance improvements in older women: effects of exercise training. *Physical Therapy*, **73**(4) (1993), 254–62.

128. J. O. Judge, M. Underwood & T. Gennosa, Exercise to improve gait velocity in older persons. *Archives of Physical Medicine and Rehabilitation*, **74**(4) (1993), 400–6.

129. E. F. Binder, K. B. Schechtman, A. A. Ehsani *et al.*, Effects of exercise training on frailty in community-dwelling older adults: results of a randomized, controlled trial. *Journal of the American Geriatrics Society*, **50**(12) (2002), 1921–8.

130. E. F. Binder, M. Brown, D. R. Sinacore *et al.*, Effects of extended outpatient rehabilitation after hip fracture: a randomized controlled trial. *JAMA: Journal of the American Medical Association*, **292**(7) (2004), 837–46.

131. M. Morey, C. Pieper & J. Cornoni-Huntley, Is there a threshold between peak oxygen uptake and self-reported physical functioning in older adults. *Medicine and Science in Sports and Exercise*, **30**(8) (1998), 1223–9.

132. G. Borg, Psychophysical basis of perceived exertion. *Medicine and Science in Sports and Exercise*, **14** (1982), 377–81.

133. L. A. Talbot, J. M. Gaines, T. N. Huynh & E. J. Metter, A home-based pedometer-driven walking program to increase physical activity in older adults with osteoarthritis of the knee: a preliminary study. *Journal of the American Geriatrics Society*, **51**(3) (2003), 387–92.

134. R. J. Petrella, J. J. Koval, D. A. Cunningham & D. H. Paterson, Can primary care doctors prescribe exercise to improve fitness? The Step Test Exercise Prescription (STEP) project. *American Journal of Preventive Medicine*, **24**(4) (2003), 316–22.

135. J. Maire, A. Faillenet-Maire, C. Grange *et al.*, A specific arm-interval exercise program could improve the health status and walking ability of elderly patients after total hip arthroplasty: a pilot study. *Journal of Rehabilitation Medicine*, **36**(2) (2004), 92–4.

136. N. Morris, G. Gass, M. Thompson & D. Conforti, Physiological responses to intermittent and continuous exercise at the same relative intensity in older men. *European Journal of Applied Physiology*, **90**(5–6) (2003) 620–625.

137. N. Morris, G. Gass, M. Thompson *et al.*, Rate and amplitude of adaptation to intermittent and continuous exercise in older men. *Medicine and Science in Sports and Exercise*, **34**(3) (2002), 471–7.

138. J. D. Posner, K. M. Gorman, L. Windsor-Landsberg *et al.*, Low to moderate intensity endurance training in healthy older adults: physiological responses after four months. *Journal of the American Geriatrics Society*, **40**(1) (1992), 1–7.

139. J. S. Stevenson & R. Topp, Effects of moderate and low intensity long-term exercise by older adults. *Research in Nursing and Health*, **13**(4) (1990), 209–18.

140. M. C. Morey, P. A. Cowper, J. R. Feussner *et al.*, Two-year trends in physical performance following supervised exercise among community-dwelling older veterans. *Journal of the American Geriatrics Society*, **39**(6) (1991), 549–54.

141. F. Naso, E. Carner, W. Blankfort-Doyle & K. Coughey, Endurance training in the elderly nursing home patient. *Archives of Physical Medicine and Rehabilitation*, **71**(3) (1990), 241–3.

142. W. R. Hiatt, E. E. Wolfel, R. H. Meier & J. G. Regensteiner, Superiority of treadmill walking exercise versus strength training for patients with peripheral arterial disease. Implications for the mechanism of the training response. *Circulation*, **90**(4) (1994), 1866–74.

143. G. C. Leng, B. Fowler & E. Ernst, Exercise for intermittent claudication (Cochrane Review). In *The Cochrane Library, Issue 3, 1999.* (Oxford: Update Software, 1998).

144. J. Brandsma, B. Robeer, S. van den Heuvel *et al.*, The effect of exercises on walking distance of patients with intermittent claudication: a study of randomised controlled trials. *Physical Therapy*, **78**(3) (1998), 278–88.

145. K. Potempa, M. Lopez, L. Braun *et al.*, Physiological outcomes of aerobic exercise training in hemiparetic stroke patients. *Stroke*, **26** (1995), 101–5.

146. M. Katz-Leurer, M. Shochina, E. Carmeli & Y. Friedlander, The influence of early aerobic training on the functional capacity in patients with cerebrovascular accident at the subacute stage. *Archives of Physical Medicine and Rehabilitation*, **84**(11) (2003), 1609–14.

147. B. Fletcher, S. Dunbar, J. Felner *et al.*, Exercise testing and training in physically disabled men with clinical evidence of coronary artery disease. *American Journal of Cardiology*, **73** (1994), 170–4.

148. M. A. Minor, J. E. Hewett, R. R. Webel, S. K. Anderson & D. R. Kay, Efficacy of physical conditioning exercise in patients with rheumatoid arthritis and osteoarthritis. *Arthritis and Rheumatism*, **32**(11) (1989), 1396–405.

149. C. H. van den Ende, J. M. Hazes, S. le Cessie *et al.*, Comparison of high and low intensity training in well controlled rheumatoid arthritis. Results of a randomised clinical trial. *Annals of the Rheumatic Diseases*, **55**(11) (1996), 798–805.

150. C. van den Ende, T. Vliet Vlieland, M. Munneke & J. Hazes, Dynamic exercise therapy in rheumatoid arthritis: a systematic review. *British Journal of Rheumatology*, **37** (1998), 677–87.

151. J. Nosworthy, C. Barter, S. Thomas & M. Flynn, An evaluation of three elements of pulmonary rehabilitation. *Australian Journal of Physiotherapy*, **38**(3) (1992), 189–93.

152. K. Pitetti, P. Snell J. Stray-Gundersen & F. Gottschalk, Aerobic training exercises for individuals who had amputation of the lower limb. *The Journal of Bone and Joint Surgery*, **69A**(6) (1987), 914–21.

153. M. Pollock & J. Wilmore, *Exercise in Health and Disease: Evaluation and Prescription for Prevention and Rehabilitation*, (Philadelphia: WB Saunders Company, 1990).

154. American College of Sports Medicine. *Guidelines for Exercise Testing and Prescription*, 4th edn (Philadelphia: Lea & Febiger, 1991).

155. M. Kallinen, S. Sipila, M. Alen & H. Suominen, Improving cardiovascular fitness by strength or endurance training in women aged 76–78 years. A population-based, randomized controlled trial. *Age and Ageing*, **31**(4) (2002), 247–54.

156. D. M. Buchner, Physical activity to prevent or reverse disability in sedentary older adults. *American Journal of Preventive Medicine*, **25**(3) (2003), 214–5.

157. J. S. Green & S. F. Crouse, The effects of endurance training on functional capacity in the elderly: a meta-analysis. *Medicine and Science in Sports and Exercise*, **27**(6) (1995), 920–6.

158. J. D. Posner, K. M. Gorman, L. N. Gitlin *et al.*, Effects of exercise training in the elderly on the occurrence and time to onset of cardiovascular diagnoses. *Journal of the American Geriatrics Society*, **38**(3) (1990), 205–10.

159. W. Haskell, Health consequences of physical activity: understanding and challenges regarding dose-response. *Medicine and Science in Sports and Exercise*, **26**(6) (1994), 649–60.

160. R. R. Pate, M. Pratt, S. N. Blair *et al.*, Physical activity and public health. A recommendation from the Centers for Disease Control and Prevention and the American College of Sports Medicine. *JAMA: Journal of the American Medical Association*, **273**(5) (1995), 402–7.

161. D. T. Badenhop, P. A. Cleary, S. F. Schaal, E. L. Fox & R. L. Bartels, Physiological adjustments to higher- or lower-intensity exercise in elders. *Medicine and Science in Sports and Exercise*, **15**(6) (1983), 496–502.

162. A. C. King, W. L. Haskell, C. B. Taylor, H. C. Kraemer & R. F. DeBusk, Group-vs. home-based exercise training in healthy older men and women. A community-based clinical trial. *JAMA: Journal of the American Medical Association*, **266**(11) (1991), 1535–42.

163. B. Penninx, S. P. Messier, W. J. Rejeski *et al.*, Physical exercise and the prevention of disability in activities of daily living in older persons with osteoarthritis. *Archives of Internal Medicine*, **161**(19) (2001), 2309–16.

164. S. R. Lord, J. A. Ward & P. Williams, Exercise effect on dynamic stability in older women: a randomised controlled trial. *Archives of Physical Medicine and Rehabilitation*, **77** (1996), 232–6.

165. S. Lord, D. Lloyd, M. Nirui, The effect of exercise on gait patterns in older women: a randomized controlled trial. *Journal of Gerontology*, **51A** (1996), M64–70.

166. J. C. Agre, L. E. Pierce, D. M. Raab, M. McAdams & E. L. Smith, Light resistance and stretching exercise in elderly women: effect upon strength. *Archives of Physical Medicine and Rehabilitation*, **69**(4) (1988), 273–6.

167. D. M. Buchner, M. E. Cress, B. J. de Lateur *et al.*, A comparison of the effects of three types of endurance training on balance and other fall risk factors in older adults. *Aging – Clinical and Experimental Research*, **9**(1–2) 1997, 112–9.

168. G. Johansson & G. B. Jarnlo, Balance training in 70-year-old women. *Physiotherapy Theory and Practice*, **7** (1991), 121–5.

169. M. E. McMurdo & L. Burnett, Randomised controlled trial of exercise in the elderly. *Gerontology*, **38**(5) (1992), 292–8.

170. E. M. Mills, The effect of low-intensity aerobic exercise on muscle strength, flexibility, and balance among sedentary elderly persons. *Nursing Research*, **43** (1994), 207–11.

171. G. Bravo, P. Gauthier, P. M. Roy *et al.*, Impact of a 12-month exercise program on the physical and psychological health of osteopenic women. *Journal of the American Geriatrics Society*, **44**(7) (1996), 756–62.

172. M. E. McMurdo & L. Rennie, A controlled trial of exercise by residents of old people's homes. *Age and Ageing*, **22**(1) (1993), 11–5.

173. M. E. McMurdo & L. M. Rennie, Improvements in quadriceps strength with regular seated exercise in the institutionalized elderly. *Archives of Physical Medicine and Rehabilitation*, **75**(5) (1994), 600–3.

174. M. E. McMurdo & R. Johnstone, A randomized controlled trial of a home exercise programme for elderly people with poor mobility. *Age and Ageing*, **24**(5) (1995), 425–8.

175. A. Papaioannou, J. D. Adachi, K. Winegard *et al.*, Efficacy of home-based exercise for improving quality of life among elderly women with symptomatic osteoporosis-related vertebral fractures. *Osteoporosis International*, **14**(8) (2003), 677–82.

176. V. B. Pothula, F. Chew, T. H. Lesser & A. K. Sharma, Falls and vestibular impairment. *Clinical Otolaryngology*, **29**(2) (2004), 179–82.

177. S. J. Herdman, Advances in the treatment of vestibular disorders. *Physical Therapy*, **77**(6) (1997), 602–18.

178. S. J. Herdman, M. C. Schubert & R. J. Tusa, Strategies for balance rehabilitation: fall risk and treatment. *Annals of the New York Academy of Science*, **942** (2001), 394–412.

179. C. D. Hall, M. C. Schubert & S. J. Herdman, Prediction of fall risk reduction as measured by dynamic gait index in individuals with unilateral vestibular hypofunction. *Otology and Neurotology*, **25**(5) (2004), 746–51.

180. H. S. Cohen & K. T. Kimball, Decreased ataxia and improved balance after vestibular rehabilitation. *Otolaryngology and Head and Neck Surgery*, **130**(4) (2004), 418–25.

181. H. S. Cohen & K. T. Kimball, Changes in a repetitive head movement task after vestibular rehabilitation. *Clinical Rehabilitation*, **18**(2) (2004), 125–31.

182. H. S. Cohen & K. T. Kimball, Increased independence and decreased vertigo after vestibular rehabilitation. *Otolaryngology and Head and Neck Surgery*, **128**(1) (2003), 60–70.

183. M. Johansson, D. Akerlund, H. C. Larsen & G. Andersson, Randomized controlled trial of vestibular rehabilitation combined with cognitive-behavioral therapy for dizziness in older people. *Otolaryngology and Head and Neck Surgery*, **125**(3) (2001), 151–6.

184. L. Yardley, S. Beech, L. Zander, T. Evans & J. Weinman, A randomized controlled trial of exercise therapy for dizziness and vertigo in primary care. *The British Journal of General Practice*, **48**(429) (1998), 1136–40.

185. F. B. Horak, C. Jones-Rycewicz, F. O. Black & A. Shumway-Cook, Effects of vestibular rehabilitation on dizziness and imbalance. *Otolaryngology and Head and Neck Surgery*, **106**(2) (1992), 175–80.

186. D. E. Krebs, K. M. Gill-Body, S. W. Parker, J. V. Ramirez & M. Wernick-Robinson, Vestibular rehabilitation: useful but not universally so. *Otolaryngology and Head and Neck Surgery*, **128**(2) (2003), 240–50.

187. O. Topuz, B. Topuz, F. N. Ardic *et al.*, Efficacy of vestibular rehabilitation on chronic unilateral vestibular dysfunction. *Clinical Rehabilitation*, **18**(1) (2004), 76–83.

188. K. Murray, S. Carroll & K. Hill, Relationship between change in balance and self-reported handicap after vestibular rehabilitation therapy. *Physiotherapy Research International*, **6**(4) (2001), 251–63.

189. N. T. Shepard & S. A. Telian, Programmatic vestibular rehabilitation. *Otolaryngology and Head and Neck Surgery*, **112**(1) (1995), 173–82.

190. D. Goldvasser, C. A. McGibbon & D. E. Krebs, Vestibular rehabilitation outcomes: velocity trajectory analysis of repeated bench stepping. *Clinical Neurophysiology*, **111**(10) (2000), 1838–42.

191. F. O. Black, C. R. Angel, S. C. Pesznecker & C. Gianna, Outcome analysis of individualized vestibular rehabilitation protocols. *American Journal of Otolaryngology*, **21**(4) (2000), 543–51.

192. S. Corna, A. Nardone, A. Prestinari *et al.*, Comparison of Cawthorne-Cooksey exercises and sinusoidal support surface translations to improve balance in patients with unilateral vestibular deficit. *Archives of Physical Medicine and Rehabilitation*, **84**(8) (2003), 1173–84.

193. M. Pavlou, A. Lingeswaran, R. A. Davies, M. A. Gresty & A. M. Bronstein, Simulator based rehabilitation in refractory dizziness. *Journal of Neurology*, **251**(8) (2004), 983–95.

194. E. Viirre & R. Sitarz, Vestibular rehabilitation using visual displays: preliminary study. *Laryngoscope*, **112**(3) (2002), 500–3.

195. L. Yardley, M. Donovan-Hall, H. E. Smith *et al.*, Effectiveness of primary care-based vestibular rehabilitation for chronic dizziness. *Annals of Internal Medicine*, **141**(8) (2004), 598–605.

196. S. L. Whitney, D. M. Wrisley, G. F. Marchetti & J. M. Furman, The effect of age on vestibular rehabilitation outcomes. *Laryngoscope*, **112**(10) (2002), 1785–90.

197. D. E. Bamiou, R. A. Davies, M. McKee & L. M. Luxon, Symptoms, disability and handicap in unilateral peripheral vestibular disorders. Effects of early presentation and initiation of balance exercises. *Scandinavian Audiology*, **29**(4) (2000), 238–44.

198. R. K. Dishman, J. F. Sallis & D. R. Orenstein, The determinants of physical activity and exercise. *Public Health Reports*, **100**(2) (1985), 158–71.

199. R. E. Rhodes, A. D. Martin, J. E. Taunton *et al.*, Factors associated with exercise adherence among older adults. An individual perspective. *Sports Medicine*, **28**(6) (1999), 397–411.

200. D. Chao, C. G. Foy & D. Farmer, Exercise adherence among older adults: challenges and strategies. *Controlled Clinical Trials*, **21**(5)(Suppl) (2000), 212S–17S.

201. K. A. Schutzer & B. S. Graves, Barriers and motivations to exercise in older adults. *Preventive Medicine*, **39**(5) (2004), 1056–61.

202. I. Ajzen, From intentions to actions: a theory of planned behaviour. In *Action Control: From Cognition to Behavior*, ed. J. Kuhl & J. Beckman, Springer, Heidelberg, Germany. (1985), pp. 11–39.

203. E. McAuley, G. J. Jerome, S. Elavsky, D. X. Marquez & S. N. Ramsey, Predicting long-term maintenance of physical activity in older adults. *Preventive Medicine*, **37**(2) (2003), 110–18.

204. C. M. Castro, A. C. King & G. S. Brassington, Telephone versus mail interventions for maintenance of physical activity in older adults. *Health Psychology*, **20**(6) (2001), 438–44.

205. K. Williams, K. Mustian & C. Kovacs, A home-based intervention to improve balance, gait and self-confidence in older adults. *Activities, Adaptation and Aging*, **27**(2) (2002), 1–16.

206. L. Clemson, R. G. Cumming & H. Kendig, The effectiveness of a community-based program for reducing the incidence of falls in the elderly: a randomized trial. *Journal of the American Geriatrics Society*, **52**(9) (2004), 1487–94.

207. M. Fransen, S. McConnell, & M. Bell, Exercise for osteoarthritis of the hip or knee. *Cochrane Database of Systematic Reviews* 2003.

208. A. K. Van der Bij, M. G. H. Laurant & M. Wensing, Effectiveness of physical activity interventions for older adults – a review. *American Journal of Preventive Medicine*, **22**(2) (2002), 120–33.

209. J. L. Helbostad, O. Sletvold & R. Moe-Nilssen, Effects of home exercises and group training on functional abilities in home-dwelling older persons with mobility and balance problems. A randomized study. *Aging – Clinical and Experimental Research*, **16**(2) (2004), 113–21.

210. J. L. Helbostad, O. Sletvold & R. Moe-Nilssen, Home training with and without additional group training in physically frail old people living at home: effect on health-related quality of life and ambulation. *Clinical Rehabilitation*, **18**(5) (2004), 498–508.

211. M. B. King, R. H. Whipple, C. A. Gruman *et al.*, The Performance Enhancement Project: improving physical performance in older persons. *Archives of Physical Medicine and Rehabilitation*, **83**(8) (2002), 1060–9.

212. J. O. Judge, R. B. Davis & S. Ounpuu, Step length reductions in advanced age: the role of ankle and hip kinetics. *Journal of Gerontology*, **51A**(6) (1996), M303–12.

213. D. M. Buchner, Physical activity and quality of life in older adults [editorial]. *JAMA: Journal of the American Medical Association*, **277**(1) (1997), 64–6.

214. D. A. Skelton, A. Young, C. A. Greig & K. E. Malbut, Effects of resistance training on strength, power, and selected functional abilities of women aged 75 and older. *Journal of the American Geriatrics Society*, **43**(10) (1995), 1081–7.

215. C. M. Dean, & R. B. Shepherd, Task-related training improves performance of seated reaching tasks after stroke: a randomized controlled trial. *Stroke*, **28**(4) (1997), 722–8.

216. R. McClellan & L. Ada, A six-week, resource-efficient mobility program after discharge from rehabilitation improves standing in people affected by stroke: placebo-controlled, randomised trial. *Australian Journal of Physiotherapy*, **50**(3) (2004), 163–7.

217. L. Daltroy, C. Robb-Nicholson, M. Iversen, E. Wright & M. Liang, Effectiveness of minimally supervised home aerobic training in patients with systemic rheumatic disease. *British Journal of Rheumatology*, **34**(11) (1995), 1064–9.

218. J. Kugler, J. E. Dimsdale, L. H. Hartley, & J. Sherwood, Hospital supervised vs. home exercise in cardiac rehabilitation: effects on aerobic fitness, anxiety, and depression. *Archives of Physical Medicine and Rehabilitation*, **71**(5) (1990), 322–5.

219. M. Hillsdon, M. Thorogood, T. Anstiss & J. Morris, Randomised controlled trials of physical activity promotion in free living populations: a review. *Journal of Epidemiology and Community Health*, **49**(5) (1995), 448–53.

220. K. Kerschan, Y. Alacamlioglu, J. Kollmitzer *et al.*, Functional impact of unvarying exercise program in women after menopause. *American Journal of Physical Medicine and Rehabilitation*, **77**(4) (1998), 326–32.

12

Medical management of older people at risk of falls

Written with Anne Tiedemann

Older people present to a wide range of healthcare specialists with problems related to or causing falls. The role of individual professions and institutions in the assessment and management of the older faller is not always apparent with frequent blurring of professional and organizational boundaries.

Only one-quarter of falls amongst community-dwelling older people are reported to any healthcare professional, but of those who do report a fall, 75% do so to their general practitioner (GP) [1]. It is therefore imperative to ensure that GPs are aware of existing evidence-based assessment tools and intervention strategies, and have available to them appropriate referral pathways to allow for more detailed assessment and intervention if required.

This chapter discusses the role of the medical practitioner in the identification and management of the older person at risk of falling. It focuses on assessments and interventions that are traditionally within the skill set of a doctor, but also acknowledges that as professional boundaries and areas of specialization change, others may undertake some of the assessments and interventions covered.

Identification of at risk populations

Identification of at risk populations is key to the delivery of effective interventions to prevent falls in older people. At present there is limited evidence to support a population-based approach to falls prevention. It is interesting to note that such interventions have developed in parallel with the individual randomized controlled trials and have not in all cases used known evidence-based approaches to prevention. Nonetheless, the limited evidence available to us in the Cochrane review of population-based interventions does suggest that population-based preventions are likely to be successful but need to be evaluated in the form of multi-centre randomized controlled trials [2]. In terms of risk identification and stratification, it is important to differentiate between measures used to simply identify people at increased risk of falling and tools used to identify risk factors amenable to intervention, and to provide a basis for tailoring a prevention strategy. At risk people can be identified on the basis of age, history of falls, place of presentation, usual place of residence, number of diseases and prescribed medications. Existing UK guidelines [3] recommend that older people presenting to their GP should be routinely asked about falls. Older people living in institutional care or presenting to the Emergency Department are well documented high-risk populations [4, 5].

A simple checklist of risk factors aligned with suggested interventions is often the most efficient way of identifying people at risk of falling, and allows for a subsequent and more detailed assessment of risk linked to appropriate and tailored interventions (Table 12.1).

Clinical assessment of the older faller

When trying to establish the cause of a fall it is important to remember that most falls occur as a result of an interaction between intrinsic and extrinsic factors, and that multiple factors increase the risk of falls [6]. There are many disease processes seen more commonly in the older population that contribute to an increased risk of falls, mainly through impairing postural stability (see Chapter 6).

A detailed history of the events surrounding a fall is essential. Corroborative information should be sought in those with limited recollection of the incident. In addition, there is a significant overlap between syncope and falls, with many older people having amnesia for the event [7, 8]. It is also important to establish cognitive ability at an early stage in the consultation as patients with cognitive impairment and dementia may provide misleading information.

Points to consider in the history include:
(i) Does the individual have amnesia for the event?
   Reason: possible syncopal, cardiac or neurological problem.
(ii) Where and at what time did the fall happen?
   Reason: postural hypotension in proximity to change in posture, falls occurring in relation to medication ingestion, mechanical falls at night with poor lighting, etc.
(iii) What was the individual doing at the time of the fall – getting up from a chair/bed, turning the head, reaching up or bending down?
   Reason: certain conditions are related to specific actions, such as postural hypotension on standing or carotid sinus syndrome related to turning of the head.
(iv) Was the fall preceded by any dizziness or palpitations?
   Reason: possible neurocardiogenic syncope, cardiac arrhythmia or vestibular problem.

Table 12.1 Suggestions for management of medical risk factors in general practice

Risk factor	GP Management	Referral/Liaison
IMPAIRED VISION (including refractive errors, macular degeneration, cataracts, glaucoma, retinopathies)	Simple visual acuity test (preferably low contrast) and fundoscopy.	Optician/optometrist ophthalmologist, occupational therapist
ORTHOSTATIC HYPOTENSION Supine blood pressure measured after minimum of 5 minutes lying down and then postural pressures checked at 1, 3 and 5 minutes after standing	Review any potential culprit medications, hydration status and consider possibility of autonomic problem. Increase fluid intake, offer compression hosiery, stop culprit medications.	If symptoms fail to settle – consider referral to cardiologist or geriatrician
FOOT DISORDERS (including corns and calluses, bunions, nail problems, ulceration)	Scalpel reduction of calluses, orthotic devices/insoles, footwear, and home footcare advice and education.	Podiatrist, orthopaedic surgeon, orthotist, boot-maker
MUSCULO-SKELETAL DISORDERS (including osteoarthritis, rheumatoid arthritis, acute soft tissue injuries)	Appropriate diagnostic evaluation, anti-inflammatory drugs, mobility aids (frames, walking sticks), education and advice on exercise and weight loss if appropriate.	Physiotherapist, orthopaedic surgeon, prosthetist, orthotist, rheumatologist, occupational therapist
PERIPHERAL NEUROPATHY	Check for evidence of B_{12} deficiency, diabetes, alcohol misuse or other causes of a peripheral neuropathy.	If cause uncertain – refer to neurologist. If diabetic, ensure regular diabetic foot review including podiatry
USE OF MEDICATIONS	Avoid all centrally acting medications where possible. Withdrawal of benzodiazepines if possible. Review need for all medications and prescribe lowest effective dose.	Pharmacist or geriatrician
VESTIBULAR DYSFUNCTION Consider Meniere's disease, benign paroxysmal positional vertigo	Avoidance of drugs with vestibular effects. Undertake Epley manoeuvre.	Consider referral to ENT surgeon for vestibular rehabilitation programme

Table 12.1 *(cont.)*

Risk factor	GP Management	Referral/Liaison
NEUROLOGICAL DISORDERS (including stroke, cerebellar disorders, Parkinson's disease)	Appropriate diagnostic evaluation, disease modifying medications.	Neurologist, geriatrician, physiotherapist, occupational therapist
PSYCHOLOGICAL FACTORS (including dementia, depression, anxiety)	Exclude acute delirium. Detect reversible causes of dementia or depression.	Neurologist, psychiatrist, psychologist, geriatrician
INCONTINENCE	Determine nature of incontinence and review any medications precipitating incontinence.	Refer for formal urodynamics and further assessment/ intervention
UNEXPLAINED FALLS, DIZZINESS AND SYNCOPE	12 lead ECG	Refer for further specialist evaluation

(v) Does the individual remember losing consciousness?

Reason: syncope suggestive of cardiac arrhythmia, neurally mediated syncope or epilepsy.

(vi) Was the individual able to get off the floor after the fall?

Reason: predictor of further falls as well as identifying a care need linked to interventions, i.e. training in how to get up from the floor, alarms or increased care levels.

(vii) Does the pattern of injury described and/or visualized fit with the details of the fall – did the individual manage to break his/her fall or were there facial/head injuries?

Reason: in syncopal episodes, the individual is rarely able to break the fall and more likely to sustain more central injuries, including facial injuries.

(viii) What injuries were sustained as a result of the fall?

Reason: low trauma fractures should trigger an assessment of bone health.

(ix) How often has the person fallen on another occasion in the last year?

Reason: one of the strongest predictors of falling again.

In addition to a detailed falls history, an accurate medical and drug history is required, including over the counter medications, herbal remedies, etc. Drugs commonly associated with an increased risk of falling include sedatives, anti-depressants and anti-psychotics (see Chapter 7). Polypharmacy (four or more regularly prescribed medications) has been consistently associated with falls, although in most cases it is primarily an indicator of underlying chronic disease [9].

Examination

Clinical examination of the older faller should be tailored to the history associated with the fall. At the end of the assessment, further evaluation and/or investigations may be required. Figure 12.1 highlights the more common and important examination findings that may provide some insight into the cause of an individual's fall.

Assessment of postural stability

Many diseases seen more frequently in the older population will present with problems relating to gait and balance, including osteoarthritis, stroke and Parkinson's disease. Gait and balance problems tend to be the most prevalent risk factors for falls, and are potentially modifiable with strength and balance training accessed through appropriately trained practitioners. Assessment of postural stability is therefore a key area in the management of an older person at risk of falling. Both the American Geriatrics Society/British Geriatrics Society/American Academy of Orthopaedic Surgeons guidelines [10] and National Institute for Clinical Excellence guidelines [3] recommend the Timed Up and Go Test (TUGT) as a simple screening tool to identify people warranting more detailed assessment of gait and balance [11]. It involves measuring the time taken for a person to rise from a chair, walk three metres at normal pace, and, with usual assistive devices, turn, return to the chair and sit down. Three retrospective studies have shown that TUGT performance can discriminate between fallers and non-fallers, and that a time of 15 or more seconds to complete the test indicates impaired functioning [12–14].

Whilst useful as a screening tool to identify older people with problems relating to postural stability, the TUGT does not provide detailed information regarding the impairments in physiological domains that contribute to falls risk. Therefore it provides little in the way of information about how to target intervention strategies. On the other hand, the Physiological Profile Assessment (discussed in Chapter 16) provides detailed quantitative information on the physiological domains contributing to postural stability. It takes 30–45 minutes to complete, requires training to undertake, record and interpret the results, and is perhaps more useful for physiotherapists or in a specialist setting. A recent addition to the physiological approach to assessing postural stability is QuickScreen, which is designed for use in primary care and in the home environment. It is likely to be of use to community therapists, nurses and GPs.

QuickScreen

QuickScreen is a brief risk assessment suitable for general practice, based on the sensorimotor functional model for falls prediction. The multifactorial aetiology

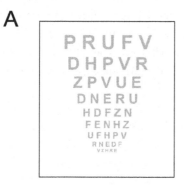

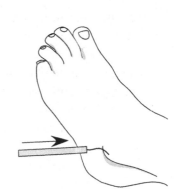

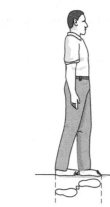

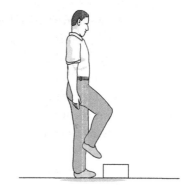

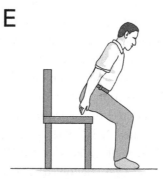

Fig. 12.1   The five tests making up QuickScreen. A: low contrast visual acuity, B: tactile sensitivity, C: near tandem stand, D: alternate step test, E: sit-to-stand.

of falls lends itself well to a sensorimotor model as it allows the clinician not only to predict which older patients are likely to fall, but also to determine which sensorimotor systems are impaired. This gives greater insight into the causes of instability and falls, and provides guidance for the tailoring of appropriate intervention strategies.

The falls assessment requires minimal equipment: a low contrast eye chart, an aesthesiometer filament for measuring touch sensation, and a small step. The assessment takes less than ten minutes to complete, and includes information which can be given to the patient to educate them about their falls risk and assist them to reduce or compensate for any identified risk factors. It is also portable so that an assessment can be performed in the home, in a GP surgery, hospital ward or residential care setting.

The five simple tests are highlighted in Figure 12.1 A–E.

(1) *Low contrast visual acuity*. Vision is assessed by the use of a low contrast visual acuity chart (Figure 12.1A). Acuity is assessed binocularly with the chart at a distance of three metres and the patient wearing their distance glasses (if applicable). The patient is asked to read aloud the letters on the chart and must be able to correctly identify all of the letters on the third line from the top to pass the test.

(2) *Tactile sensitivity*. Peripheral sensation is measured by using a tactile sensitivity test at the ankle. A Semmes-Weinstein-type pressure aesthesiometer containing a nylon filament is applied to the centre of the lateral malleolus of the ankle on the patient's dominant side (Figure 12.1B). The patient must keep their eyes closed and indicate to the tester if they are able to feel the monofilament. A total of three trials are given and the patient must be able to feel at least two of the three trials to pass the test.

(3) *Near tandem stand*. The near tandem stand test is a measure of lateral stability. It is a modification of the tandem stand test, which has previously been shown to be too difficult for many older people to carry out and hence inappropriate for a clinical screen. For this test, the subject is asked to stand in a near tandem position, with their bare feet parallel and separated laterally by 2.5 cm, and the heel of the front foot 2.5 cm anterior to the great toe of the back foot (Figure 12.1C). The subject is required to stand in this position for ten seconds with their eyes closed. If a score of five seconds or less is obtained, a second trial is allowed. The subject must stand in this position for ten seconds without moving their feet or opening their eyes in order to pass the test.

(4) *Alternate step test*. The alternate step test is a modified version of the stool stepping task, which is one of the 14 components of the Berg Balance Scale [15]. It is a practical measure of the requirements of walking and stair

climbing, and is also a measure of medio-lateral balance. This test involves placing the whole foot (shoes removed) onto a step (which is 19 cm high and 40 cm deep) and alternating right and left feet, four times for each foot, as fast as possible (Figure 12.1D). The time taken (measured in seconds) to complete the eight foot taps is recorded and the patient must complete the task within 10 seconds to pass the test.

(5) *Sit-to-stand test.* The sit-to-stand test is predominantly a measure of lower-limb strength [16, 17], and involves standing up and sitting down five times from a seated position in a 45 cm high chair, with the arms folded in front of the body (Figure 12.1E). The bare-footed subject is asked to perform the five repetitions as quickly as possible, finishing in the seated position. The time taken to complete the task, measured in seconds, is noted. To pass the test, the subject must complete the task within 12 seconds.

Two additional questions are asked regarding a history of falls and number of prescribed medications.

The criteria for identifying impairments that increase the risk of falls were determined from prospective cohort studies of community-dwelling older people [18]. Figure 12.2 shows the QuickScreen form with suggested interventions based on identified physiological deficits, and a falls risk score based on the number of identified risk factors in the screen [19].

The increased risks relating to multiple risk factors were derived from a validation study of 200 community-dwelling people who comprised the control group of a falls prevention randomized controlled trial.

Gait and balance problems

Where gait and balance problems are identified, it may be possible to modify or substantially reduce the risk through an exercise intervention, and more specifically strength and balance training. Specific exercise interventions are discussed in detail in Chapters 10 and 11. However, when offering evidence-based interventions to older people it is important to offer a choice in the mode of delivery of that intervention. Exercise is a prime example in which choice is often limited by service constraints, with group exercise or one-to-one physiotherapy the more common means of delivery. We have looked at the implementation of an evidence-based approach to strength and balance training, and the effect of offering patients choice in the way they take up their exercise. Figure 12.3 shows the results of offering choice to consecutive falls clinic attendees at King's College Hospital, London. Patients are assessed using the Physiological Profile Assessment and their falls risk categorized as low, moderate or high. Those at moderate risk are asked whether they would prefer to exercise at home or in a group setting and the results to date show that

---

QuickScreen Falls Risk Assessment

Patient: _____   Date: _____

MEASURE	RISK FACTOR PRESENT? (please circle)	ACTION
Previous falls		
One/more in previous year	Yes/No	

MEASURE	RISK FACTOR PRESENT?	ACTION
Medications		
Four or more, excluding vitamins	Yes/No	
Any psychotropic?	Yes/No	

Recommendation: Review current medications.

MEASURE	RISK FACTOR PRESENT?	ACTION
Vision		
Low contrast visual acuity test – unable to see all of line 16	Yes/No	

Recommendation: Give vision information sheet. Examine for glaucoma, cataracts and suitability of spectacles. Refer if necessary.

MEASURE	RISK FACTOR PRESENT?	ACTION
Peripheral sensation		
Tactile sensitivity test – unable to feel 2 out of the 3 trials	Yes/No	

Recommendation: Give sensation loss information sheet. Check for diabetes.

MEASURE	RISK FACTOR PRESENT?	ACTION
Strength/reaction time/balance		
Near tandem stand test – unable to stand for 10 secs	Yes/No	
Alternate step test – unable to complete in 10 secs	Yes/No	
Sit-to-stand test – unable to complete in 12 secs	Yes/No	

Recommendation: Give strength/balance information sheet. Refer to community exercise class or home exercise programme if appropriate to individual level of functioning.

Number of risk factors	0	1	2	3	4	5+
Total risk increase	1	1.4	2.1	4.7	8.7	12

The patient has_____ times the risk of falling as someone with no risk factors.

Fig. 12.2   The QuickScreen form.

when given the option, many older people prefer to exercise in their own home environment. Patients in the high-risk group continue to be offered one-to-one physiotherapy, either in the home or hospital setting, whilst low-risk patients are encouraged to use leisure services as a way of accessing strength and balance training.

	No/Mild Balance impairment *Low/no/mild falls risk score on PPA*	Moderate balance impairment *Moderate/marked falls risk score on PPA but balance is **adequate** for safe independent exercise*	Severe balance impairment *High falls risk score on PPA and balance **inadequate** for safe independent exercise*
Able to participate independently. Prefers home/individual approach to exercise	Leisure card for general exercise Walking groups Advice on exercise 22 patients	Otago home exercise programme 66 patients	One-to-one strength and balance training with physiotherapist/assistant 5 patients
Unable to participate independently or elects to undertake exercise in group setting	Exercise groups in community including chronic disease exercise groups. Largely driven by leisure services 1 patient	Exercise groups in hospital and community setting. Exercise groups in care homes. Largely driven by health services 28 patients	One-to-one strength and balance training with physiotherapist/assistant/health care assistant 9 patients

Fig. 12.3   Number of patients and form of exercise intervention undertaken according to patient choice and level of balance impairment.

Using the Otago Exercise Programme as the intervention [20], it has been possible to train exercise instructors to deliver strength and balance training in the home environment, leisure services and healthcare services. A repeat Physiological Profile Assessment undertaken on 50 consecutive patients going through the programme has shown statistically significant improvements in the Physiological Profile Assessment score, which is equally apparent for the home and group based programmes. This approach is being rolled out to a population of 50 000 people aged 65+ through the Southwark and Lambeth Integrated Care Pathway for Fallers (SLIPS), and represents a service delivery model which has taken the existing evidence and applied it in the context of the normal service setting.

In addition to strength and balance training for people with postural instability, it is possible that further medical intervention may be required for older people with degenerative joint disease of the large weight-bearing joints as they may well benefit from a joint replacement.

Vision problems

Vision has long been shown to be a risk factor for falls, but it is only in recent years that a single vision intervention has been shown to prevent falls [21, 22]. Older people should be encouraged to have their eyesight checked by an optician on a regular basis in order to detect any remediable cause of decline in visual function. A quick visual screen is often undertaken in the GP surgery and the most commonly used means of assessment is the traditional high contrast

Snellen chart. However, low contrast visual acuity tests have been shown to be a better predictor of falls in both community and residential home populations, and are recommended when considering a person's falls risk [18, 23, 24]. Low contrast visual acuity is tested in a standard manner, which is by asking patients to read the smallest line of letters on the chart they can see from a set distance (usually three metres). A Snellen fraction score of greater than 6/20 indicates significantly impaired low contrast visual acuity.

Where a visual deficit is identified, a diagnosis should be sought and an appropriate intervention offered. Refractive errors can be dealt with by the use of prescription spectacles. There is evidence to suggest that by expediting cataract extraction (surgery within one month), the rate of falls can be reduced, as can the number of fractures, when compared to a routine wait for surgery (12 months) [22].

Unexplained falls, dizziness and syncope

Not all falls are caused directly by gait and balance problems. It is individuals presenting with recurrent falls and no obvious cause that require further detailed specialist assessment, and access to specific investigative and diagnostic facilities. Recent studies have started to unravel the ragbag symptom of a 'drop attack' into a number of individual diseases associated with distinct pathologies, including carotid sinus syndrome, neurocardiogenic (vasovagal) syncope, sick sinus syndrome, micturition or cough syncope, and orthostatic hypotension. The overlap between syncope and 'drop attacks' has also been clearly shown, whereby people deny loss of consciousness despite this being witnessed first hand [25].

The European College of Cardiology have produced a useful clinical algorithm to assist with the assessment and diagnosis of possible syncope [26] as well as issuing treatment guidelines.

In a recent study by Parry and Kenny [27], a definitive diagnosis was ascertained in almost 90% of 93 consecutive patients presenting to an emergency department with three or more 'drop attacks' in the previous six months. Carotid sinus hypersensitivity and vestibular disorders were the most commonly diagnosed problems. In this study, the 12 lead ECG and 24 hour tape were shown to have a very low diagnostic yield, with patients requiring a more complex investigative approach.

Neurocardiogenic syncope

Neurocardiogenic or vasovagal syncope represents the most common form of neurally mediated syncope, and is characterized by a failure of the autonomic nervous system to maintain a pulse and blood pressure sufficient to ensure adequate cerebral perfusion [28, 29]. The underlying pathophysiological mechanism behind this form of syncope is thought to relate to excessive peripheral venous pooling leading to reduced peripheral venous return, a hypercontractile cardiac state with a paradoxical reflex bradycardia and a further decrease in vascular resistance [30, 31]. An excellent overview of this condition by Blair Grubb was published in the *New England Journal of Medicine* in 2005 [32].

Tilt table testing is the recommended investigation to make the diagnosis of neurocardiogenic syncope and formal protocols are available in the literature [26]. A positive test needs to document a significant change in haemodynamic status in the presence of symptoms comparable to those previously experienced by the individual at the time of an episode of collapse. Treatment usually involves avoidance of the precipitating factor – dehydration, extreme heat, prolonged standing, etc. However, there are individuals with neurocardiogenic syncope who have recurrent episodes of collapse and no associated warning symptoms. Treatment options include beta blockers [33], midodrine [34, 35] or paroxetine [36]. Cardiac pacing has also been considered although the evidence for this has been inconsistent [37–39].

Orthostatic hypotension

As discussed in Chapter 6, orthostatic hypotension has not been found to be a strong risk factor for falls in large population studies. However, few clinicians would doubt that symptomatic postural hypotension can lead to falls and the intermittent nature of the problem makes it difficult to establish a direct causal link. In a large series from the UK, orthostatic hypotension was found to account for 14% of all causes of syncope referred to a dedicated syncope unit [40].

Orthostatic hypotension is triggered by peripheral venous pooling, leading to a reduction in venous return and reduced cardiac filling pressures. The healthy response to reduced filling pressures in order to maintain a normal cardiac output is to peripherally vasoconstrict and increase heart rate. Failure to mount an appropriate response can be caused by vasodilator medications and/or autonomic failure associated with conditions commonly seen in advancing years, including diabetes and chronic renal failure. Orthostatic hypotension is also observed in people taking diuretics causing volume depletion.

Formal testing involves the patient lying initially in the supine position for a minimum of five minutes before lying blood pressure is recorded. Subsequent readings are taken on assuming the upright position at one, three and five minutes using a standard sphygmomanometer, although continuous beat-to-beat monitoring is more accurate.

Treatment of symptomatic orthostatic hypotension firstly involves a review of any potential culprit medication. Other measures include increasing fluid and salt intake, compression hosiery, and use of the alpha agonist midodrine [41].

Carotid sinus syndrome

Carotid sinus syndrome can be defined as an abnormal haemodynamic response to massage of the carotid sinus [8]. It is seen more commonly in old age and is characterized clinically by unexplained dizziness and/or syncope. There are three sub-types of the carotid sinus syndrome – cardioinhibitory, vasodepressor and mixed. The pathophysiology of the carotid sinus syndrome is far from clear and any plausible mechanism must adequately explain the clinically observed sub-types of the syndrome.

Sub-types

The *cardioinhibitory* response is characterized by a period of more than three seconds of asystole following carotid sinus massage. This is usually seen within a few seconds of onset of massage and tends to be self limiting, although atropine and full resuscitation facilities should be readily accessible. The *vasodepressor* response is identified by a fall in systolic blood pressure of greater than 50 mm Hg in the absence of a significant bradycardia. The *mixed* type is a combination of both responses. The drop in blood pressure is seen within seconds of massage and as such is difficult to detect without the use of continuous non-invasive blood pressure monitoring.

Method of testing

A useful protocol to follow is the Newcastle protocol [42]. Any individual (particularly an older person) who has unexplained episodes of collapse, loss of consciousness, dizziness or 'drop attacks' should be considered for carotid sinus studies and head-up tilt table testing. A history of a stroke, transient ischaemic attack or myocardial infarction within the last three months is a contra-indication to undertaking carotid sinus massage. Those with carotid artery bruits should undergo carotid dopplers before undertaking the study to exclude significant carotid artery disease, and if proceeding in the presence of carotid artery disease, the risks and benefits need to be discussed with the individual.

Surface ECG monitoring, non-invasive beat-to-beat monitoring of blood pressure and immediate access to resuscitation facilities should be available. Patients are initially tested in the supine position with the neck slightly extended. Massage is applied over the point of maximal carotid impulse, medial to the sternomastoid muscle at the level of the upper border of the thyroid cartilage. Firm longitudinal massage is applied for five seconds, initially on the right, and after a 60 second interval repeated on the left. The procedure is then repeated with the patient tilted upright to 70 degrees.

Carotid sinus studies are not without risk of complications, including both transient and permanent neurological damage [43–46]. Of the four series published, the highest reported rate of any neurological complication was 0.9% and this corresponded with 0.1% of all cases having persistent neurological deficits [46]. It is possible that the difference in complication rates documented at different sites relates more to methodological issues and possibly case mix rather than any true difference, as differences in definition are apparent in the existing literature.

Treatment

Symptomatic carotid sinus hypersensitivity (syndrome) of the cardioinhibitory sub-type should be treated with dual chamber pacing [47]. Atrial pacing is contraindicated in view of the high incidence of atrioventricular block during baroreflex stimulation. Ventricular pacing fails to control symptoms in many patients due to either aggravation of coexisting vasodepression or the development of the pacemaker syndrome.

Treatment of the vasodepressor response has proved less successful and almost certainly reflects a limited understanding of the underlying mechanisms producing the response. In a recent study, patients with vasodepressor carotid sinus syndrome were shown to have an impaired responsiveness to vasoconstrictive stimuli when compared to healthy old and younger subjects [48]. A review of prescribed medications is the first step, particularly looking for drugs with vasodilator and/or vagal activity. In a recent pilot study, Moore *et al.* have reported an improvement in symptomatology with the alpha agonist midodrine [49]. Surgical dennervation remains a therapeutic option for symptomatic vasodepression resistant to other forms of therapy, but it is of course not without risk and is rarely undertaken.

Cardiac arrhythmias

Both brady and tachy arrhythmias have the potential to cause a fall in older people. A 12 lead ECG is essential in the investigation of an arrhythmic syncope and Kapoor has suggested that up to 11% of syncopal patients will have a diagnosis assigned from their ECG [50]. This is in direct conflict with the recent paper by Parry *et al.* [27] who found routine ECG to have a negligible diagnostic yield. An entirely normal ECG in someone with syncopal attacks is unlikely to lead to an arrhythmia as the cause of the episodes of collapse [41]. The 24 hour ECG has been the mainstay clinical investigation for those with intermittent palpitations, dizziness and syncope, but has a very low diagnostic yield [27]. Patient-activated recorders and implantable loop recorders are becoming the preferred investigative mechanisms for those in whom an intermittent cardiac arrhythmia is suspected. Implantable loop recorders are small devices (Figure 12.4) inserted subcutaneously under local anaesthetic that can store up to 45 minutes of retrospective ECG recording when triggered by the individual.

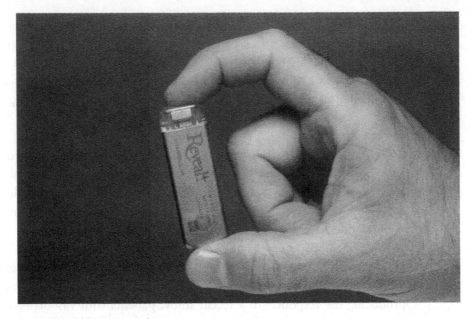

Fig. 12.4   An implantable loop recorder.

The device can remain *in situ* for up to 18 months with reported diagnostic yields of up to 40% [51].

Medication review

Review of medication is a core part of the assessment of an older person and should be undertaken on a regular basis for those having repeat prescriptions. National recommendations in the UK suggest that all older people should have their medication reviewed at least yearly and for those on four or more medications, at least six monthly [52]. Given the association between certain medications and falls, a medication review should also form a basic part of the medical assessment of the older faller.

As discussed in Chapter 7, the number of prescribed medications has been shown to be a predictor of falls, with an increased risk associated with the use of four or more medications. However, a recent study has suggested that the use of multiple medications is likely to represent underlying chronic disease, and it is the underlying disease process and possibly even the functional consequences that are the predictor of increased falls risk [9].

The purpose of a medication review is to ensure that people are on medications from which they stand to benefit and that there are no untoward or intolerable effects from taking those medications. The evidence-base for appropriate prescribing in older people is strong, and as more evidence emerges as to pharmacological interventions for more and more diseases, so the number of drugs available for prescription increases. Polypharmacy could therefore be considered a redundant term and the focus should be on appropriate prescribing. Older people should have access to the best pharmacological agents available, and a rational discussion with the patient is often required to weigh up the risks and benefits of different medications and numbers of drugs prescribed.

Centrally acting medications

When considering an association between medications and the risk of falls, it is the centrally acting medications that have been consistently shown be a predictor of risk, with some studies demonstrating a two- to three-fold increase in falls associated with their use [53, 54].

Not only is there evidence to link centrally acting medications to falls, but also evidence of the beneficial effects of withdrawing centrally acting medications on the subsequent risk of falls. Campbell *et al.* assessed the benefits of withdrawing centrally acting medications as part of a 2×2 factorial randomized controlled trial [55]. Subjects were recruited through their local GP practice. A 14-week structured withdrawal programme and a follow-up period of 44 weeks showed a 66% reduction in falls in the medication withdrawal group, when compared to those remaining on medication. A total of 70% of the control group fell in the follow-up period, which highlights the high-risk nature of this population. Of those in the medication withdrawal arm, 67% were on a benzodiazepine, 33% on an antidepressant and 17% were prescribed a major tranquillizer. Whilst the benefits in terms of reducing falls risk appear to be substantial, one should not overlook the difficulties involved in undertaking a withdrawal programme. In the trial the recruitment rate was just 19% and within one month of the end of the study, 47% of subjects were back on their centrally acting medication(s).

There is now little justification for the regular prescription of benzodiazepines as a hypnotic agent unless there is a clear pattern of addiction and/or a failure to successfully complete a withdrawal programme. Non-pharmacological approaches to the management of sleep disorders, depression and anxiety should be considered, particularly in populations at high risk of side effects from medications, including falls and fractures.

Non-pharmacological approaches to managing sleep disorders, anxiety and depression

Psychosocial treatments have been shown to be effective for the treatment of sleep disorders, anxiety and depression, with electroconvulsive therapy as a treatment option for refractive major depression [56]. There is now a great deal of evidence that a range of psychosocial therapies conducted by appropriately trained psychologists are effective in treating anxiety, depression and insomnia in the general population [57–60]. There is increasing evidence that such approaches are also efficacious in older people [56–58].

Many behavioural interventions for insomnia have been undertaken, and several reviews and meta-analyses of their effectiveness have been conducted [57–59]. Nowell et al. [57] reviewed over 30 trials and concluded that stimulus control, i.e. instructional procedures designed to curtail incompatible sleep behaviours and regulate sleep-wake schedules, is an effective strategy for improving sleep quality. Other effective strategies identified from the review include sleep restriction, relaxation and cognitive behaviour therapy [57]. Similarly, Murtagh and Greenwood [59] and Morin et al. [58] found from their meta-analyses that psychological interventions produce reliable and durable benefits in the treatment of insomnia, as determined by reduced sleep onset latency, increased sleep time, fewer nocturnal awakenings and improved sleep quality ratings. Morin et al. also suggest that although psychological treatments may be more expensive and time consuming than pharmacotherapy, they may be more cost-effective in the long term.

Another alternative to pharmacological therapy for sleep disturbances is the prescription of exercise, which has been found to have beneficial effects on sleep patterns in several studies [61–64]. Two randomized controlled trials have produced promising results in nursing home and community-dwelling older people. King et al. [63] evaluated the effect of a weekly, 30-minute moderate intensity exercise programme, involving light aerobics and brisk walking in 67 sedentary older community-dwelling subjects with moderate sleep complaints. Compared with the control group, the exercise group exhibited significant improvements in sleep quality and duration after the 16 weeks of exercise.

Physical activity also has a role to play in enhancing sleep among residents of aged care facilities. An investigation by Alessi et al. [64] assessed sleep quality and agitation in incontinent nursing home residents who were randomized to receive either: (i) daytime physical activity and a night-time programme aimed at noise reduction (the intervention group); or (ii) a night-time noise reduction programme only (the control group). Subjects who received the daytime activity experienced significantly improved sleep duration compared to those who received the night-time programme alone. Furthermore, seven out of the 15 intervention subjects had a decrease in observed agitation, compared to only one of the 14 control subjects.

Kanda et al. [65] found that after bathing, older people in their study were more likely to report good sleep and quicker sleep onset, verified by less frequent body movements in the first three hours of sleep. Older people may also benefit by simply being informed that they require less sleep than when they were younger and that early waking in not unusual in older people [66].

A large number of randomized clinical trials have established the efficacy of selected psychosocial interventions, including cognitive behavioural therapy, and brief psychodynamic treatment for depression in older people [56, 61]. From their extensive review of this topic, Niederehe and Schneider concluded that in clinical practice, psychosocial treatments should be used in combination with pharmacological treatments and this ought to be considered standard care [56].

There are fewer studies on the effectiveness of treatments for later life anxiety disorders, and recommendations are based on findings from studies undertaken on younger persons and older non-symptomatic volunteers. The psychosocial treatments for anxiety that hold promise include relaxation methods, rational-emotive training and anxiety management training [56].

To maximize treatment efficacy, Niederehe and Schneider recommend that comprehensive treatment 'packages' for the treatment of anxiety and depression should be developed which integrate both psychological and biological components. These packages, however, should go beyond simply having the patient see the physician for medications and someone else for psychotherapy, but involve interdisciplinary collaboration in the primary care setting with the inclusion of family members as key players in the overall treatment strategy [56].

Other specific medications to consider in a review

Medication review has been an integral part of several randomized controlled trials [5, 67–71] which have taken a multifaceted approach to the prevention of falls. Whilst it is not possible to delineate the precise contribution of the change in medication to the reduction in falls, most would agree that it is an essential part of a comprehensive geriatric assessment. In the PROFET study [5], 10.5% of the intervention group were referred to their GP for a further review of medication and the majority of these referrals related to benzodiazepine use. Tinetti *et al.* [68] were able to significantly reduce the number of prescribed medications following intervention in a group of community-dwelling older people. They also saw a reduction in sedative/hypnotic use during the one-year follow-up period. In a recent study by Davison *et al.* [67], 77 (53%) of the intervention group were felt to be on a medication possibly contributing to risk of falling.

Vitamin D supplementation

Vitamin D insufficiency is common in older people, particularly those who are housebound or who reside in nursing homes [72, 73]. In addition to increasing bone turnover and increasing the risk of osteoporosis [74], there is also evidence that inadequate vitamin D causes muscle weakness [75], and is associated with increased postural sway [76] and impaired psychomotor function [77], thereby increasing the risk of both falls and fractures. Recent studies have found that vitamin D supplementation can reduce postural sway [76] and improve strength [77]. Although there are some inconsistent findings in the literature, there is some evidence that vitamin D may reduce the risk of falls [78] and fractures [79].

Given the high prevalence of vitamin D insufficiency and the evidence of a preventative effect of vitamin D on falls and fractures, it has been recommended that identification of vitamin D insufficiency and advice regarding vitamin D intake should become routine clinical practice in falls clinics. However, Dhesi *et al.* [80] have argued that because identification of hypovitaminosis D requires a blood test and there are no accurate clinical predictors of inadequate vitamin D, a more pragmatic approach may be to provide vitamin D supplements to *all* older people attending a falls clinic. Although excessive intake of vitamin D can lead to toxic effects, this generally occurs with doses of 40 000 iu per day, whereas the treatments levels of 800 iu per day would be unlikely to cause toxicity [81]. Therefore, in the absence of individual contraindications, there does seem to be a sound rationale for routine vitamin D supplementation in older people at risk of falls.

In addition to its effects on muscle and nervous tissue, vitamin D is important for bone health. The assessment and management of osteoporosis is outside the scope of this book but suffice to say if we are to realistically achieve reductions in fracture rates at a population level, then falls and bone health need to be considered in parallel.

Conclusion

The multifactorial aetiology of falls is such that input and expertize from disciplines including medicine is often required to prevent falls. Identification of at risk populations needs to be considered and those at high risk often present via the general practice route. It is unrealistic to expect GPs to become experts in the assessment and prevention of falls in older people, but there is a place for basic clinical assessment, including medication review, simple tests of postural stability, gait, balance and vision. Centrally acting medications should be avoided or actively withdrawn where possible and alternate non-pharmacological approaches considered in high-risk individuals.

Postural instability caused by various combinations of ageing, physical inactivity and disease remains the most common cause of falls in older people, and access to strength and balance training programmes is important for these individuals. An additional environmental assessment may also be required.

Not all falls relate directly to postural instability, and those individuals with unexplained falls, syncope or dizziness should be referred for specialist assessment, investigations and intervention.

REFERENCES

1. H. J. Graham & J. Firth, Home accidents in older people: role of primary health care team. *British Medical Journal*, **305** (1992), 30–2.
2. R. McClure, C. Turner, N. Peel *et al.*, Population-based interventions for the prevention of fall-related injuries in older people [Review]. *The Cochrane Database of Systematic Reviews* (2005), CD004441.
3. National Institute for Clinical Excellence, Clinical practice guideline for the assessment and prevention of falls in older people. (National Institute for Clinical Excellence, 2004).
4. L. Z. Rubenstein, K. Z. Josephson & A. S. Robbins, Falls in the nursing home. *Annals of Internal Medicine*, **121** (1994), 442–51.
5. J. Close, M. Ellis, R. Hooper *et al.*, Prevention of falls in the elderly trial (PROFET): a randomised controlled trial. *The Lancet*, **353** (1999), 93–7.
6. M. E. Tinetti, T. F. Williams & R. Mayewski, Fall risk index for elderly patients based on number of chronic disabilities. *American Journal of Medicine*, **80** (1986), 429–34.
7. A. B. Dey, N. R. Stout & R. A. Kenny, Cardiovascular syncope is the most common cause of drop attacks in the elderly. *Pacing and Clinical Electrophysiology*, **20** (1997), 818–19.
8. R. A. Kenny & G. Traynor, Carotid sinus syndrome – clinical characteristics in elderly patients. *Age and Ageing*, **20** (1991), 449–54.
9. D. A. Lawlor, R. Patel & S. Ebrahim, Association between falls in elderly women and chronic diseases and drug use: cross sectional study. *British Medical Journal*, **327** (2003), 712–17.
10. American Geriatrics Society, British Geriatric Society, American Academy of Orthopaedic Surgeons Guideline for the prevention of falls in older persons. *Journal of the American Geriatrics Society*, **49** (2001), 664–72.
11. D. Podsialdo & S. Richardson, The timed "up and go": a test of basic functional mobility for frail elderly persons. *Journal of the American Geriatrics Society*, **39** (1991), 142–8.
12. A. Shumway-Cook, M. Baldwin, N. L. Polissar *et al.*, Predicting the probability for falls in community-dwelling older adults. *Physical Therapy*, **77** (1997), 812–19.
13. D. J. Rose, C. J. Jones & N. Lucchese, Predicting the probability of falls in community-residing older adults using the 8-foot up-and-go: a new measure of functional mobility. *Journal of Aging and Physical Activity*, **10** (2002), 466–75.
14. K. B. Gunter, K. N. White, W. C. Hayes & C. M. Snow, Functional mobility discriminates nonfallers from one-time and frequent fallers. *Journal of Gerontology*, **55** (2000), M672–6.
15. K. O. Berg, S. L. Wood-Dauphinee, J. I. Williams *et al.*, Measuring balance in the elderly: validation of an instrument. *Canadian Journal of Public Health*, **83** (1992), S7–11.
16. M. Csuka & D. J. McCarty, Simple method for measurement of lower extremity muscle strength. *American Journal of Medicine*, **78** (1985), 77–81.

17. S. R. Lord, S. M. Murray, K. Chapman *et al.*, Sit-to-stand performance depends on sensation, speed, balance, and psychological status in addition to strength in older people. *Journal of Gerontology*, **57A** (2002), M539–43.

18. S. R. Lord, J. A. Ward, P. Williams *et al.*, Physiological factors associated with falls in older community-dwelling women. *Journal of the American Geriatrics Society*, **42** (1994), 1110–17.

19. S. R. Lord, A. Tiedemann, K. Chapman *et al.*, The effect of an individualized fall prevention program on fall risk and falls in older people: a randomized controlled trial. *Journal of the American Geriatrics Society*, **53** (2005), 1296–304.

20. A. J. Campbell, M. C. Robertson, M. M. Gardner *et al.*, Randomised controlled trial of a general practice programme of home based exercise to prevent falls in elderly women. *British Medical Journal*, **315** (1997), 1065–9.

21. S. Brannan, C. Dewar, J. Sen *et al.*, A prospective study of the rate of falls before and after cataract surgery. *British Journal Ophthalmology*, **87** (2003), 560–2.

22. R. H. Harwood, A. J. E. Foss, F. Osborn *et al.*, Falls and health status in elderly women following first eye cataract surgery: a randomised controlled trial. *British Journal Ophthalmology*, **89** (2005), 53–9.

23. S. R. Lord, R. D. Clark & I. W. Webster, Visual acuity and contrast sensitivity in relation to falls in an elderly population. *Age and Ageing*, **20** (1991), 175–81.

24. J. H. Verbaken & A. W. Johnston, Clinical contrast sensitivity testing; the current status. *Clinical and Experimental Optometry*, **69** (1986), 204–12.

25. A. J. Davies & R. A. Kenny, Falls presenting to the accident and emergency department: types of presentation and risk factor profile. *Age and Ageing*, **25** (1996), 362–6.

26. M. Brignole, P. Alboni, D. Benditt *et al.*, Guidelines on management (diagnosis and treatment) of syncope. *European Heart Journal*, **22** (2001), 1256–306.

27. S. W. Parry & R. A. Kenny, Drop attacks in older adults: systematic assessment has a high diagnostic yield. *Journal of the American Geriatrics Society*, **53** (2005), 74–8.

28. R. F. J. Shepherd & J. T. Shepherd, Control of the blood pressure and circulation in man. In *Autonomic Failure: a Text Book of Clinical Disorders of the Autonomic Nervous System*, 4th edn, ed. C. Mathias & R. Bannister. (Oxford: Oxford University Press, 1999).

29. B. Grubb & B. Karas, Clinical disorders of the autonomic nervous system associated with orthostatic intolerance: an overview of classification, clinical evaluation, and management. *Pacing and Clinical Electrophysiology*, **22** (1999), 798–810.

30. D. Kosinski & B. Grubb, Pathophysiological aspects of neurocardiogenic syncope: current concepts and new perspectives. *Pacing and Clinical Electrophysiology*, **18** (1995), 716–24.

31. K. Lurie & D. Benditt, Syncope and the autonomic nervous system. *Journal Cardiovascular Electrophysiology*, **7** (1996), 760–76.

32. B. P. Grubb, Neurocardiogenic syncope. *New England Journal of Medicine*, **352** (2005), 1004–10.

33. R. Sheldon, The Prevention of Syncope Trial (POST) results. *Late breaking Clinical Trials*, *Heart Rhythm*, (San Francisco, 2004).

34. H. Kaufmann, D. Saadia & A. Voustianiouk, Midodrine in neurally mediated syncope: a double-blind, randomised, crossover study. *Annals of Neurology*, **52** (2002), 342–5.

35. A. Perez-Lugones, R. Schweikert, S. Pavia *et al.*, Usefulness of midodrine in patients with severely symptomatic neurocardiogenic syncope: a randomized control study. *Journal Cardiovascular Electrophysiology*, **12** (2001), 935–8.

36. E. D. Girolamo, C. D. Iorio, P. Sabatini *et al.*, Effects of paroxetine hydrochloride, a selective serotonin reuptake inhibitor, on refractory vasovagal syncope: a randomized, double-blind, placebo-controlled study. *Journal American College Cardiology*, **33** (1999), 1227–30.

37. R. Sutton, M. Brignole, C. Menozzi *et al.*, Dual-chamber pacing in treatment of neurally mediated tilt-positive cardioinhibitory syncope: pacemaker versus no therapy: a multicenter randomized study. *Circulation*, **102** (2000), 294–9.

38. S. J. Connolly, R. Sheldon, K. E. Thorpe *et al.*, Pacemaker therapy for the prevention of syncope in patients with recurrent severe vasovagal syncope: Second Vasovagal Pacemaker Study (VPS II): a randomized trial. *Journal of the American Medical Association*, **289** (2003), 2224–9.

39. A. Raviele, F. Giada, C. Menozzi *et al.*, Vasovagal Syncope and Pacing Trial Investigators. A randomized, double-blind, placebo-controlled study of permanent cardiac pacing for the treatment of recurrent tilt-induced vasovagal syncope. The Vasovagal Syncope and Pacing Trial (SYNPACE). *European Heart Journal*, **25** (2004), 1741–8.

40. S. McIntosh, D. Da Costa & R. A. Kenny, Outcome of an integrated approach to the investigation of dizziness, falls and syncope in elderly patients referred to a 'syncope' clinic. *Age and Ageing*, **22** (1993), 53–8.

41. J. Jankovic, J. L. Gilden, B. C. Hiner *et al.*, Neurogenic orthostatic hypotension: a double-blind, placebo-controlled study with midodrine. *American Journal of Medicine*, **95** (1993), 38–48.

42. R. Kenny, D. O'Shea & S. Parry, The Newcastle protocols for head-up tilt table testing in the diagnosis of vasovagal syncope, carotid sinus hypersensitivity, and related disorders. *Heart*, **83** (2000), 564–9.

43. A. Davies & R. Kenny, Frequency of neurological complications following carotid sinus massage. *American Journal Cardiology*, **81** (1998), 1256–7.

44. N. Munro, S. McIntosh, J. Lawson *et al.*, Incidence of complications after carotid sinus massage in older patients with syncope. *Journal American Geriatrics Society*, **42** (1994), 1248–51.

45. E. Puggioni, V. Guiducci, M. Brignole *et al.*, Results and complications of carotid sinus massage performed according to the "method of symptoms". *American Journal Cardiology*, **89** (2002), 599–601.

46. D. Richardson, R. Bexton, F. Shaw *et al.*, Complications of carotid sinus massage – a prospective series of older people. *Age and Ageing*, **29** (2000), 413–17.

47. R. A. Kenny, Syncope in the elderly: diagnosis, evaluation, and treatment. *Journal of Cardiovascular Electrophysiology*, **14** (2003), S74–7.

48. A. A. Mangoni, E. Ouldred, T. Y. Allain *et al.*, Paradoxical vasodilation during lower body negative pressure in patients with vasodepressor carotid sinus syndrome. *Journal of the American Geriatrics Society*, **51** (2003), 853–7.

49. A. Moore, M. Watts, T. Sheehy *et al.*, Treatment of vasodepressor carotid sinus syndrome with midodrine: a randomized, controlled pilot study. *Journal of the American Geriatrics Society*, **53** (2005), 114–8.

50. W. Kapoor, Diagnostic evaluation of syncope. *American Journal Medicine*, **90** (1991), 91–106.

51. A. P. Fitzpatrick, Ambulatory electrocardiographic (AECG) monitoring for evaluation of syncope. In *The Evaluation and Treatment of Syncope: a Handbook for Clinical Practice*, ed. D. Benditt, J.-J. Blanc, M. Brignole *et al.* (New York: Futura Publishing, 2003), pp. 63–70.

52. Department of Health, *National Service Framework for Older People*. (London: Department of Health, 2001).

53. A. J. Campbell, M. J. Borrie & G. F. Spears, Risk factors for falls in a community-based prospective study of people 70 years and older. *Journal of Gerontology*, **44** (1989), M112–17.

54. Y. B. Yip & R. G. Cumming, The association between medications and falls in Australian nursing-home residents. *Medical Journal of Australia*, **160** (1994), 14–18.

55. A. J. Campbell, M. C. Robertson, M. M. Gardner *et al.*, Psychotropic medication withdrawal and a home-based exercise program to prevent falls: a randomized, controlled trial. *Journal of the American Geriatrics Society*, **47** (1999), 850–3.

56. G. Niederehe & L. Schneider, Treatments for depression and anxiety in the aged. In *A Guide to Treatments that Work*, ed. P. Nathan & J. Gorman. (New York: Oxford University Press, 1998).

57. P. Nowell, D. Buysse, C. Morin *et al.*, Effective treatments for selective sleep disorders. In *A Guide to Treatments that Work*, ed. P. Nathan & J. Gorman. (New York: Oxford University Press, 1998).

58. C. Morin, J. Culbert & S. Schwartz, Nonpharmacological interventions for insomnia: a meta-analysis of treatment efficacy. *American Journal of Psychiatry*, **151** (1994), 1172–80.

59. D. Murtagh & K. Greenwood, Identifying effective psychological treatments for insomnia: a meta-analysis. *Journal of Consulting and Clinical Psychology*, **63** (1995), 79–89.

60. C. Brown & H. Schulberg, The efficacy of psychosocial treatments in primary care: a review of randomized clinical trials. *General Hospital Psychiatry*, **17** (1995), 414–24.

61. C. Alessi, J. Schnelle, P. MacRae *et al.*, Does physical activity improve sleep in impaired nursing home residents? *Journal of the American Geriatrics Society*, **43** (1995), 1098–102.

62. M. Vitiello, P. Prinz & R. S. Schwartz, The subjective sleep quality of healthy older men and women is enhanced by participation in two fitness training programs: a non-specific effect. *Sleep Research*, **23** (1994), 148.

63. A. King, R. Oman, G. Brassington *et al.*, Moderate-intensity exercise and self-rated quality of sleep in older adults. A randomized controlled trial. *Journal of the American Medical Association*, **277** (1997), 32–7.

64. C. A. Alessi, E. J. Yoon, J. F. Scnelle *et al.*, A randomized controlled trial of a combined physical activity and environmental intervention in nursing home residents: do sleep and agitation improve? *Journal of the American Geriatrics Society*, **47** (1999), 784–91.

65. K. Kanda, Y. Tochihara & T. Ohnaka, Bathing before sleep in the young and in the elderly. *European Journal of Applied Physiology and Occupational Physiology*, **80** (1999), 71–5.

66. K. Morgan, Sleep, insomnia and mental health. *Reviews in Clinical Gerontology*, **2** (1992), 246–53.

67. J. Davison, J. Bond, P. Dawson *et al.*, Patients with recurrent falls attending Accident and Emergency benefit from multifactorial intervention – a randomised controlled trial. *Age and Ageing*, **34** (2005), 162–8.

68. M. E. Tinetti, D. I. Baker, G. McAvay *et al.*, A multifactorial intervention to reduce the risk of falling among elderly people living in the community. *New England Journal of Medicine*, **331** (1994), 821–7.

69. L. Z. Rubenstein, A. S. Robbins, K. R. Josephson *et al.*, The value of assessing falls in an elderly population. A randomized clinical trial. *Annals of Internal Medicine*, **113** (1990), 308–16.

70. W. A. Ray, J. A. Taylor, K. G. Meador *et al.*, A randomized trial of a consultation service to reduce falls in nursing homes. *Journal of the American Medical Association*, **278** (1997), 557–62.

71. F. E. Shaw, J. Bond, D. A. Richardson *et al.*, Multifactorial intervention after a fall in older people with cognitive impairment and dementia presenting to the accident and emergency department: randomised controlled trial. *British Medical Journal*, **326** (2003), 73.

72. F. M. Gloth, 3rd, Osteoporosis in long term care. Part 1 of 2. Recognizing bone and beyond. *Review Director*, **12** (2004), 175–6.

73. P. Sambrook, I. Cameron, R. Cumming *et al.*, Vitamin D deficiency is common in frail institutionalised older people in northern Sydney. *Medical Journal of Australia*, **176** (2002), 560.

74. M. Peacock, G. Liu, M. Carey *et al.*, Bone mass and structure at the hip in men and women over the age of 60 years. *Osteoporosis International*, **8** (1998), 231–9.

75. S. Boonen, R. Lysens & G. Verbeke, Relationship between age associated endocrine deficiencies and muscle function in elderly women: a cross-sectional study. *Age and Ageing*, **27** (1998), 449–54.

76. M. Pfiefer, B. Begerow, H. Minne *et al.*, Effects of a short-term vitamin D and calcium supplementation on body sway and secondary hyperparathyroidism in elderly women. *Journal of Bone and Mineral Research*, **15** (2000), 1113–18.

77. J. Dhesi, L. Bearne, C. Monitz *et al.*, Neuromuscular and psychomotor function in elderly subjects who fall and the relationship with vitamin D status. *Journal of Bone and Mineral Research*, **17** (2002), 891–7.

78. H. Bischoff, H. Stahelin, W. Dick *et al.*, Effects of vitamin D and calcium supplementation on falls: a randomized controlled trial. *Journal of Bone and Mineral Research*, **18** (2003), 343–51.

79. M. C. Chapuy, M. E. Arlot, F. Duboeuf *et al.*, Vitamin D_3 and calcium to prevent hip fractures in the elderly women. *New England Journal of Medicine*, **327** (1992), 1637–42.

80. J. K. Dhesi, C. Moniz, J. C. Close *et al.*, A rationale for vitamin D prescribing in a falls clinic population. *Age and Ageing*, **31** (2002), 267–71.

81. R. Vieth, Vitamin D supplementation, 2,5-hydroxyvitamin D concentrations and safety. *American Journal of Clinical Nutrition*, **69** (1999), 842–56.

13

Assistive devices and falls prevention

As discussed in Chapter 1, falls result from the interaction between intrinsic risk factors (i.e. those pertaining to the individual, such as poor vision and reduced strength) and extrinsic risk factors (i.e. those relating to environmental hazards). The interface between the individual and their environment is also important, and can be modified by a range of physical assistive devices, which are used by at least one-quarter of older people [1]. Devices to be addressed in this chapter include footwear, foot orthoses, walking aids, other physical assistive devices, spectacles, hip protectors, aids to prevent 'long lies' and restraints. The potential impact of each of these devices on falls and/or fall injury is discussed.

Footwear

Footwear has an important role in protecting the foot from extremes of temperature, moisture and mechanical trauma. However, since the development and widespread popularity of fashion footwear in the 1600s, the functional aspect of footwear has largely been supplanted by cosmetic requirements. In both males and females of all ages, shoe selection is primarily based on aesthetic considerations, many of which are incompatible with optimal function of the lower extremity [2]. This is of particular importance in older people, as certain types of footwear, by modifying the interface between the sole of the foot and the ground, may have a significantly detrimental impact on postural stability and possibly predispose to falls [3].

Unfortunately, evidence to support the suggestion that certain types of shoes increase the risk of falls is meagre. A number of studies have assessed footwear in older people who have fallen, and have implicated a wide range of shoe features which may have been responsible, such as narrow heels, slippery soles, inadequate fixation, poorly fitting shoes and soft heel counters [4–8]. However, the wearing of inadequate footwear is a common finding in this age group [9, 10], as many older people base their footwear selection primarily on comfort rather than safety [9, 11]. Stronger evidence comes from case-control or cohort studies, in which the footwear of fallers is compared to non-fallers. Four such studies have recently been undertaken, with varying results. Kerse *et al.* [12] assessed footwear in 606 older people in residential care, and found that wearing slippers rather than shoes increased the risk of fractures during the 12-month follow-up period. However, there was no association between footwear and falls once potential confounders were accounted for. Keegan *et al.* [13] examined risk factors for various fall-related fractures in people aged over 45 years. They found that medium-high heeled shoes and shoes with a narrow heel significantly increased the likelihood of all types of fracture, while slip-on shoes and sandals increased the risk of foot fractures as a result of a fall. A study of 4281 people aged over 66 years by Larsen *et al.* [14] found that those who had fallen in the last 24 hours were four times more likely to have been wearing socks or slippers without a sole. Finally, a nested case-control study of 654 people aged over 65 years by Koepsell *et al.* [15] found that going barefoot or wearing stockings was associated with a ten-fold increased risk of falling, with athletic shoes being associated with the lowest risk. Further evaluation of footwear characteristics from this study found that increased heel height was associated with an increased risk of falling, whereas greater sole contact area was associated with a decreased risk [16]. Although each of these studies suggests that there is some relationship between footwear, falls and fractures, the lack of a standard protocol when assessing footwear makes comparisons difficult.

Nevertheless, a number of features of shoe design have been implicated as having an impact on balance (see Figure 13.1). The main features thought to play a role in affecting stability are heel height, the cushioning properties of the midsole, slip resistance of the outersole and method of fixation. Two additional features, the height of the heel collar and midsole geometry, have not been widely evaluated in the context of postural stability, but rather in relation to overuse injuries in sports people. However, given that a number of authors have recommended the wearing of high-top boots or shoes with broad heels as a means of improving stability in older people [9, 17–19], these features warrant further investigation. Finally, there is some emerging evidence that foot orthoses may play a role in improving balance in older people. Each of these components is discussed in more detail in the following sections.

Heel height

High heels first became widely used in the early 1600s and despite minor fluctuations in their popularity, still remain a dominant feature in female footwear [20, 21]. However, the use of heel elevation in footwear design is by no

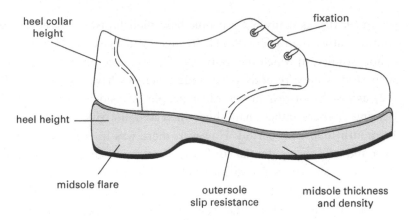

Fig. 13.1   Shoe features thought to influence postural stability in older people.

means restricted to women's shoes, as a number of boots worn by men also feature a raised heel (e.g. safety footwear, 'cowboy' boots). Research into the effects of heel elevation has tended to focus on postural and kinematic alterations, due to the proposed relationship between wearing high heels and the development of overuse symptoms in the foot, knee, hip and lower spine. These studies have revealed that heel elevation leads to a reduction in lumbar lordosis [22–25], increased loading on the forefoot [26–30], alterations in the function of the big toe joint during the propulsive phase of gait [31, 32], decreased stride length [33], increased energy consumption [34], increased arch height [35], and altered motion of the ankle and knee joints [24, 29, 34, 36, 37–41]. These alterations have generally been interpreted as detrimental to normal lower extremity function. However, kinematic differences between inexperienced and experienced wearers of high heels suggests that some habituation occurs over time which may act to minimize these adverse effects [42–44].

A number of authors have suggested that the changes in function produced by high heeled footwear may be responsible for instability and falling in older people [9, 17, 18, 45–47]. High heels are thought to contribute to instability by affecting the position of the centre of mass and by altering the position of the foot when walking [29, 48]. Three recent reports have highlighted the detrimental impact of high heels on balance. Brecht *et al.* [49] reported that balance performance on a moving platform was significantly worse in a heeled cowboy boot compared to a tennis shoe and suggested that heel elevation may make the wearer more susceptible to falling backwards. We have also found that balance ability in older women is detrimentally affected by high heels [50]. In our study, older women's balance was tested (using measures of postural sway and forward leaning ability) when subjects were barefoot, in their own shoes and in high heeled shoes (heel height 6 cm). The worst balance performances occurred when women wore high heeled shoes. Arnadottir and Mercer [51] found that performance on the functional reach test, the Timed Up and Go Test and the ten metre walk test was impaired in elderly women when wearing dress shoes (mean heel height 5 cm), compared to barefoot or when wearing walking shoes (mean heel height 1 cm). In contrast to these findings, Lindemann *et al.* [52] found no differences in balance when 26 older women wore shoes with a range of heel heights. The highest heel used in this study was 4 cm, suggesting that there may be a critical height at which heel elevation becomes problematic for balance. Further research therefore needs to be undertaken to ascertain the optimum heel elevation for women's shoes, as many older women report that they feel safer in a slight heel. Heel elevation may have some beneficial effects in older people with Parkinson's disease to facilitate forward propulsion [53]. Habitual wearers of high heeled shoes may have experienced some changes to the extensibility of posterior soft tissue structures (e.g. calf muscle tightening), which may contribute to greater comfort and possibly safety while wearing these shoes. This is yet to be investigated in research studies. However, it would appear that heel elevation greater than 6 cm should be avoided.

Midsole cushioning

The use of expanded polymer foam materials in the construction of footwear midsoles is widely accepted as a means of enhancing the level of comfort the shoe can provide to the wearer and as such is commonly recommended as a beneficial feature in footwear for older people [19, 54]. However, research undertaken by Robbins and colleagues suggests that the use of thick, soft materials in footwear midsoles leads to instability as the midsole material induces a state of 'sensory insulation', thereby reducing sensory input to the central nervous system regarding foot position [55].

To test this hypothesis, Robbins and colleagues (among others) have conducted a number of studies which have evaluated balance ability when older people wear footwear which varies according to the thickness and softness of the midsole material. They found that shoes with thick, soft midsoles have a detrimental effect on the ability of older people to maintain balance when walking on a beam [55], to detect the position of their ankle joint when standing on different surface inclinations [56] and to detect the position of their foot when walking [57]. The detrimental influence of thick soles was further supported by Sekizawa *et al.* [58], who evaluated foot position sense when subjects stood on a sloped surface and found that subjects underestimated the position of their foot in dorsiflexion when wearing shoes with thick soles (5 cm at heel, 3 cm at forefoot). Contrary to these findings, we recently found that midsole hardness was not associated with stability in older women [78], however, the materials used for the shoes in our study were not as soft as those used by Robbins and colleagues.

Nevertheless, the suggestion that soft shoes may have detrimental effects on balance has been supported by the investigations of Finlay [9], who reported an association between wearing soft slippers and falls, and Frey and Kubasak [5], who found that a large number of older people that fell were wearing cushioned running shoes at the time. Furthermore, older subjects have been found to sway more on soft floors than hard floors [59], and we have shown that body sway when standing on foam is a good indicator of falls risk [60, 61]. It would therefore appear that the interaction between sensory feedback and stability proposed by Robbins and colleagues is plausible, and may contribute to falls among otherwise healthy older people. Large scale prospective investigations are required to clarify whether a direct causal relationship exists between cushioning footwear and falls in older people. However, it may be prudent to advise against the wearing of shoes with very soft soles unless there is a specific therapeutic need for extra cushioning.

Slip resistance of footwear outersoles

Accidental falls caused by slipping are a common concern in older people, particularly in countries where snow- and ice-covered pavements are implicated in a large number of injuries to older people during the winter months [62, 63]. It has been estimated that over one million injuries caused by slipping are treated by hospitals in the United Kingdom every year [64], and the majority of these slipping incidents result in damage to the lumbar spine [65]. However, while a number of investigations have attributed falls in older people to slipping or tripping on unstable surfaces such as cracked paths, bathroom tiles or snow, few studies in the gerontology or rehabilitation literature have focused on the role of the shoe outersole in these accidents. Much of the work in this area has been performed in the context of occupational safety, due to the high number of injuries in the workplace resulting from slipping on factory floors [64, 66].

In an attempt to decrease the high incidence of slipping accidents, considerable investigative effort has been directed towards the development of slip resistant factory floors and footwear soles. However, progress towards a complete understanding of slip resistance is slow, due to the inability of testing apparatus to accurately simulate the wide variations in normal gait [65, 67] and the practical dilemma created by the fact that people walk over a wide range of surfaces during a normal day. Nevertheless, a number of authors have suggested that older people should be advised to avoid shoes with slippery soles – the assumption being that a textured, slip resistant sole may prevent slip-related accidents [9, 17, 18, 45–47]. Such a recommendation may not be appropriate in all situations as a number of cases have been reported in which falls are attributed to excessive slip resistance of the shoe when walking on a pavement or performing a household task [7, 68]. However, it would appear that falls related to excessive slip resistance are far less common than those resulting from inadequate slip resistance.

Gait analysis studies have revealed that slipping is most likely to occur when the heel first strikes the ground [62, 69, 70], and therefore, the geometry and texture of the heel section of a shoe may play an important role in preventing slipping accidents. We have recently shown that casual shoes vary considerably in their slip resistance properties [71]. Using a specially designed force plate apparatus, two types of shoes were tested: lace-up Oxford-style shoes and women's fashion shoes. The Oxford shoes were modified to produce four different heel configurations: the unmodified Oxford shoe had a flat heel with no flaring or sole texture; the second shoe was modified by flaring the heel laterally by 30 degrees; the third shoe was modified by grinding a 10 degree bevel into the rear section of the heel; and the fourth shoe had a 'non-slip' textured material adhered to the sole. The women's fashion shoes were modified to produce a narrow heel and a broad heel, and each of these shoes were tested with and without a 'non-slip' textured material applied to the sole. All shoes were tested on dry and wet bathroom tiles, concrete, vinyl flooring material and terra cotta. Testing revealed that the Oxford shoes offered greater slip resistance than the women's fashion shoes. The addition of a textured sole material had no effect on slip resistance on wet surfaces, and broadening the heel of women's shoes offered little additional benefit. The most slip resistant shoe was the Oxford shoe with the 10 degree heel bevel, which is consistent with previous reports in the occupational safety literature. A bevel is thought to improve slip resistance by increasing the surface area of the plantar aspect of the sole at heel contact [72]. A comparison of the shoes is shown in Figure 13.2.

In addition to the heel geometry, the hardness of the heel material may also play a role in slip resistance, although the effect depends on the characteristics of the surface. A number of laboratory experiments have shown that softer materials offer better slip resistance on dry ice [70, 71], presumably because compression of the heel at heel strike provides a greater contact area. However, when walking on wet ice, very hard sole materials with sharp cleats offer better slip resistance, as scratching the surface increases surface roughness [72].

Although heel modification has been found to be of benefit under experimental conditions, it remains to be seen whether such footwear modifications can help prevent slipping in older people. Further research is required to simulate the actual slipping event in an older person on a range of commonly

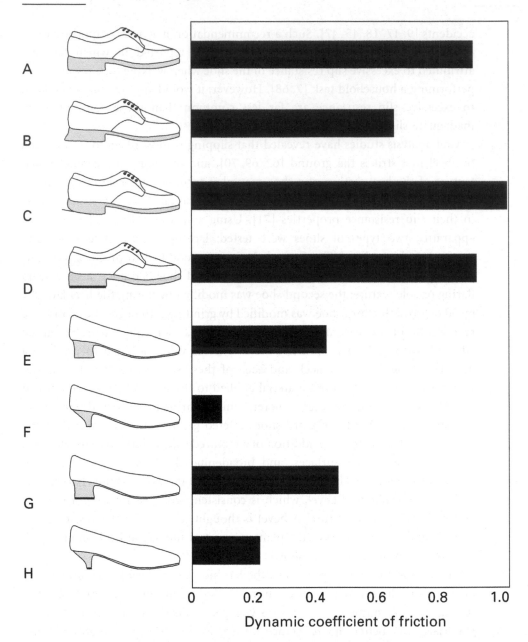

Dynamic coefficient of friction

Fig. 13.2   Slip resistance of different casual shoes. Shoe A: a 'standard' Oxford shoe with no sole flaring (heel surface area = 56 cm²). Shoe B: Oxford shoe with a 30 degree sole flare (heel surface area = 74 cm²). Shoe C: Oxford shoe with a 10 degree bevel ground into the posterior region of the heel. Shoe D: standard Oxford shoe with the addition of a non-slip textured sole. Shoe E: women's fashion shoe with a broad heel and no sole texture. Shoe F: women's fashion shoe with a narrow heel and no sole texture. Shoe G: Women's fashion shoe with a broad heel and a non-slip textured sole. Shoe H: Women's fashion shoe with a narrow heel and a non-slip textured sole. The minimum 'safe' dynamic coefficient of friction is 0.4. Diagram adapted from Menz *et al.* [71].

encountered surfaces. However, the practical difficulties in conducting these experiments are considerable. The main problem is that research subjects inevitably change their gait pattern in anticipation of walking on a slippery floor [73–75], so results obtained from laboratory experiments may not be indicative of the mechanisms responsible for a slip in real life situations. Thus, although some advances have been made in the understanding of slip resistance in occupational safety research, difficulties arise in applying these findings to falls prevention in older people. Nevertheless, the widely reported recommendation of avoiding very slippery-soled shoes would appear to be appropriate in most circumstances.

Heel collar height

High heel collars are commonly found in safety footwear and in shoes designed for specific sporting activities, such as football and basketball [73, 74]. Subsequently, much of the literature regarding the effects of heel collar height evaluates the ability of the shoe to prevent ankle sprains. Two main theories have been suggested to explain why high heel collars may be of benefit in ankle sprain prophylaxis. Firstly, the mere presence of the material surrounding the ankle region is thought to provide mechanical stability to the ankle and subtalar joints in the frontal plane, such that rapid excursions of the foot into eversion or inversion are restricted by the shoe [75–77]. Secondly, the presence of the high heel collar may provide additional tactile stimulation, thereby improving proprioceptive feedback of ankle position [73].

Stability around the heel is widely regarded as a desirable feature when recommending footwear for unstable older people, despite a lack of supporting evidence [9, 17–19, 54]. We recently assessed the balance ability of older women when barefoot, and in shoes with a standard collar height (Oxford-style shoe) and a raised collar height (eight-laced 'Doc Marten' boot). The results revealed that subjects performed better in the high collared shoe, presumably because the high heel collar provides greater ankle stability and increased proprioceptive feedback compared to standard footwear [78].

The use of high heel collars as a means of improving stability in older people warrants further investigation, as both peripheral sensory loss [60] and ankle muscle weakness [79] have been found to contribute to falling. Given that ankle support has been found to improve mechanical stability and ankle position sense in younger people [76, 80], shoes with high heel collars may be able to compensate for age-associated declines in sensory and motor function of the foot and ankle. However, such shoes must not be too restrictive, as a certain amount of foot flexibility is required to adapt to uneven terrain when walking [81, 82].

Midsole flaring

The term *midsole flare* refers to the difference between the width of the midsole at the level of the upper and its width at the level of the outersole. A number of authors have suggested that a large midsole flare is of benefit in older people as it provides a broader base of support, thereby enhancing the stability of the shoe [9, 17–19, 45]. These recommendations appear to have been developed in response to the recognition of narrow heels (such as those found in most high heeled footwear) provoking instability in older people. No studies have directly evaluated the effect of midsole flaring on balance ability, although associations between narrow heels and falls [16], and narrow heels and fall-related fractures [13] have been recently reported. The association with fractures suggests that if a fall does occur, the loss of balance when wearing narrow heels may result in greater sideways impact.

Theoretically, midsole flaring should improve mechanical stability by increasing the surface contact area of the shoe-ground interface [83, 84]. However, studies have also found that large midsole flares may make the foot pronate (roll inwards) more during gait [85, 86], and there is the possibility that a large midsole flare may make the wearer susceptible to tripping by contacting the contralateral limb during the swing phase of gait. Whether these proposed detrimental effects of midsole flaring have significant ramifications for stability in older people is uncertain. Therefore, no absolute recommendations can yet be developed regarding the benefits or otherwise of midsole flaring in footwear for older people. However, given that recent work suggests that impaired lateral stability is associated with falls [87], and that people who wear shoes with narrow heels are more likely to fall [16] and suffer fractures [13], any attempt to improve the control of lateral movements of the centre of mass may be beneficial.

Fixation

The method used to attach the shoe to the foot may also play a role in falls risk. It is a common clinical observation that many elderly people wear shoes with inadequate fixation, such as slippers, moccasins and soft canvas slip-on shoes [9, 10]. These types of shoes promote a shuffling gait pattern and may become separated from the foot when walking, thereby acting as an external tripping hazard. In a recent study of 95 older people who had been admitted to hospital following a fall-related hip fracture, we found that those who suffered a trip were three times more likely to be wearing shoes without laces, zips or Velcro fastening [8]. Two of the subjects who suffered a trip and were wearing these types of shoes specifically blamed their footwear for the fall. One reported that her slipper 'got stuck', causing her to lose balance, while another stated that her moccasin 'slipped off' her foot, causing her to trip over it. The association recently reported between the wearing of slip-on shoes and fall-related foot fracture adds further weight to this suggested mechanism [13]. Although it is difficult to confirm that the shoes were responsible for the fall, it would seem prudent to recommend that older people wear shoes that are firmly fitted to their feet.

Foot orthoses

Sensory receptors on the sole of the foot play an important role in maintaining balance by providing the brain with information about foot position and changes in plantar pressure distribution. This is evidenced by numerous studies which have demonstrated balance deficits in subjects with sensory neuropathy [88, 89], and when the feet of healthy subjects are anaesthetized [90]. In response to these observations, there has been some preliminary work undertaken to determine whether the sensory role of plantar mechanoreceptors can be harnessed to develop novel interventions to improve balance. Theoretically, placing textured insoles under the foot may provide additional tactile sensory input that can be used by the brain to compensate for deficits in other systems contributing to balance.

While a number of studies have indicated that different types of foot orthoses may improve balance in sportspeople [91–93], the mechanisms that may be responsible for this have only recently been investigated. Hosoda et al. [94] compared responses to platform perturbation in healthy subjects when wearing two types of footwear (flat leather soled sandals and 'health sandals' containing an insole with numerous small raised projections), and reported shorter reflex latencies when the health sandals were worn. Similarly, Waddington and Adams [95] evaluated the effect of textured rubber insoles (7 mm deep nodules at $4/cm^2$) on the ability of healthy young subjects to detect ankle inversion, and found that inserting an insole into the shoe provided similar movement detection to the barefoot condition. The authors concluded that textured insoles may be able to compensate for the loss of sensitivity produced by wearing soft-soled footwear, presumably by enhancing sensory feedback. Maki et al. [96] measured responses to platform perturbation in young and older people, with and without a specially designed plastic tube attached to the perimeter of the sole of the foot. This 'plantar facilitation' reduced the incidence of multiple stepping responses when the platform was displaced in the antero-posterior direction. This suggested that the enhanced sensory input provided by the insoles during the initial protective step response was utilized by the brain to stabilize posture, rendering an additional step unnecessary. More recently,

Priplata *et al.* [97] demonstrated significant reductions in sway variables when older people stood on randomly vibrating insoles, and suggested that the introduction of tactile 'noise' could ameliorate age-related impairments in balance control. Although these results provide interesting insights into the role of peripheral sensory input on the stabilization of posture, a great deal more research is required before insoles can be considered an effective falls prevention strategy in older people. The issue of comfort may also be a practical constraint, as people with sensitive feet or those who suffer from foot pain may not welcome the additional stimulation provided by the insoles.

Compliance issues

Despite the recognition that certain footwear features may be suboptimal from the perspective of balance and falls, it may nevertheless be difficult to convince older people to change their footwear. Fashion exerts a very powerful influence over footwear selection [98, 99], so much so that advising older people to change their footwear for health reasons has been called 'an exercise in eternal futility' [100]. Indeed, a recent survey of healthcare providers found that emergency department physicians rarely offered intervention or referral regarding footwear for elderly fallers, as they viewed 'patient stubbornness and vanity' as major barriers to compliance [101]. Unfortunately, many of the features considered detrimental to balance (such as high heels and lack of fixation) have long been considered fashionable and are likely to remain so. Therefore, while advising older people on the potential hazards of certain types of footwear may be a potentially useful falls prevention activity, it is important to consider that compliance issues will limit the efficacy of such an intervention.

In summary, the available evidence indicates that footwear may influence postural stability in either a beneficial or detrimental manner. Shoes alter the interface between the sole of the foot and the ground, both mechanically and neurophysiologically. Although many questions remain unanswered regarding the influence of specific design features on postural stability and falls, it would seem reasonable to suggest that older people should be advised against the wearing of high heeled shoes, shoes with very soft soles and shoes with slippery soles. Conversely, postural stability may be improved by: the wearing of shoes with thin, flat, broad, bevelled heels constructed with a firm material; textured soles to improve traction; laces to provide adequate fixation; and possibly the addition of ankle support by the use of a high heel collar. The theoretically optimal safe shoe for older people is shown in Figure 13.3. However, because no experimental studies of footwear have examined falls as an outcome, the level of evidence for these recommendations as a falls prevention strategy is low [102]. The potential for foot orthoses and insoles to improve balance also warrants further investigation.

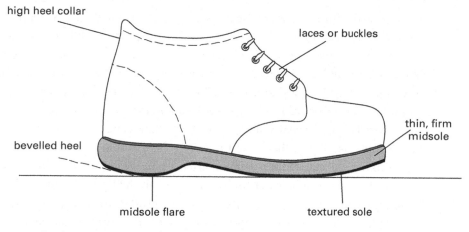

high heel collar

laces or buckles

thin, firm midsole

bevelled heel

midsole flare

textured sole

Fig. 13.3   The theoretical optimal 'safe' shoe.

Walking aids

Walking aids are commonly recommended to older people as a means of increasing their walking ability and decreasing their risk of falling. The prescription of a walking aid, however, is not a straightforward procedure. While appropriate for many older people, walking aids should ideally be prescribed by a health professional, after an assessment of the person's gait [103]. Commonly used walking aids are outlined in Box 13.1.

> **Box 13.1 Types of walking aids.**
>
> | | |
> |---|---|
> | Sticks | Single sticks (wooden or metal) |
> | | Quad sticks (four-pronged) |
> | Crutches | Axillary (fit under axilla, weight taken on hands) |
> | | Canadian (weight taken through hands and forearms) |
> | | Forearm support |
> | Frames | Forearm support frames (large wheeled frames on which the forearms are placed) |
> | | Rollator frames (smaller wheeled frames which are pushed using hands) |
> | | Pick-up frames (without wheels, the person picks up the frame and places it in front of them and then steps up to it) |

Indications and possible role in falls prevention

The main indications for a walking aid are excessive pain on weight bearing, decreased leg muscle strength and/or control, instability, shortness of breath, poor vision and poor distal lower-limb proprioception. These deficits may either be associated with acute events such as surgery or major illness, or with chronic conditions leading to a more gradual decline in physical abilities. As outlined earlier, many of these deficits have been found to increase an individual's risk of falling. Thus, walking with an appropriate walking aid may reduce the risk of falling by compensating for these risk factors and thus lessening their potential to contribute to a fall. Walking aids may have the additional benefit of marking frailty so that others take care when walking near the person using the aid in public. Some older people also report that an aid may even be useful in self-defence [104].

A walking aid can reduce pain experienced in weight bearing by decreasing load on the joints of the lower limbs, as up to half the body weight can be taken through a walking aid [105]. This may be of great benefit to people suffering from arthritis, and following lower limb fractures or joint replacements.

A walking aid may assist in maximizing the safety and independence of gait for a person who has difficulty generating and/or coordinating appropriate force in the lower-limb musculature. Substantial extensor torque is required to support the body weight against gravity. This extension of the hip, knee and ankle during stance phase is central to independent gait [106], and has been described as an essential component of walking [107]. Use of a walking aid can compensate for an inability to keep the leg extended against gravity. The hip abductors also play a crucial role in walking; large amounts of hip abductor muscle contraction are required during stance phase to keep the pelvis horizontal. The use of a walking aid decreases the hip abductor muscle force requirements [105], especially if held in the contralateral hand [108]. The ankle plantarflexors are also very important in normal walking, primarily in generating eccentric force to restrain forward motion of the lower limb [109]. A contralateral walking stick can compensate for poor plantarflexor muscle strength or control [105, 110]. In these instances the aid will enable the person to compensate for this lack of lower-limb strength and/or control by using the upper-limb musculature.

If a person is unsteady while standing and walking they may also benefit from a walking aid. A walking stick can effectively increase their base of support [105], which may increase stability and assist the person to feel more confident. Walking with a frame allows the person to use their upper limbs to assist the lower limbs in maintaining an upright posture, thereby compensating for poor postural control.

People with chronic airflow limitation and other respiratory or cardiac conditions leading to a shortness of breath, may find a wheeled walking aid useful. Studies have shown that such a walking aid increases the distance that people with chronic airflow limitation can walk, probably by allowing them to fix their shoulder girdle to enable the use of accessory muscles of respiration to assist with breathing [111, 112]. A recent study among inpatients found some additional benefits of using a gutter frame rather than a rollator frame [113].

A walking aid may also be of assistance when sensory information is impaired, such as following amputation or peripheral nerve damage [105], or in individuals with poor vision. Jeka and Lackner [114] have shown that light finger touch of a firm support can dramatically increase standing stability in young people, and we have found that such tactile information is also beneficial for balance in older people who fall and people with diabetic neuropathy [115]. This indicates that in addition to providing a mechanical support, a walking aid can provide the person with information about their position in and movement through the environment.

Several studies [116–120] have found that use of a walking aid is associated with a higher risk of falling. In the majority of cases, it is likely that the use of a walking aid is merely a marker for a gait/balance impairment, i.e. it is really the impairment that causes the increased risk of falls not the use of the walking aid per se.

No studies have yet found that walking aid prescription alone can decrease fall rates. However, several studies have used walking aid prescription and/or training in the use of aids as a component in a multi-faceted intervention programme which did have an impact on fall rates [121, 122].

Prescription principles

A walking aid is best prescribed by a health professional after an assessment of gait, muscle strength, balance and pain. Older people should be discouraged from purchasing or borrowing walking aids without such an assessment [123]. An inappropriate walking aid may actually make walking more difficult than no aid [124].

Several authors have suggested methods for prescribing walking aids [125–128]. As different walking aids have different characteristics, the person's abilities and environment need to be taken into account when prescribing an aid. For example, a rollator frame may be difficult to manoeuvre in a small bathroom, a pick-up frame may be unsafe for someone who is unable to stand unsupported while moving it forwards, and the stability of a quad stick may encourage a person to bear excessive weight through their upper limb. A person may also need to use different aids when walking outdoors from when indoors [129].

An individual's use of a walking aid should be reviewed at regular intervals as their needs are likely to change over time. A further assessment may reveal that the person no longer needs the aid or requires a different aid. The user must also be taught how to maintain the aid. For example, worn ferrules are commonly found on walking aids used in the community [123]. These pose an easily avoidable risk to the user.

A large number of walking aids are commercially available. These vary considerably on a number of aspects of their design, which enables further tailoring of the aid to an individual's needs. For example, when choosing a walking frame, aspects to consider include: weight, base area, manoeuvrability, handle design, foldability, brake design and attachments, such as seats and baskets [126]. A tray may also be a useful addition to a frame, enabling the individual to carry items independently [130]. The skill required to use a particular aid also should be considered. For example, attentional demands have been found to be greater with a pick-up frame than with a rollator frame [131]. This indicates the more complex nature of the task of walking with a pick-up frame and probably reflects its greater apparent variation from the biomechanical requirements of normal walking.

The height of a walking aid may also affect its usefulness. If a walking aid is too low it may cause excessive lateral flexion of the spine, which may decrease gait efficiency and cause pain. If it is too high, the person may be required to elevate their shoulder to hold the aid, which may also lead to pain. The usual height of an aid allows the elbow to be in 15–30 degrees of flexion. If the elbow is flexed more than 30 degrees (i.e. the aid is higher) the person is likely to put less weight on the aid. If the aid is lower the person will tend to put more weight on it [132, 133].

A walking aid should be prescribed after an assessment of the person's physical problems, analysis of the causes of these, and the interaction of physical, environmental and psychosocial factors, rather than on a preconceived idea of what is appropriate for a certain condition [126, 134]. Creative thinking by the healthcare professional may also be required in walking aid prescription. For example, a person with Parkinson's disease who suffers from 'freezing' while walking, may benefit from a stick with a horizontal bar close to its distal end to either step over [135] or touch [136], or a frame with a piece of horizontal string which the person aims to kick.

Limitations

There are several limitations of and disadvantages to the use of walking aids. These can be summarized as: adverse effects on the upper limbs, deterioration of motor function, energy consumption, social stigma and possible increased risk of falling.

Walking with an aid has the potential to cause pain in joints of the arm, particularly the shoulder. The upper limb joints are subject to unaccustomed compressive forces as a result of bearing weight on the arms. In addition,

Crosbie and Nicol [137] and Crosbie [138] found that the upper limb musculature is required to generate large amounts of force, which also leads to compressive forces over joints. However, they also found that the loads imposed on the upper limbs can be reduced by modifications to the gait pattern used when walking with crutches ('alternate step' rather than 'step to') [137] and by a modification to the crutch design (by angling and retracting the crutch shaft to bring the arm closer to the trunk) [138].

As with any motor skill, walking involves the coordination of different muscle actions. It can be argued that walking with a walking aid is a fundamentally different skill from walking unaided. During aided gait, as the arms are assisting the legs in maintaining an upright position against gravity, the nature of the task is changed. The differing demands of the two tasks are reflected in the different ways the tasks are performed. For example, when walking with a frame the hip remains in a flexed position throughout the gait cycle [137] unlike unaided gait [139]. It is therefore possible that once an older person has learnt to walk with a walking aid, it may be difficult for them to walk unaided. They may need training and practice to relearn the skill of walking unaided [107]. In addition, if a person then becomes reliant on the use of a walking aid, they may actually be more unsafe when they attempt to stand, walk or reach outside of their base of support without hand support. This will interfere with their ability to carry out activities of daily living independently and is likely to increase their risk of falling.

Some people may be required by medical practitioners to fully unload a lower limb due to a complicated fracture or surgery. If the person is able, they may hop with crutches or a frame. When compared with unaided gait, this procedure has been associated with increased energy consumption, an increased heart rate [140, 141] and an increased oxygen cost [141, 142]. This increase appears to be greater for walking with a pick-up frame than for walking with crutches [142]. This may put undue stress on the already compromised cardiovascular systems of some older people.

Some older people may also be reluctant to use a walking aid due to negative social stigma associated with the use of assistive devices [104, 143, 144]. The health professional needs to be conscious of these issues when suggesting that an older person requires an aid.

As discussed above, while it seems likely that the appropriate use of a walking aid could contribute to falls prevention, no study has yet demonstrated that this is the case. In fact, the use of walking aids has been associated with an increased risk of falling [116–120]. As some people may fall as a direct consequence of the use of an aid (e.g. by tripping over the aid, catching the aid on furniture or as a result of a poorly maintained aid) care needs to be taken to minimize this. A walking aid may also impede the compensatory lateral stepping mechanism, which can ordinarily assist in avoiding a fall in response to a perturbation [145]. However, it seems likely that most falls among older people who use walking aids result from impaired gait and the use of a walking aid is merely an indicator of this impairment.

Alternatives to walking aids

Use of a walking aid basically enables the individual to continue to walk despite problems, such as pain, decreased muscle strength and poor balance. The walking aid serves to compensate for these problems. Other strategies (such as exercise programmes, motor training, pain relief) to address these problems should be considered instead of, or in addition to, the prescription of the aid. As was outlined in Chapter 11, many older people have the potential to improve their strength, balance and gait. In a recent study among inpatients soon after hip fracture, we found that those who had undertaken a two-week weight-bearing exercise programme (i.e. more relevant to the task of walking) required a less supportive walking aid than those who had undertaken a two-week bed exercise programme [146].

Other physical assistive devices

A number of other devices have been designed to assist the older person to interact with their environment more safely and easily, and thus maintain independence. Assistive devices can be classified as those designed to assist with: physical disabilities, hearing impairments, visual impairments, tactile impairments and cognitive impairments [147]. Physical devices include: bath seats and benches, handheld showers, toilet surrounds, modified cutlery [148], modified cooking equipment [149], shower chairs, bath mats [150], orthoses [151–153], bath treads and lifts [154], long-handled shoehorns, reachers, sponges, sock-aids [155], remote controls for televisions, cordless phones [156], lift chairs [156, 157], adaptive shoelaces [158], wheelchairs, and motorized scooters [129].

Several authors have outlined prescription principles for physical assistive devices [127, 154, 158, 159]. Many assistive devices are best prescribed by an occupational therapist following a visit to the person's home to assess their needs in their own environment [155, 160]. Follow-up visits may be necessary as the individual's needs are likely to change over time [161]. Indeed, even people with cognitive impairments have the potential to increase their use of assistive devices after intervention from an occupational therapist [148].

Several clinical trials have now found value in the prescription and use of assistive devices. Hart *et al.* [149] conducted a randomized controlled trial of 79 community dwellers aged 85 and over with some disability, but not using any assistive devices prior to the study intervention. Following assessment by an occupational therapist, subjects in the intervention group were issued with a raised toilet seat, a teapot tipper, a tap turner, a shoehorn and elastic laces, and a double-handled saucepan. The observed degree of difficulty in completing relevant tasks was subsequently reduced. In a randomized controlled trial of a home visit from an occupational therapist after discharge from hospital among people who had suffered a stroke, Corr and Bayer [162] found that the intervention group who used more aids were less likely to be readmitted to hospital.

Further investigation is required to assess the effects of these improvements on falls. Promisingly, occupational therapy assessment and provision of appropriate aids was a key component of a randomized controlled trial which showed a significant decrease in falls among people who had previously presented to the emergency department following a fall [163]. One other trial [121] which included provision and training in the use of aids during home visits also showed an effect on falls, whereas a study which focused purely on environmental aspects did not have such positive results [164].

Spectacles

Impaired vision can have substantially adverse effects on the ability to read, enjoy recreational pastimes and undertake activities of daily living [165–167] as well as directly affect balance and predispose older people to falls (see Chapter 4). Despite this, several surveys have found that many older people who wear glasses with outdated prescriptions or no glasses at all would benefit from wearing new glasses with correct prescriptions [165–167]. This indicates that older people are not aware of their declining vision, and/or do not perceive the benefits of regular vision assessments and updated glasses outweigh the risks to safety and lifestyle. Reduced access to eye care may also comprise an important barrier for some frail older people.

Irrespective of the correction for distance vision, multifocal glasses may pose a significant risk of falling for older people. Multifocal (bifocal, trifocal or progressive lens) glasses are prescribed to correct for presbyopia (an inability to focus on close objects), which is the most prevalent form of visual impairment in older people [168, 169]. These glasses have benefits for tasks that require changes in focal length, including everyday tasks of driving, shopping and cooking. However, multifocals also have disadvantages. There are many anecdotal reports that multifocals constitute a danger for older people, particularly when walking on stairs [170] and in those with disabilities that affect gait [171]. Bifocal glasses have optical defects, such as prismatic jump at the top of the

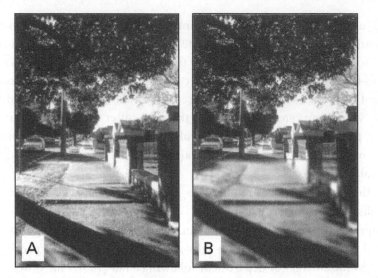

Fig. 13.4   Simulated view of a street scene as viewed through A: single-lens distance glasses and B: bifocal glasses. The footpath misalignment is clearly seen in A, but is blurred in B.

reading segment, that causes an apparent displacement of fixed objects [169, 172]. The lower lenses of all types of multifocal glasses blur distant objects in the lower visual field and this factor, in particular, may represent a significant problem for older people [170, 173]. Figure 13.4 shows a simulated view of a street scene as viewed through single-lens distance and multifocal glasses.

Multifocal glasses may predispose older people to falls because viewing the environment through their lower lenses impairs the important visual capabilities (contrast sensitivity and depth perception) for detecting environmental hazards, particularly in challenging or unfamiliar environments. As indicated in Chapter 4, several studies have shown that contrast sensitivity and depth perception are among the strongest visual risk factors for falls and fall-related fractures in older people [174–180]. Further, most falls in older people occur while walking [181, 182]. Studies have found that when walking, people view the environment at distances approximating two steps ahead [183]. For multifocal wearers, the lower lenses of their glasses (with focal lengths of 0.6m) substantially blur their lower visual fields, impairing contrast sensitivity and depth perception at the critical focal distances required for detecting and discriminating floor-level objects (approximately 1.5 to 2m) [183].

We recently conducted a study that was designed to assess the effects of multifocal glasses on vision and falls in older people [184]. In this prospective cohort study of 156 participants aged 63–90 years, 56% were regular wearers of multifocal glasses. These participants performed significantly worse in both distant depth perception and edge-contrast sensitivity tests in conditions which forced them to view test stimuli through the lower segments of their glasses. Multifocal glasses wearers had significantly greater odds of falling in the one-year follow-up period than non-multifocal glasses wearers (OR = 2.27, 95% CI = 1.04−4.97), when adjusting for age and known physiological risk factors for falls. Multifocal glasses wearers were also more likely to fall when outside their homes (OR = 2.54, 95% CI = 1.19−5.77) and when walking up or down stairs ($p < 0.001$). The population attributable risks of regular multifocal glasses use were 35% for any falls and 41% for falls outside the home.

As many older people are at an increased risk of falls due to impairments that limit their ability to detect and correct postural disturbances resulting from trips [185], they may benefit from wearing single-lens glasses when walking. This would appear to be particularly important when walking up or down stairs and in unfamiliar settings outside the home. Public health initiatives would assist in raising awareness in older people and their carers of the importance of regular eye examinations and use of appropriate prescription glasses.

Hip protectors

It may be possible to decrease the likelihood that a fall will result in a fracture by changing the interaction between the faller and the surface on which they fall. This can be undertaken by modifying the surface onto which the person falls or by placing a barrier between the person and the hard surface onto which they fall. Hip protectors are designed to fulfil this latter role.

Hip protectors are worn by the individual and are designed both to absorb energy and to transfer load from the bone to the surrounding soft tissues [186]. The original hip protectors designed in Denmark [187] have a firm outer shell and an inner foam section. Another version is made of dense plastic without an outer shell [188]. The protector is either removable and fits into pockets in special underwear or non-removable and built into underwear. Early research into hip protectors led to international enthusiasm about the potential for preventing hip fractures in high-risk groups, such as nursing home residents, with a relatively low cost intervention and minimal side effects. The original Danish model was tested in a randomized controlled study among 701 residents of a nursing home [187]. The risk of fracture was significantly decreased in the intervention group (relative risk 0.44). Although eight members of the intervention group suffered hip fractures, none were wearing the hip protectors at the time of fracture. A further study in Sweden [189] tested a different model of hip protector. They also found a decreased fracture rate among residents of a randomly selected nursing home who were offered hip protectors, compared with a control nursing home (relative risk 0.33).

However, further research into the efficacy and practicality of hip protector use has not been as positive. It is now thought that the results from the early trials may have over estimated the efficacy of hip protectors, partly due to incorrect analysis given their cluster-randomized designs [190]. Subsequent trials with individual randomization have not shown such positive results. The Cochrane review on this topic [190] finds that 'pooling of data from five individually randomized trials conducted in nursing/residential care settings (1426 participants) showed no statistically significant reduction in hip fracture incidence (hip protectors 37/822 (4.5%), controls 40/604 (6.6%), relative risk = 0.83, 95% CI = 0.54–1.24) and that two individually randomized studies that recruited community-dwelling elderly people 'did not achieve a statistically significant reduction in the incidence of hip fractures (27/484 (5.6%) in hip protector group vs. 24/482 (5.0%) in controls, relative risk = 1.11, 95% CI = 0.65–1.90).' A more recent cluster-randomized trial [191] among residents of 127 aged care facilities (4117 occupied beds) also failed to find an effect on fracture rates of hip protectors (rate ratio for the intervention group compared to the control group of 1.05 (95% CI = 0.77–1.43).

When worn correctly, hip protectors probably work well to prevent hip fractures. The majority of fractures in intervention groups of hip protector studies occur while the hip protector is not actually being worn or is incorrectly positioned [190]. A recent study compared protected and unprotected falls among high-risk nursing home residents and found the risk of hip fracture was reduced to less than one-third in protected falls compared with unprotected falls [192].

Compliance seems to be the major limitation to efficacy of hip protectors. Many of the trials included in the Cochrane review [190] had compliance rates of less than 40% by the end of the studies. For example, the recent O'Halloran *et al.* study [191] found initial acceptance of the hip protectors was 37.2% (508/1366) with adherence falling to 19.9% (272/1366) at 72 weeks. Several studies found that many potential participants declined to be involved in the study (e.g. 79% declined in Birks *et al.* [193]). A systematic review [194] found very variable acceptance (37%–72%, median 68%) and compliance with hip protectors (20%–92%, median 56%). Key reasons for poor compliance were: not being comfortable (too tight/ poor fit); the extra effort needed to wear the device; urinary incontinence; and physical difficulties/illnesses. In some settings, cost may be a barrier to hip protector use [195]. Hip protectors do not decrease the risk of other fractures, e.g. pelvic fractures [190], but have been found to reduce fear of falling [196].

Despite their limitations, hip protectors can be useful clinically as a hip fracture prevention strategy among those at high risk of falls who are willing and able to wear them. More work is required to establish the optimum design for hip protectors [190, 195].

Aids to prevent 'long lies'

Up to half of all older people who fall without suffering injuries are unable to get up from the floor unaided [197]. As well as additional emotional distress, this can result in a number of serious medical problems, as outlined in Chapter 1. If possible, older people should be taught how to get up off the floor [198, 199].

For persons unable to get up from the floor independently, one way of preventing long lies is the use of personal alarm systems. These involve the older person having an alert button within reach at all times, i.e. worn on a cord around the neck or kept in a pocket. If the person falls and requires assistance, the alarm allows them to notify those nearby and/or an operator who can arrange for appropriate assistance to be provided. Although not evaluated in research trials, many older people and their families report feeling reassured once such a system is installed. Unfortunately, the cost of these systems may be prohibitive to some older people. Less costly alternatives are mobile or cordless phones carried by the older person at all times.

If an older person is at risk of not being able to get off the floor following a fall, steps should also be taken to minimize the consequences of the time spent on the floor [200]. For example, a blanket can be kept on or near the floor in commonly used rooms of the house to prevent hypothermia while waiting for help to arrive [198].

Restraints

Physical restraints were traditionally used to prevent a person falling as well as to control disruptive or potentially dangerous behaviours. While restraints are still used for this purpose in residential care and acute care settings [201], their use has been reduced in the past decade [202]. Many items and actions constitute restraint including: wrist or leg cuffs to stop the person moving one or more limbs by fixing them to an object; vests or jackets to stop a person sitting up in bed or getting out of a chair; tables to stop the person getting out of a chair; bed rails; use of low chairs or beds to prevent the person standing up; as well as certain medications (chemical restraints).

The use of restraints is highly controversial. It is clear that the widespread use of restraints impinges on the person's autonomy and personal freedom, with associated philosophical and legal ramifications. Inappropriate restraint use could also lead to a deterioration in motor functioning if physical activity levels are insufficient to maintain muscle strength. Some restraints may also increase the risk of injury (e.g. skin damage from cuff, fall while attempting to climb over bedrail). Several authors have found that the use of restraints does not even decrease the risk of fall injury [203–207].

In recent years, programmes have been introduced and legislation has been enacted in many countries to minimize the use of restraints [208]. Werner *et al.* [209] reported the successful removal of restraints in 92% of previously restrained residents in a long term care setting. Similarly, Levine *et al.* [210] reported being able to reduce the prevalence of physical restraint use in a large nursing facility from 39% to 4% over a three year period without a change in the rate of falls or accident-related injuries. Evans *et al.* [211] found that greater restraint reduction was achieved in residential aged care facilities when a consultation service was provided in addition to education. Restraint use can probably be reduced more easily in purpose-built facilities, where the person is safe to walk around freely. In poorly designed facilities, people may be restrained to prevent them becoming lost or injuring themselves on unsafe equipment, or other environmental factors.

Restraint reduction requires that alternatives to restraint use are fully investigated prior to the introduction of a restraint [208]. Instead of, or in addition to, restraint use, an individual's risk factors for falls should be minimized as per other chapters in this book, i.e. appropriate medication use, medical conditions identified and treated, appropriate footwear use, exercise for physical risk factors [212], and environmental safety optimized. In addition, many physical, psychological and spiritual strategies to increase a person's comfort and contentment have been suggested (see Box 13.2).

Box 13.2 Alternatives to restraints (adapted from Letizia *et al.* [208]).

Individual risk factor assessment and reduction: medications, medical conditions, footwear, factors amenable to exercise or training.

Other physical measures: bed alarms, motion detectors.

Ensure provision for basic needs (hunger, thirst, toileting).

Exercise and activities, diversional therapy, relaxation techniques, rocking chairs, music, television.

Psychological measures: talking and listening to patients, frequent orientation, explanation of procedures, providing companionship.

Supervision/staffing: intensive staffing, one-to-one staffing using a sitter at the bedside, organization of family visiting schedules, varied staff assignment.

Spiritual needs: visits from pastoral care staff and clergy.

Environmental measures: careful determination of patient/staff location, safety optimized.

However, there is also evidence that in certain circumstances, restraints may play a role in fall injury prevention [213]. For example, a restraint may be

14. E. R. Larsen, L. Mosekilde & A. Foldspang, Correlates of falling during 24 h among elderly Danish community residents. *Preventive Medicine*, **39** (2004), 389–98.

15. T. D. Koepsell, M. E. Wolf, D. M. Buchner *et al.*, Footwear style and risk of falls in older adults. *Journal of the American Geriatrics Society*, **52** (2004), 1495–501.

16. A. F. Tencer, T. D. Koepsell, M. E. Wolf *et al.*, Biomechanical properties of shoes and risk of falls in older adults. *Journal of the American Geriatrics Society*, **52** (2004), 1840–6.

17. J. E. Edelstein, If the shoe fits: footwear considerations for the elderly. *Physical and Occupational Therapy in Geriatrics*, **5** (1987), 1–16.

18. J. E. Edelstein, Foot care for the aging. *Physical Therapy*, **68** (1988), 1882–6.

19. L. Sudarsky, Geriatrics: gait disorders in the elderly. *New England Journal of Medicine*, **322** (1990), 1441–6.

20. C. C. Frey, F. Thompson, J. Smith, M. Sanders & H. Horstman, American Orthopedic Foot and Ankle Society women's shoe survey. *Foot and Ankle*, **14** (1993), 78–81.

21. L. Mitchell, *Stepping Out – Three Centuries of Shoes* (Sydney: Powerhouse Publishing, 1997).

22. T. Bendix, S. S. Sorenson & K. Klausen, Lumbar curve, trunk muscles, and line of gravity with different heel heights. *Spine*, **9** (1984), 223–7.

23. K. A. Opila, S. S. Wagner, S. Schiowitz & J. Chen, Postural alignment in barefoot and high-heeled stance. *Spine*, **13** (1988), 542–7.

24. B. J. DeLateur, R. M. Giaconi, K. Questad, M. Ko & J. F. Lehmann, Footwear and posture – compensatory strategies for heel height. *American Journal of Physical Medicine and Rehabilitation*, **70** (1991), 246–54.

25. M. E. Franklin, T. C. Chenier, L. Brauninger, H. Cook & S. Harris, Effect of positive heel inclination on posture. *Journal of Orthopaedic and Sports Physical Therapy*, **21** (1995), 94–9.

26. B. W. Gastwirth, T. D. O'Brien, R. M. Nelson, D. C. Manger & S. A. Kindig, An electrodynographic study of foot function in shoes of varing heel heights. *Journal of the American Podiatric Medical Association*, **81** (1991), 463–72.

27. R. E. Snow, K. R. Williams G. B. Holmes, Jr, The effects of wearing high heeled shoes on pedal pressures in women. *Foot and Ankle*, **13** (1992), 85–92.

28. J. P. Corrigan, D. P. Moore & M. M. Stephens, Effect of heel height on forefoot loading. *Foot and Ankle*, **14** (1993), 148–52.

29. R. E. Snow & K. R. Williams, High heeled shoes: their effect on centre of mass position, posture, three dimensional kinematics, rearfoot motion and ground reaction forces. *Archives of Physical Medicine and Rehabilitation*, **75** (1994), 568–76.

30. M. Nyska, C. McCabe, K. Linge & L. Klenerman, Plantar forefoot pressures during treadmill walking with high-heel and low-heel shoes. *Foot and Ankle International*, **17** (1996), 662–6.

31. R. E. Sussman & J. C. D'Amico, The influence of the height of the heel on the first metatarsophalangeal joint. *Journal of the American Podiatric Medical Association*, **74** (1984), 504–8.

32. I. D. McBride, U. P. Wyss, T. D. Cooke *et al.*, First metatarsophalangeal joint reaction forces during high-heel gait. *Foot and Ankle*, **11** (1991), 282–8.

33. H. H. Merrifield, Female gait patterns in shoes with different heel heights. *Ergonomics*, **14** (1971), 411–17.

34. C. J. Ebbeling, J. Hamill & J. A. Crussemeyer, Lower extremity mechanics and energy cost of walking in high-heeled shoes. *Journal of Orthopaedic and Sports Physical Therapy*, **19** (1994), 190–6.

35. R. P. Schwartz & A. L. Heath, Preliminary findings from a roentgenographic study of the influence of heel height and empirical shank curvature on osteo-articular relationships of the normal female foot. *Journal of Bone and Joint Surgery*, **46A** (1959), 324–34.

36. P. D. Gollnick, C. M. Tipton & P. V. Karpovich, Electromyographic study of walking on high heels. *Research Quarterly*, **35** (Suppl) (1964), 370–8.

37. G. Gehlsen, S. J. Braatz & N. Assmann, Effects of heel height on knee rotation and gait. *Human Movement Science*, **5** (1986), 149–55.

38. R. W. Soames & A. A. Evans, Female gait patterns: the influence of footwear. *Ergonomics*, **30** (1987), 893–900.

39. K. A. Opila-Correia, Kinematics of high-heeled gait. *Archives of Physical Medicine and Rehabilitation*, **71** (1990), 304–9.

40. C. Reinschmidt & B. M. Nigg, Influence of heel height on ankle joint moments in running. *Medicine and Science in Sports and Exercise*, **27** (1995), 410–16.

41. D. C. Kerrigan, M. K. Todd & P. O. Riley, Knee osteoarthritis and high-heeled shoes. *The Lancet*, **351** (1998), 1399–401.

42. K. A. Opila-Correia, Kinematics of high-heeled gait with consideration for age and experience of wearers. *Archives of Physical Medicine and Rehabilitation*, **71** (1990), 905–9.

43. K. H. Lee, A. Matteliano, J. Medige & T. Smiehorowski, Electromyographic changes of leg muscles with heel lift: therapeutic implications. *Archives of Physical Medicine and Rehabilitation*, **68** (1987), 298–301.

44. K. H. Lee, J. C. Shieh, A. Matteliano & T. Smiehorowski, Electromyographic changes of leg muscles with heel lifts in women: therapeutic implications. *Archives of Physical Medicine and Rehabilitation*, **71** (1990), 31–3.

45. M. J. Gibson, R. O. Andres, B. Isaacs, T. Radebaugh & J. Worm-Petersen, The prevention of falls in later life. *Danish Medical Bulletin*, **34** (Suppl 4) (1987), 1–24.

46. L. Rubenstein, A. Robbins, B. Schulman *et al.*, Falls and instability in the elderly. *Journal of the American Geriatrics Society*, **36** (1988), 266–78.

47. M. E. Tinetti & M. Speechly, Prevention of falls among the elderly. *New England Journal of Medicine*, **320** (1989), 1055–9.

48. M. J. Adrian & P. V. Karpovich, Foot instability during walking in shoes with high heels. *Research Quarterly*, **37** (1966), 168–75.

49. J. S. Brecht, M. W. Chang, R. Price & J. Lehmann, Decreased balance performance in cowboy boots compared with tennis shoes. *Archives of Physical Medicine and Rehabilitation*, **76** (1995), 940–6.

50. S. R. Lord & G. M. Bashford, Shoe characteristics and balance in older women. *Journal of the American Geriatrics Society*, **44** (1996), 429–33.

51. S. A. Arnadottir & V. S. Mercer, Effects of footwear on measurements of balance and gait in women between the ages of 65 and 93 years. *Physical Therapy*, **80** (2000), 17–27.

52. U. Lindemann, S. Scheibe, E. Sturm *et al.*, Elevated heels and adaptation to new shoes in frail elderly women. *Zeitschrift für Gerontologie und Geriatrie,* **36** (2003), 29–34.

53. F. Surdyk & P. Kostyniuk, Heel rise: an aid in ambulation for Parkinsonian patients who lose their balance backward. *American Journal of Corrective Therapy,* **23** (1969), 107.

54. J. Hogan-Budris, Choosing foot materials for the elderly. *Topics in Geriatric Rehabilitation,* **7** (1992), 49–61.

55. S. E. Robbins, G. J. Gouw & J. McClaran, Shoe sole thickness and hardness influence balance in older men. *Journal of the American Geriatrics Society,* **40** (1992), 1089–94.

56. S. E. Robbins, E. Waked & J. McClaran, Proprioception and stability: foot position awareness as a function of age and footwear. *Age and Ageing,* **24** (1995), 67–72.

57. S. E. Robbins, E. Waked, P. Allard, J. McClaran & N. Krouglicof, Foot position awareness in younger and older men: the influence of footwear sole properties. *Journal of the American Geriatrics Society,* **45** (1997), 61–6.

58. K. Sekizawa, M. A. Sandrey, C. D. Ingersoll, M. L. Cordova, Effects of shoe sole thickness on joint position sense. *Gait and Posture,* **13** (2001), 221–8.

59. M. S. Redfern, P. L. Moore & C. M. Yarsky, The influence of flooring on standing balance among older persons. *Human Factors,* **39** (1997), 445–55.

60. S. R. Lord, R. D. Clark & I. W. Webster, Physiological factors associated with falls in an elderly population. *Journal of the American Geriatrics Society,* **39** (1991), 1194–200.

61. S. R. Lord, D. McLean & G. Stathers, Physiological factors associated with injurious falls in older people living in the community. *Gerontology,* **38** (1992), 338–46.

62. R. Gronqvist, J. Roine, E. Jarvinen & E. Korhonen, An apparatus and a method for determining the slip resistance of shoes and floors by simulation of human foot motions. *Ergonomics,* **32** (1989), 979–95.

63. U. Bjornstig, J. Bjornstig & A. Dahlgren, Slipping on ice and snow – elderly women and young men are typical victims. *Accident Analysis and Prevention,* **29** (1997), 211–15.

64. D. P. Manning, I. Ayers, C. Jones, M. Bruce & K. Cohen, The incidence of underfoot accidents during 1985 in a working population of 10000 Merseyside people. *Journal of Occupational Accidents,* **10** (1988), 121–30.

65. D. P. Manning, Slipping and the penalties inflicted generally by the law of gravitation. *Journal of Social and Occupational Medicine,* **38** (1988), 123–7.

66. J. Bell, Slip and fall accidents. *Occupational Health and Safety,* December (1995), 40–41, 57.

67. L. Strandberg, The effect of conditions underfoot on falling and over-exertion accidents. *Ergonomics,* **28** (1985), 131–47.

68. A. Gabell, M. A. Simons & Nayak, Falls in the healthy elderly: predisposing causes. *Ergonomics,* **28** (1985), 965–75.

69. P. J. Perkins & M. P. Wilson, Slip-resistance testing of shoes – new developments. *Ergonomics,* **26** (1983), 73–82.

70. M. Tisserand, Progress in the prevention of falls caused by slipping. *Ergonomics,* **28** (1985), 1027–42.

71. H. B. Menz, S. R. Lord & A. S. McIntosh, Slip resistance of casual footwear: implications for falls in older adults. *Gerontology,* **47** (2001), 145–9.

72. D. Lloyd & M. G. Stevenson, Measurement of slip resistance of shoes on floor surfaces. Part 2. Effect of a bevelled heel. *Journal of Occupational Health and Safety*, **5** (1989), 229–35.

73. O. Petrov, K. Blocher & R. Bradbury, Footwear and ankle stability in the basketball player. *Clinics in Podiatric Medicine and Surgery*, **5** (1988), 275–90.

74. J. A. Denton, Athletic shoes. In *Clinical Biomechanics of the Lower Extremities*, ed. R. Valmassy. (St Lois: Mosby, 1996), pp. 453–63.

75. G. Johnson, D. Dowson & V. Wrights, A biomechanical approach to the design of football boots. *Journal of Biomechanics*, **9** (1976), 581–5.

76. R. A. Ottaviani, J. A. Ashton-Miller, S. U. Kothari & E. M. Wojtys, Basketball shoe height and maximal muscular resistance to applied ankle inversion and eversion moments. *American Journal of Sports Medicine*, **23** (1995), 418–23.

77. A. Stacoff, J. Steger, E. Stussi & C. Reinschmidt, Lateral stability in sideward cutting movements. *Medicine and Science in Sports and Exercise*, **28** (1996), 350–8.

78. S. R. Lord, G. M. Bashford, A. Howland & B. Munro, Effects of shoe collar height and sole hardness on balance in older women. *Journal of the American Geriatrics Society*, **47** (1999), 681–4.

79. R. H. Whipple, L. I. Wolfson & P. M. Amerman, The relationship of knee and ankle weakness to falls in nursing home residents: an isokinetic study. *Journal of the American Geriatrics Society*, **35** (1987), 13–20.

80. S. E. Robbins, E. Waked & R. Rappel, Ankle taping improves proprioception before and after exercise. *British Journal of Sports Medicine*, **29** (1995), 242–7.

81. N. Matsusaka, Control of the medial-lateral balance in walking. *Acta Orthopedica Scandinavica*, **57** (1986), 555–9.

82. H. Gauffin & H. Tropp, Postural control in single limb stance strategies for correction. *Journal of Human Movement Studies*, **26** (1994), 267–78.

83. P. Hoogvliet, W. A. V. Duyl, J. V. D. Bakker, P. G. H. Mulder & H. J. Stam, A model for the relation between the displacement of the ankle and the centre of pressure in the frontal plane, during one leg stance. *Gait and Posture*, **6** (1997), 39–49.

84. P. Hoogvliet, W. A. V. Duyl, J. V. D. Bakker, P. G. H. Mulder & H. J. Stam, Variations in foot breadth: effect on aspects of postural control during one-leg stance. *Archives of Physical Medicine and Rehabilitation*, **78** (1997), 284–9.

85. T. E. Clarke, E. C. Frederick & C. L. Hamill, The effects of shoe design parameters on rearfoot control in running. *Medicine and Science in Sports and Exercise*, **15** (1983), 376–81.

86. B. M. Nigg & M. Morlock, The influence of lateral heel flare of running shoes on pronation and impact forces. *Medicine and Science in Sports and Exercise*, **19** (1987), 294–302.

87. S. R. Lord, M. W. Rogers, A. Howland & R. Fitzpatrick, Lateral stability, sensorimotor function and falls in older people. *Journal of the American Geriatrics Society*, **47** (1999), 1077–81.

88. G. G. Simoneau, J. S. Ulbrecht, J. A. Derr, M. B. Becker & P. R. Cavanagh, Postural instability in patients with diabetic sensory neuropathy. *Diabetes Care*, **17** (1994), 1411–21.

89. P. Boucher, N. Teasdale, R. Courtemanche, C. Bard & M. Fleury, Postural stability in diabetic polyneuropathy. *Diabetes Care*, **18** (1995), 638–45.

90. M. Magnusson, H. Enbom, R. Johansson & I. Pyykko, Significance of pressor input from the human feet in anterior-posterior postural control. *Acta Otolaryngologica*, **110** (1990), 182–8.

91. L. C. Orteza, W. D. Vogelbach & C. R. Denegar, The effects of molded and unmolded orthotics on balance and pain while jogging following inversion ankle sprain. *Journal of Athletic Training*, **27** (1992), 80–4.

92. K. Guskiewicz & D. Perrin, Effect of orthotics on postural sway following inversion ankle sprain. *Journal of Orthopaedic and Sports Physical Therapy*, **23** (1996), 326–31.

93. D. E. Stude & D. K. Brink, Effects of nine holes of simulated golf and orthotic intervention on balance and proprioception in experienced golfers. *Journal of Manipulative and Physiological Therapeutics*, **20** (1997), 590–601.

94. M. Hosoda, O. Yoshimaru, K. Takayanagi *et al.*, The effects of various footwear types and materials, and of fixing of the ankles by footwear, on upright posture control. *Journal of Physical Therapy Science*, **9** (1997), 47–51.

95. G. Waddington & R. Adams, Textured insole effects on ankle movement discrimination while wearing athletic shoes. *Physical Therapy in Sport*, **1** (2000), 119–28.

96. B. E. Maki, S. D. Perry, R. G. Norrie & W. E. McIlroy, Effect of facilitation of sensation from plantar foot-surface boundaries on postural stabilization in young and older adults. *Journal of Gerontology*, **54A** (1999), M281–7.

97. A. A. Priplata, J. B. Niemi, J. D. Harry, L. A. Lipsitz & J. J. Collins, Vibrating insoles and balance control in elderly people. *The Lancet*, **362** (2003), 1123–4.

98. K. Seale, Women and their shoes: unrealistic expectations? *American Academy of Orthopedic Surgeons Instructional Course Lectures*, **44** (1995), 379–84.

99. P. Joyce, Women and their shoes: attitudes, influences and behaviour. *British Journal of Podiatry*, **3** (2000), 111–15.

100. W. Rossi, The frustration of "sensible" shoes. *Journal of the American Podiatry Association*, **70** (1980), 257–8.

101. R. H. Fortinsky, M. Iannuzzi-Sucich, D. I. Baker *et al.*, Fall-risk assessment and management in clinical practice: views from healthcare providers. *Journal of the American Geriatrics Society*, **52** (2004), 1522–6.

102. American Geriatrics Society, Guideline for the prevention of falls in older persons. *Journal of the American Geriatrics Society*, 49 (2001), 664–72.

103. A. A. Ogle, Canes, crutches, walkers, and other ambulation aids. *Physical Medicine and Rehabilitation: State of the Art Reviews*, **14** (2000), 485–92.

104. F. Aminzadeh & N. Edwards, Exploring seniors' views on the use of assistive devices in fall prevention. *Public Health Nursing*, **15** (1998), 297–304.

105. A. Deathe, K. Hayes & D. Winter, The biomechanics of canes, crutches and walkers. *Critical Reviews in Physical and Rehabilitation Medicine*, **5** (1993), 15–29.

106. D. Winter, Overall principle of lower limb support during stance phase of gait. *Journal of Biomechanics*, **13** (1980), 923–7.

107. J. Carr & R. Shepherd, *Neurological Rehabilitation: Optimizing Motor Performance* (Oxford: Butterworth-Heinemann, 1998).

108. D. A. Neumann, Hip abductor muscle activity as subjects with hip prostheses walk with different methods of using a cane. *Physical Therapy*, **78** (1998), 490–501.

109. D. Sutherland, C. Cooper & D. Daniel, The role of the ankle plantar flexors in normal walking. *The Journal of Bone and Joint Surgery*, **62-A** (1980), 354–63.

110. A. Moseley, A. Wales, R. Herbert, K. Shurr & S. Moore, Observation and analysis of hemiplegic gait: stance phase. *Australian Journal of Physiotherapy*, **39** (1993), 259–67.

111. S. Wesmiller & L. Hoffman, Assistive device for ambulation in oxygen dependent patients with COPD. *Journal of Cardiopulmonary Rehabilitation*, **14** (1994), 122–6.

112. P. Honeyman, P. Barr & D. Stubbing, Effect of a walking aid on disability, oxygenation, and breathlessness in patients with chronic airflow limitation. *Journal of Cardiopulmonary Rehabilitation*, **16** (1996), 63–7.

113. A. M. Yohannes & M. J. Connolly, Early mobilization with walking aids following hospital admission with acute exacerbation of chronic obstructive pulmonary disease. *Clinical Rehabilitation*, **17** (2003), 465–71.

114. J. Jeka & J. Lackner, Fingertip contact influences human postural control. *Experimental Brain Research*, **100** (1994), 495–502.

115. M. W. Rogers, D. L. Wardman, S. R. Lord & R. C. Fitzpatrick, Passive tactile sensory input improves stability during standing. *Experimental Brain Research*, **136** (2001), 514–22.

116. M. E. Tinetti, M. Speechley & S. F. Ginter, Risk factors for falls among elderly persons living in the community. *New England Journal of Medicine*, **319** (1988), 1701–7.

117. A. J. Campbell, M. J. Borrie & G. F. Spears, Risk factors for falls in a community-based prospective study of people 70 years and older. *Journal of Gerontology*, **44** (1989), M112–17.

118. J. Teno, D. P. Kiel & V. Mor, Multiple stumbles: a risk factor for falls in community-dwelling elderly. A prospective study. *Journal of the American Geriatrics Society*, **38** (1990), 1321–5.

119. M. E. Tinetti, J. Doucette, E. Claus & R. Marottoli, Risk factors for serious injury during falls by older persons in the community. *Journal of the American Geriatrics Society*, **43** (1995), 1214–21.

120. D. K. Kiely, D. P. Kiel, A. B. Burrows & L. A. Lipsitz, Identifying nursing home residents at risk for falling. *Journal of the American Geriatrics Society*, **46** (1998), 551–5.

121. T. Nikolaus & M. Bach, Preventing falls in community-dwelling frail older people using a home intervention team (HIT): results from the randomised falls-HIT trial. *Journal of the American Geriatrics Society*, **51** (2003), 300–5.

122. J. Jensen, L. Lundin-Olsson, L. Nyberg & Y. Gustafson, Fall and injury prevention in older people living in residential care facilities: a cluster randomized trial. *Annals of Internal Medicine*, **136** (2002), 733–41.

123. C. Simpson & L. Pirrie, Walking aids: a survey of suitability and supply. *Physiotherapy*, **77** (1991), 231–4.

124. S. F. Tyson & A. Ashburn, The influence of walking aids on hemiplegic gait. *Physiotherapy Theory and Practice*, **10** (1994), 77–86.

125. J. Breuer, Assistive devices and adapted equipment for ambulation programs for geriatric patients. *Physical and Occupational Therapy in Geriatrics*, **1** (1981), 51–77.

126. J. Hall, A. Clarke & R. Harrison, Guide lines for prescription of walking frames. *Physiotherapy*, **76** (1990), 118–20.

127. P. Holliday & G. Fernie, Assistive devices: aids to independence. In *Physiotherapy with Older People*, ed. B. Pickles, A. Compton, C. Cott *et al.* (London: W.B. Saunders, 1995), pp. 360–81.

128. C. Prajapati, C. Watkins, H. Cullen *et al.*, The 'S' test – a preliminary study of an instrument for selecting the most appropriate mobility aid. *Clinical Rehabilitation*, **10** (1996), 314–18.

129. J. York, Mobility methods selected for use in home and community environments. *Physical Therapy*, **69** (1989), 736–47.

130. R. Farley & J. Roy, Equipment review: the Edinburgh Homewalker – design and field trial. *British Journal of Occupational Therapy*, **59** (1996), 22.

131. D. Wright & T. Kemp, The dual-task methodology and assessing the attentional demands of ambulation with walking devices. *Physical Therapy*, **72** (1992), 306–15.

132. A. B. Deathe, R. D. Pardo, D. A. Winter, K. C. Hayes & J. Russell-Smyth, Stability of walking frames. *Journal of Rehabilitation Research and Development*, **33** (1996), 30–5.

133. C. L. Lu, B. Yu, J. R. Basford, M. E. Johnson & K. N. An, Influences of cane length on the stability of stroke patients. *Journal of Rehabilitation Research and Development*, **34** (1997), 91–100.

134. C. Wilkin, Pragmatics in the issuing of sticks and frames. *Physiotherapy*, **82** (1996), 331–5.

135. J. Pearce, A walking aid for Parkinsonian patients [letter]. *The Lancet*, **342** (1993), 62.

136. J. Blau, Seymour stick [letter]. *The Lancet*, **342** (1993), 250.

137. W. J. Crosbie & A. C. Nicol, Aided gait in rheumatoid arthritis following knee arthroplasty. *Archives of Physical Medicine and Rehabilitation*, **71** (1990), 299–303.

138. W. J. Crosbie, Kinematics of walking frame ambulation. *Clinical Biomechanics*, **8** (1993), 31–6.

139. D. A. Winter, A. E. Patla, J. S. Frank & S. E. Walt, Biomechanical walking pattern changes in the fit and healthy elderly. *Physical Therapy*, **70** (1990), 340–7.

140. I. Baruch & K. Mossberg, Heart-rate response of elderly women to nonweight-bearing ambulation with a walker. *Physical Therapy*, **63** (1983), 1782–7.

141. A. Annesley, M. Almada-Norfleet, D. Arnall & M. Cornwall, Energy expenditure of ambulation using the Sure-Gait crutch and the standard axillary crutch. *Physical Therapy*, **70** (1990), 18–23.

142. C. Holder, E. Haskvitz & A. Weltman, The effects of assistive devices on the oxygen cost, cardiovascular stress, and perception of nonweight-bearing ambulation. *Journal of Orthopaedic and Sports Physical Therapy*, **18** (1993), 537–42.

143. K. L. Rush & L. L. Ouellet, Mobility aids and the elderly client. *Journal of Gerontological Nursing*, **23** (1997), 7–15.

144. K. Pippin & G. R. Fernie, Designing devices that are acceptable to the frail elderly: a new understanding based upon how older people perceive a walker. *Technology and Disability*, **7** (1997), 93–102.

145. H. Bateni, E. Heung, J. Zettel, W. E. McLlroy & B. E. Maki, Can use of walkers or canes impede lateral compensatory stepping movements? *Gait and Posture*, **20** (2004), 74–83.

146. C. Sherrington, S. Lord & R. Herbert, A randomised trial of weight-bearing versus non-weight-bearing exercise for improving physical ability in inpatients after hip fracture. *Australian Journal of Physiotherapy*, **49** (2003), 15.

147. W. Mann, D. Hurren & M. Tomita, Comparison of assistive device use and needs of home-based older persons with different impairments. *American Journal of Occupational Therapy*, **47** (1993), 980–7.

148. S. Nochajski, M. Tomita & W. Mann, The use and satisfaction with assistive devices by older persons with cognitive impairments: a pilot intervention study. *Topics in Geriatric Rehabilitation*, **12** (1996), 38–53.

149. D. Hart, A. Bowling, M. Ellis & A. Silman, Locomotor disability in very elderly people: value of a programme for screening and provision of aids for daily living. *British Medical Journal*, **301** (1990), 216–20.

150. L. Clemson & R. Martin, Usage and effectiveness of rails, bathing and toileting aids. *Occupational Therapy in Health Care*, **10** (1996), 41–59.

151. E. Isakov, J. Mizrahi, I. Onna & Z. Susak, The control of genu recurvatum by combining the Swedish knee-cage and an ankle-foot brace. *Disability and Rehabilitation*, **14** (1992), 187–91.

152. R. Berenter & D. Kosai, Various types of orthoses used in podiatry. *Clinics in Podiatric Medicine and Surgery*, **11** (1994), 219–29.

153. S. Hesse, A. Gahein-Sama & K.-H. Mauritz, Technical aids in hemiparetic patients: prescription, costs and usage. *Clinical Rehabilitation*, **10** (1996), 328–33.

154. W. Mann, D. Hurren, M. Tomita & B. Charvat, Use of assistive devices for bathing by elderly who are not institutionalised. *Occupational Therapy Journal of Research*, **16** (1996), 261–86.

155. M. Finlayson & K. Havixbeck, A post-discharge study on the use of assistive devices. *Canadian Journal of Occupational Therapy*, **59** (1992), 201–7.

156. W. Mann, D. Hurren & M. Tomita, Assistive devices used by home-based elderly persons with arthritis. *American Journal of Occupational Therapy*, **49** (1995), 810–20.

157. B. J. Munro, J. R. Steele, G. M. Bashford, M. Ryan & N. Britten, A kinematic and kinetic analysis of the sit-to-stand transfer using an ejector chair: implications for elderly rheumatoid arthritic patients. *Journal of Biomechanics*, **31** (1998), 263–71.

158. R. Schemm & L. Gitlin, How occupational therapists teach older patients to use bathing and dressing devices in rehabilitation. *American Journal of Occupational Therapy*, **52** (1998), 276–82.

159. L. Gitlin & D. Burgh, Issuing assistive devices to older patients in rehabilitation: an exploratory study. *American Journal of Occupational Therapy*, **49** (1995), 994–1000.

160. P. Clarke & J. Gladman, A survey of predischarge occupational therapy home assessment visits for stroke patients. *Clinical Rehabilitation*, **9** (1995), 339–42.

161. H. V. Sorensen, S. Lendal, K. Schultz-Larsen & T. Uhrskov, Stroke rehabilitation: assistive technology devices and environmental modifications following primary rehabilitation in hospital – a therapeutic perspective. *Assistive Technology*, **15** (2003), 39–48.

162. S. Corr & A. Bayer, Occupational therapy for stroke patients after hospital discharge – a randomised controlled trial. *Clinical Rehabilitation*, **9** (1995), 291–6.

163. J. Close, M. Ellis, R. Hooper *et al.*, Prevention of falls in the elderly trial (PROFET): a randomised controlled trial. *The Lancet*, **353** (1999), 93–7.

164. M. Stevens, C. D. J. Holman, N. Bennett & N. deKlerk, Preventing falls in older people: outcome evaluation of a randomized controlled trial. *Journal of the American Geriatrics Society*, **49** (2001), 1448–55.

165. K. Attebo, R. Q. Ivers & P. Mitchell, Refractive errors in an older population: the Blue Mountains Eye Study. *Ophthalmology*, **106** (1999), 1066–72.

166. J. M. Tielsch, A. Sommer, K. Witt, J. Katz & R. M. Royall, Blindness and visual impairment in an American urban population: the Baltimore Eye Survey. *Archives of Ophthalmology*, **108** (1990), 286–90.

167. C. I. Jack, T. Smith, C. Neoh, M. Lye & J. N. McGalliard, Prevalence of low vision in elderly patients admitted to an acute geriatric unit in Liverpool: elderly people who fall are more likely to have low vision. *Gerontology*, **41** (1995), 280–5.

168. S. P. Donahue, Loss of accommodation and presbyopia. In *Ophthalmology*, ed. M. Yanoff & J. S. Duker. (London: Mosby, 1999).

169. C. J. Patorgis, Presbyopia. In *Diagnosis and Management in Vision Care*, ed. J. F. Amos, (Stoneham: Butterworth, 1987).

170. R. Bettigole, Reducing the risk of falls among the elderly [letter]. *New England Journal of Medicine*, **332** (1995), 269.

171. M. El-Arabi & O. Rashed, Bifocal glasses. *Bulletin of the Ophthalmology Society of Egypt*, **64** (1971), 249–52.

172. S. D. Elder, *The Practice of Refraction* (London: Churchill, 1963).

173. M. E. Tinetti, Preventing falls in elderly persons. *New England Journal of Medicine*, **348** (2003), 42–9.

174. R. Q. Ivers, R. G. Cumming, P. Mitchell & K. Attebo, Visual impairment and falls in older adults: the Blue Mountains Eye Study. *Journal of the American Geriatrics Society*, **46** (1998), 58–64.

175. M. Nevitt, S. Cummings, S. Kidd & D. Black, Risk factors for recurrent non-syncopal falls. *Journal of the American Medical Association*, **261** (1989), 2663–8.

176. S. R. Lord, R. D. Clark & I. W. Webster, Visual acuity and contrast sensitivity in relation to falls in an elderly population. *Age and Ageing*, **20** (1991), 175–81.

177. M. R. de Boer, S. M. Pluijm, P. Lips *et al.*, Different aspects of visual impairment as risk factors for falls and fractures in older men and women. *Journal of Bone and Mineral Research*, **19** (2004), 1539–47.

178. S. R. Lord & J. Dayhew, Visual risk factors for falls in older people. *Journal of the American Geriatrics Society*, **49** (2001), 508–12.

179. D. T. Felson, J. J. Anderson & M. T. Annan, Impaired vision and hip fracture. The Framingham study. *Journal of the American Geriatrics Society*, **37** (1989), 495–500.

180. S. R. Cummings, M. C. Nevitt, W. S. Browner *et al.*, Risk factors for hip fracture in white women. Study of Osteoporotic Fractures Research Group. *New England Journal of Medicine*, **332** (1995), 767–73.

181. R. Norton, A. J. Campbell, T. Lee-Joe, E. Robinson & M. Butler, Circumstances of falls resulting in hip fractures among older people. *Journal of the American Geriatrics Society*, **45** (1997), 1108–12.

182. W. P. Berg, H. M. Alessio, E. M. Mills & C. Tong, Circumstances and consequences of falls in independent community-dwelling older adults. *Age and Ageing*, **26** (1997), 261–8.

183. A. E. Patla & J. N. Vickers, Where and when do we look as we approach and step over an obstacle in the travel path? *Neuro Report*, **8** (1997), 3661–5.

184. S. R. Lord, J. Dayhew & A. Howland, Multifocal glasses impair edge-contrast sensitivity and depth perception and increase the risk of falls in older people. *Journal of the American Geriatrics Society*, **50** (2002), 1760–6.

185. M. D. Grabiner & D. W. Jahnigen, Modeling recovery from stumbles: preliminary data on variable selection and classification efficacy. *Journal of the American Geriatrics Society*, **40** (1992), 910–13.

186. N. Mills, The biomechanics of hip protectors. *Proceedings of the Institution of Mechanical Engineers. Part H. Journal of Engineering in Medicine*, **210** (1996), 259–66.

187. J. B. Lauritzen, M. M. Petersen & B. Lund, Effect of external hip protectors on hip fractures. *The Lancet*, **341** (1993), 11–13.

188. R. B. Wallace, J. E. Ross, J. C. Huston, C. Kundel & G. Woodworth, Iowa FICSIT trial: the feasibility of elderly wearing a hip joint protective garment to reduce hip fractures. *Journal of the American Geriatrics Society*, **41** (1993), 338–40.

189. A. Ekman, H. Mallmin, K. Michaelsson & S. Ljunghall, External hip protectors to prevent osteoporotic hip fractures [letter]. *The Lancet*, **350** (1997), 563–4.

190. M. Parker, L. Gillespie & W. Gillespie, Hip protectors for preventing hip fractures in the elderly. *Cochrane Database of Systematic Reviews*, (3) (2004), CD001255.

191. P. O'Halloran, G. Cran, T. Beringer *et al.*, A cluster randomised controlled trial to evaluate a policy of making hip protectors available to residents of nursing homes. *Age and Ageing*, **33** (2004), 582–8.

192. L. Forsen, A. Sogaard, S. Sandvig *et al.*, Risk of hip fracture in protected and unprotected falls in nursing homes in Norway. *Injury Prevention*, **10** (2004), 16–20.

193. Y. Birks, J. Porthouse, C. Addie *et al.*, Randomized controlled trial of hip protectors among women living in the community. *Osteoporosis International*, **15** (2004), 701–6.

194. N. van Schoor, W. Deville, L. Bouter & P. Lips, Acceptance and compliance with external hip protectors: a systematic review of the literature. *Osteoporosis International*, **13** (2002), 917–24.

195. I. D. Cameron, Hip protectors: prevent fractures but adherence is a problem [editorial]. *British Medical Journal*, **324** (2002), 375–6.

196. I. Cameron, B. Stafford, R. Cumming *et al.*, Hip protectors improve falls self efficacy. *Age and Ageing*, **29** (2000), 57–62.

197. M. E. Tinetti, W. L. Liu & E. B. Claus, Predictors and prognosis of inability to get up after falls among elderly persons. *Journal of the American Medical Association*, **269** (1993), 65–70.

198. A. C. Reece & J. M. Simpson, Preparing older people to cope after a fall. *Physiotherapy*, **82** (1996), 227–35.

199. M. R. Hofmeyer, N. B. Alexander, L. V. Nyquist, J. L. Medell & A. Koreishi, Floor-rise strategy training in older adults. *Journal of the American Geriatrics Society,* **50** (2002), 1702–6.

200. J. M. Simpson, R. Harrington & N. Marsh, Guidelines for managing falls among elderly people. *Physiotherapy,* **84** (1998), 173–7.

201. M. E. Tinetti, W. Liu & S. F. Ginter, Mechanical restraint use and fall-related injuries among residents of skilled nursing facilities. *Annals of Internal Medicine,* **116** (1992), 369–74.

202. A. F. Minnick, L. C. Mion, R. Leipzig, K. Lamb & R. M. Palmer, Prevalence and patterns of physical restraint use in the acute care setting. *Journal of Nursing Administration,* **28** (1998), 19–24.

203. M. E. Watson & P. A. Mayhew, Identifying fall risk factors in preparation for reducing the use of restraints. *MEDSURG Nursing,* **3** (1994), 25–8.

204. E. Capezuti, L. Evans, N. Strumpf & G. Maislin, Physical restraint use and falls in nursing home residents. *Journal of the American Geriatrics Society,* **44** (1996), 627–33.

205. L. Z. Rubenstein, K. R. Josephson & D. Osterweil, Falls and fall prevention in the nursing home. *Clinics in Geriatric Medicine,* **12** (1996), 881–902.

206. E. Capezuti, N. E. Strumpf, L. K. Evans, J. A. Grisso & G. Maislin, The relationship between physical restraint removal and falls and injuries among nursing home residents. *Journal of Gerontology,* **53A** (1998), M47–52.

207. J. Basante, E. Bentz, J. Heck-Hackley *et al.,* Falls risk among older adults in long-term care facilities: a focused literature review. *Physical and Occupational Therapy in Geriatrics,* **19** (2001), 63–85.

208. M. Letizia, C. Babler & A. Cockrell, Repeating the call for restraint reduction. *MEDSURG Nursing,* **13** (2004), 9–13.

209. P. Werner, J. Cohen-Mansfield, V. Koroknay & J. Braun, The impact of a restraint-reduction program on nursing home residents. *Geriatric Nursing,* **15** (1994), 142–6.

210. J. M. Levine, V. Marchello & E. Totolos, Progress toward a restraint-free environment in a large academic nursing facility. *Journal of the American Geriatrics Society,* **43** (1995), 914–18.

211. L. K. Evans, N. E. Strumpf, S. L. Allen-Taylor *et al.,* A clinical trial to reduce restraints in nursing homes. *Journal of the American Geriatrics Society,* **45** (1997), 675–81.

212. J. F. Schnelle, P. G. MacRae, K. Giacobassi *et al.,* Exercise with physically restrained nursing home residents: maximizing benefits of restraint reduction. *Journal of the American Geriatrics Society,* **44** (1996), 507–12.

213. F. K. Ejaz, S. J. Folmar, M. Kaufmann, M. S. Rose & B. Goldman, Restraint reduction: can it be achieved? *Gerontologist,* **34** (1994), 694–9.

214. V. Dibartolo, 9 steps to effective restraint use. *RN,* **61** (1998), 23–4.

14

Modifying the environment to prevent falls

This chapter outlines commonly suggested environmental modification strategies, and reviews the literature evaluating falls prevention programmes that have involved environmental modification as an individual intervention or as part of multi-faceted programmes. It discusses potential barriers to home modification, issues related to hazard removal and design strategies for minimizing older people's risk of falling in public places. Approaches for addressing environmental risk factors within institutions are discussed in Chapter 15.

Environmental modification strategies

Table 8.1 in Chapter 8 presents a list of environmental falls risk factors that have been suggested in the literature. These posited risk factors are replicated in Table14.1 along with potential solutions.

Environmental modification as an individual intervention

Environmental modification is seen by many as an attractive falls prevention strategy. The homes of most older people have many environmental hazards [1–3] and the majority of these are amenable to modification. Correction and/or removal of potential hazards is a one-off intervention that can be carried out relatively cheaply. Indeed, cost-effectiveness modelling has predicted that spending AUD$244 per person on a programme involving home assessment by an occupational therapist and subsequent modifications, would save $92 per person and $916 per fall prevented, over a ten year period [4]. However, this study assumes that such a programme could prevent 25% of falls. Reductions of this magnitude have yet to be demonstrated in controlled studies.

Early investigations indicated that home modification might be an effective falls prevention strategy for the general population of older people. One study involved assessment of the homes of older volunteers by 'home safety advisers',

Table 14.1 Possible strategies to address environmental hazards

Risk factor	Solution
General	
Lighting (too low, excessive glare, uneven)	Ensure even, high, non-glare levels of illumination
	Use of night lights
Slippery floor surfaces	Non-slip floor surfaces
	Avoid excessive use of floor polish
Loose rugs	Removal or fixing down of loose rugs
Upended carpet edges	Repair of upended carpet edges and other uneven floor coverings
Raised door sills	Modification
Obstructed walkways	Clear walkways obstructed by furniture or other objects
Cord across walkways	Change cord path
Shelves or cupboards too high or too low	Avoid use of shelves or cupboards which are very high or low
Spilt liquids	Wipe up spilt liquids immediately
Pets	Take care with pets
	Training or restraint of dangerous pets
Furniture	
Low chairs	Chair raisers
Low or elevated bed height	Bed blocks or leg modification
Unstable furniture	Repair or removal of unstable furniture
Use of ladders and step ladders	Avoid use of ladders and step ladders
Bathroom/toilet/laundry	
Lack of grab rails shower/bathtub/toilet	Installation of grab rails shower/bathtub/toilet
Hob on shower recess	Removal of hob on shower recess
	Shower outside of shower recess area on a chair
Low toilet seat	Toilet seat raisers
Outdoor toilet	Use of commode instead of outdoor toilet
Slippery surfaces	Use of non-slip mats and strips
Use of bath oils	Avoid use of bath oils
Stairs	
No or inadequate handrails	Installation of appropriate handrails
Non-contrasting steps	Contrasting strips on step treads
Stairs too steep, tread too narrow	Modification of stair and surrounding design
Distracting surroundings	
Unmodifiable stairs or individual unable to manage stairs	Installation of ramps

Table 14.1 *(cont.)*

Risk factor	Solution
Outdoors	
Sloping, slippery, obstructed or uneven pathways, ramps and stairways	Re-design or modify pathways, ramps and stairways
Rushing caused by inadequate time allowed for pedestrian crossings	Longer cycles in traffic lights
Crowds	Care in crowds
	Use of walking aid to highlight frailty
Certain weather conditions (leaves, snow, ice, rain)	Removal of fallen leaves, water, snow, ice
	Care in dangerous weather conditions
Lack of places to rest	More places to rest provided
Unsafe garbage bin use	Re-design or provide assistance with garbage bins

and subsidized floor treatments (with non-slip material) and grab rail installation [5]. The 305 people who agreed to have modifications (90% of those visited) reported a 58% reduction in the number of falls experienced in the twelve months following the environmental modifications. Similarly, Plautz *et al.* [6] evaluated an intervention that involved home safety assessments and modifications, such as removing clutter, installing handrails, grab bars and non-skid strips, and securing rugs and electrical cords. This involved an average of ten person hours of unskilled labour and US$93 worth of materials. Reported falls for the six months after the intervention were reduced by 60% compared with the six months prior to the intervention. The results of such 'before and after' study designs, however, should be viewed with caution due to the lack of control groups, no investigator blinding and the use of volunteer subjects [7].

A third early study conducted in Norway evaluated the effects of a community-intervention programme as a fracture prevention strategy [8]. The intervention comprised environmental assessment and modification, and promotion of safe footwear use in winter. The investigators found decreased rates of fall-related fractures in the intervention municipality and increased fracture rates in a reference municipality where the programme was not carried out.

There have been six subsequent randomized controlled trials of home assessment and modification reporting falls as the major outcome measure [9–14]. These are summarized in Table 14.2. These studies have reported inconsistent findings, with only two showing a significant reduction in falls in the primary analysis [13, 14].

Two studies involved general community populations of older people. In the first of these, Stevens *et al.* [9] found that home assessment, education regarding

Table 14.2 Summary of randomized controlled trials addressing environmental risk factors for falls in community-dwelling older people

Study	Participants	Intervention	Main Outcomes	Comments
Stevens et al. [9]	• n = 1737 • aged 70+	• Home assessment by trained nurse assessor, education about home hazards and free installation of safety devices, i.e. grab rails, repair of flooring, etc. • Compliance: 13%–78%	• Not effective in reducing falls RR = 1.11 (95% CI = 0.82–1.50)	• Significant but limited effect on reducing home hazards • No training component
Day et al. [10]	• n = 1090 • mean age: 76.1 (SD = 5.5)	• Home assessment by trained assessor, advice, and provision of materials and labour for providing modifications, i.e. rails, grab bars, etc. • Compliance: 76%	• Not effective in reducing falls RR = 0.92 (95% CI = 0.78–1.08)	• Home hazards were significantly reduced in the intervention group • No training component
Cumming et al. [11]	• n = 530 • aged 65+	• Home assessment by OT and supervision of home modifications • Compliance: 19%–75%	• Not effective in previous non-fallers RR = 1.03 (95% CI = 0.75–1.41) Effective in previous fallers RR = 0.54 (95% CI = 0.50–0.83)	• Falls reduced to a similar degree outside the home in previous fallers • Advice provided on safe mobility and footwear • Home modifications may not have been the effective component of the intervention

Table 14.2 (cont.)

Study	Participants	Intervention	Main Outcomes	Comments
Pardessus et al. [12]	• n = 60 • aged 65+	• Home assessment by OT, advice regarding modifications and how to live safely with fixed hazards • Compliance: not described	• Not effective in reducing falls RR = 0.87 (95% CI = 0.50–1.49)	• Underpowered for falls as an outcome measure
Nikolaus and Bach [13]	• n = 360 • mean age: 81.5 (SD = 6.4)	• Home assessment by OT and physiotherapist, advice regarding modifications and training in use of assistive devices • Compliance 33%–83%	• Effective in reducing falls IRR = 0.69 (95% CI = 0.51–0.97) • Effective in previous multiple fallers IRR = 0.63 (95% CI = 0.43–0.94)	• Training in the use of mobility and technical aids provided
Campbell et al. [14]	• n = 391 • mean age: 83.6 (SD = 4.8)	• Home safety assessment and recommendations delivered by OT • Compliance 90% (complied with one or more recommendations)	• 41% fewer falls in home safety group vs. control group • IRR = 0.59 (95% CI = 0.42–0.83)	• No difference in reduction of falls at home compared to those way from home

OT: occupational therapist, RR: relative risk, CI: confidence interval, IRR: incidence rate ratio home hazards and installation of home safety devices did not significantly reduce falls or falls injuries. The authors considered that although significant, the intervention resulted in only a small number of environmental changes – a reduction in unsafe steps by 16%, unsafe floor rugs and mats by 14%, rooms with trailing cords by 26%, and unsafe chairs by 12% [2]. In addition, a number of structural hazards detected in the household assessment were not amenable to modification.

The second general community study involved 1090 subjects aged 70 years and over, and used a factorial design to assess the independent and combined effects of interventions aimed at vision improvement, home hazard reduction and group exercise [10]. The home hazard reduction intervention comprised home assessment by a trained assessor, advice, and the provision of materials and labour for providing modifications. Home hazards were significantly reduced in the intervention group. However, this did not result in a significant reduction in falls.

Four studies have targeted interventions more closely to at-risk groups [11–14]. Cumming *et al.* [11] conducted a study among 530 community dwellers, most of who had been recently hospitalized. The intervention group received a home visit by an occupational therapist who assessed the home for environmental hazards and facilitated any necessary home modifications. There was a borderline significant reduction in falls in the intervention group as a whole ($p = 0.05$). There was a significant reduction in the rate of falls among those who had fallen in the year prior to the study. However, falls in this group were also significantly reduced *outside* of the home, suggesting that the home modifications may not have been the major factor in the reduction in fall rates. Other aspects of the occupational therapy intervention, which included advice on footwear and behaviour, may have played an important role.

The study by Pardessus *et al.* [12] involved home assessment and modification in 60 people aged 65 years and over who had been hospitalized following a fall. At a one-year follow-up, there were no differences in fall rates or hospitalization between the control and intervention groups. The small sample size (n = 60) suggests that this study was not sufficiently powered to detect differences between the groups with respect to falls as an outcome measure.

Two randomized controlled trials specifically addressing home modification have reported a significant reduction in falls. The Falls-HIT trial [13] involved 361 people with mobility limitations who had recently been discharged from hospital. The intervention consisted of home assessment and recommendations in addition to training in the use of mobility aids. At a one-year follow-up, the intervention group had 31% fewer falls than the control group, with subgroup analysis revealing that the intervention was particularly effective in those with a history of multiple falls. More recently, Campbell *et al.* [14] assessed the efficacy of a home safety programme on falls in people aged 75 years and over with severe visual impairment (visual acuity of 6/24 or worse). The intervention consisted of an occupational therapy home assessment and a follow-up recommendation letter, along with facilitation of equipment purchase and installation. At the 12-month follow-up, there were 41% fewer falls in those who received the home safety intervention compared to the control group. However, there was no difference in the reduction of falls at home compared to those outside the home. This suggests, as with the study by Cumming *et al.* [11], that the efficacy of the intervention was partly due to the changes made to the environment and partly due to the general falls prevention advice provided by the occupational therapist.

A number of multi-faceted falls prevention strategies, including both intrinsic and extrinsic components (including home hazard reduction), have now been assessed with randomized controlled trials. Several of these have been found to be effective [15–18] although others have not [19–21]. Using pooled data from these trials, a Cochrane systematic review concluded that these multifactorial interventions are effective in reducing falls in older people [22]. A complementary Cochrane review of 15 studies (including multi-faceted studies), however, concluded that home environment modification is not effective in reducing injuries in older people [23].

The design of multifactorial studies does not allow assessment of the effects of individual strategies or their relative contributions to the success or otherwise of the interventions. In contrast, the factorial design used in the study by Day *et al.* [10] provides a mechanism for contrasting the effectiveness of intervention strategies. They found that as a single intervention strategy, group-based exercise was effective in reducing falls (relative risk = 0.82, 95% CI = 0.70–0.97), whereas home hazard management (relative risk = 0.92, 95% CI = 0.78–1.08) and vision improvement (relative risk = 0.89, 95% CI = 0.75–1.04) were not. The combined effect of the three interventions was greater than for exercise alone (relative risk = 0.67, 95% CI = 0.51–0.88), as was the effect of home hazard management in addition to exercise (relative risk = 0.76, 95% CI = 0.60–0.95).

Barriers to environmental modification

Compliance with suggested modifications is a key issue for successful implementation of environmental falls prevention strategies. Studies have reported compliance rates for home and lifestyle safety modifications ranging from 13% [2] to 90% [5].

There are a number of potential barriers to a person adopting recommended environmental modifications. It has been reported that older people do not welcome recommendations by health professionals to reduce home hazards such as moving furniture, tacking down carpets or improving lighting. This may be because many older people are concerned about the stigmatizing effects of safety measures, and feel that their view of their health and independence is being challenged [24]. Education programmes may assist in overcoming this barrier. It has been found that compared with individual approaches, group education can increase the likelihood of compliance in adopting home modifications, especially with low cost interventions [25]. As part of a successful multi-faceted falls prevention intervention, Clemson et al. [26] used small group sessions using a self-efficacy enhancement approach. They reported that 70% of programme participants adhered to at least 50% of the home visit recommendations.

Low financial status of older people is another limiting factor in implementing home modifications [24]. Community programmes, which provide subsidized housing modifications to older people on low incomes, offer a means of addressing this potential barrier. For example, the low intervention costs to participants is likely to have contributed to the high take-up rate of suggested modifications (90%) in the study by Thompson [5].

Public places and design issues

The issue of how to design and build public environments and buildings to accommodate the needs of older people is becoming more important as the world's population ages. Environments should be designed to safely provide for the needs of a range of users (i.e. with varying physical abilities) across all weather conditions.

Possible interventions in public places include: better design and maintenance of pavements and other surfaces; prevention of accumulation of ice and snow; prompt cleaning up of spilt liquids; widespread implementation of contrasting edges on stairs; and increased provision of resting places and grab rails. The effects of such interventions are difficult to assess but the implementation of ongoing falls surveillance by public authorities, as suggested by Sattin [27], could assist in this process.

Garner [28] has outlined a range of strategies by which local authorities can minimize the risk of falls in the community. She proposes two checklists for identifying hazards that warrant modification. The first is for assessing the adequacy of footpaths, steps and stairs, ramps, and roadways (including design, materials, construction, condition, obstructions and maintenance). The second is for assessing safety in shopping centres, malls and arcades (including assessments of entrances, steps, stairs and ramps, lighting, floor surfaces, furniture and fixtures, rest rooms, cleaning and lifts, and escalators). The initiation and sustainability of this approach may require policy and design changes, and the establishment of access and safety committees to oversee this.

Changes to floor surfaces may have the potential to reduce fall injury rates. For example, there is evidence that wooden carpeted floors are associated with fewer falls injuries than other flooring materials [29, 30]. More research is required to develop surfaces with optimal levels of friction. These surfaces should have sufficient friction to minimize slips but not so much as to impede walking (i.e. to cause feet and shoes to drag on the surface). A number of countries are now developing building standards for slip resistance of surfaces to be used in different settings [31]. There have also been some preliminary investigations performed to develop energy-absorbing floors and surfaces to reduce impact associated with falls [32].

Conclusion

Reducing hazards in the home appears not to be an effective falls prevention strategy in the general older population and those at low risk of falls. However, home hazard reduction is effective if targeted to older people with a history of falls and mobility limitations. The effectiveness of home safety interventions may depend on/be maximized by improved transfer abilities or other behavioural changes. Environmental assessment and modification by trained individuals also appears to contribute to the success of multi-faceted falls prevention programmes in at-risk groups. Solutions to potential barriers to an individual's adoption of home modifications, such as education and financial assistance, need to be considered and addressed. Further implementation and evaluation of evidenced-based building standards is required to improve the safety of public places with regard to falls risk.

REFERENCES

1. S. E. Carter, E. M. Campbell, R. W. Sanson-Fisher, S. Redman & W. J. Gillespie, Environmental hazards in the homes of older people. *Age and Ageing*, **26** (1997), 195–202.

2. M. Stevens, C. D. J. Holman & N. Bennett, Preventing falls in older people: impact of an intervention to reduce environmental hazards in the home. *Journal of the American Geriatrics Society*, **49** (2001), 1442–7.

3. T. M. Gill, C. S. Williams, J. T. Robison & M. E. Tinetti, A population-based study of environmental hazards in the homes of older persons. *American Journal of Public Health*, **89** (1999), 553–6.

4. R. D. Smith & D. Widiatmoko, The cost-effectiveness of home assessment and modification to reduce falls in the elderly. *Australian and New Zealand Journal of Public Health*, **22** (1998), 436–40.

5. P. G. Thompson, Preventing falls in the elderly at home: a community-based programme. *Medical Journal of Australia*, **164** (1996), 530–2.

6. B. Plautz, D. E. Beck, C. Selmar & M. Radetsky, Modifying the environment: a community-based injury-reduction programme for elderly residents. *American Journal of Preventive Medicine*, **12** (1996), 33–8.

7. I. D. Cameron, S. Kurrle & R. G. Cumming, Preventing falls in the elderly at home: a community-based programme [letter]. *Medical Journal of Australia*, **165** (1996), 459–60.

8. B. Ytterstad, The Harstad injury prevention study: community based prevention of fall-fractures in the elderly evaluated by means of a hospital-based injury recording system in Norway. *Journal of Epidemiology and Community Health*, **50** (1996), 551–8.

9. M. Stevens, C. D. J. Holman, N. Bennett & N. deKlerk, Preventing falls in older people: outcome evaluation of a randomized controlled trial. *Journal of the American Geriatrics Society*, **49** (2001), 1448–55.

10. L. Day, B. Fildes, I. Gordon *et al.*, A randomized factorial trial of falls prevention among older people living in their own homes. *British Medical Journal*, **325** (2002), 128–33.

11. R. G. Cumming, M. Thomas, G. Szonyi *et al.*, Home visits by an occupational therapist for assessment and modification of environmental hazards: a randomized trial of falls prevention. *Journal of the American Geriatrics Society*, **47** (1999), 1397–402.

12. V. Pardessus, F. Puisieux, C. Di Pompeo *et al.*, Benefits of home visits for falls and autonomy in the elderly: a randomised trial study. *American Journal of Physical Medical Rehabilitation*, **81** (2002), 247–52.

13. T. Nikolaus & M. Bach, Preventing falls in community-dwelling frail older people using a home intervention team (HIT): results from the randomised falls-HIT trial. *Journal of the American Geriatrics Society*, **51** (2003), 300–5.

14. A. J. Campbell, M. C. Robertson, S. J. La Grow *et al.*, Randomised controlled trial of prevention of falls in people aged ≥75 with severe visual impairment: the VIP trial. *British Medical Journal*, **331** (2005), 817.

15. M. C. Hornbrook, V. J. Stephens, D. J. Wingfield *et al.*, Preventing falls among community-dwelling older persons: results from a randomized trial. *The Gerontologist*, **34** (1994), 16–23.

16. M. E. Tinetti, D. I. Baker, G. McAvay *et al.*, A multifactorial intervention to reduce the risk of falling among elderly people living in the community. *New England Journal of Medicine*, **331** (1994), 821–7.

17. E. H. Wagner, A. Z. LaCroix, L. Grothaus *et al.*, Preventing disability and falls in older adults: a population-based randomized trial. *American Journal of Public Health*, **84** (1994), 1800–6.

18. J. Close, M. Ellis, R. Hooper *et al.*, Prevention of falls in the elderly trial (PROFET): a randomised controlled trial. *The Lancet*, **353** (1999), 93–7.

19. D. Fabacher, K. Josephson, F. Pietruszka *et al.*, An in-home preventive assessment programme for independent older adults. *Journal of the American Geriatrics Society*, **42** (1994), 630–8.

20. L. Z. Rubenstein, A. S. Robbins, K. R. Josephson, B. L. Schulman & D. Osterweil, The value of assessing falls in an elderly population. A randomized clinical trial. *Annals of Internal Medicine*, **113** (1990), 308–16.

21. N. J. Vetter, P. A. Lewis & D. Ford, Can health visitors prevent fractures in elderly people? *British Medical Journal*, **304** (1992), 888–90.

22. L. D. Gillespie, W. J. Gillespie, M. C. Robertson *et al.*, Interventions for preventing falls in elderly people (Cochrane Review). *The Cochrane Library*, **4** (2003), CD000340.

23. R. A. Lyons, L. V. Sander, A. L. Weightman *et al.*, Modification of the home environment for the reduction of injuries. *The Cochrane Database of Systematic Reviews*, **4** (2003), CD003600.

24. B. R. Connell, Role of the environment in falls prevention. *Clinics in Geriatric Medicine*, **12** (1996), 859–80.

25. J. W. Ryan & A. M. Spellbring, Implementing strategies to decrease risk of falls in older women. *Journal of Gerontological Nursing*, **22** (1996), 25–31.

26. L. Clemson, R. G. Cumming, H. Kendig *et al.*, The effectiveness of a community-based program for reducing the incidence of falls in the elderly: a randomized trial. *Journal of the American Geriatrics Society*, **52** (2004), 1487–94.

27. R. W. Sattin, Falls among older persons: a public health perspective. *Annual Review of Public Health*, **13** (1992), 489–508.

28. E. Garner, *Preventing Falls in Public Places: Challenge and Opportunity for Local Government* (Lismore: New South Wales, North Coast Public Health Unit, 1996).

29. F. Healey, Does flooring type affect risk of injury in older in-patients? *Nursing Times*, **90** (1994), 40–1.

30. A. H. R. W. Simpson, S. Lamb, P. J. Roberts, T. N. Gardner & J. G. Evans, Does the type of flooring affect the risk of hip fracture? *Age and Ageing*, **33** (2004), 242–6.

31. R. Bowman, What we must do to reduce pedestrian slips and falls. *Third National Conference on Injury Prevention and Control*, Brisbane, Australia, 1999.

32. J. A. Casalena, A. Badre-Alam, T. C. Ovaert, P. R. Cavanagh & D. A. Streit, The Penn State Safety Floor. Part II. Reduction of fall-related peak impact forces on the femur. *Journal of Biomechanical Engineering*, **120** (1998), 527–32.

15

Prevention of falls in hospitals and residential aged care facilities

Many of the risk factors and prevention strategies outlined in previous chapters are also relevant to falls among hospital patients, and residents of hostels and nursing homes. This chapter discusses risk factors for falling which seem to be particularly important within hospitals and residential aged care facilities. There have been many programmes developed which aim to reduce falls in institutional settings and a number of these have now been evaluated in randomized controlled trials (RCTs). This chapter outlines the results of trials conducted to date and discusses programme features likely to be important for preventing falls in institutional settings.

Incidence and risk factors

Hospitals

Falls among inpatients are a key issue for hospitals. Falls in hospitals increase morbidity, prolong hospital stays, and strain the resources of the healthcare system, family and community. Up to one-quarter of people fall during their time in a rehabilitation hospital [1] or ward [2]. These figures are even higher for particular diagnoses. Up to 40% of stroke patients fall while in a rehabilitation unit [3].

Many falls in hospitals occur around patients' bedside and ward area, with up to 43% of falls occurring from (or near) patients' beds [4]. Peak periods for patient falls coincide with peak periods of patient activity. A number of studies have found falls to be associated with getting in and out of beds and chairs, walking, and toileting [4]. One study [5] found that 80% of patients who fell were confused, had gait disturbance and were attempting to toilet alone.

In recent years a large number of authors have sought to document risk factors for falls in hospitals. Oliver et al. [6] recently conducted a systematic review of these and identified 28 papers on risk factors, but excluded 15 of these from further analysis due to methodological limitations. Risk factors that emerged consistently in these studies include gait instability, agitated confusion, urinary incontinence/frequency, a history of falls and prescription of 'culprit' drugs (especially sedative/hypnotics).

Residential aged care facilities

Falls incidence rates are as much as three times higher among older people in residential aged care settings than among community-dwelling older people [7]. This equates to an average annual rate of 1.5 falls per nursing home bed [7].

In a prospective study involving 18 855 residents of 272 nursing homes, Kiely *et al.* [8] found that the most important predictor of falling was a history of previous falls. Residents with a fall history were three times more likely to fall during the follow-up period than residents without such a history. Other independent risk factors were wandering behaviour, use of a cane or walker, deterioration in performing activities of daily living, age greater than 87 years, unsteady gait, independence in performing transfers, not requiring a wheelchair and male gender. Interestingly, fall rates varied greatly among the nursing homes studied and this was independent of patient-specific factors. This indicates the importance of broader design and management issues in falls prevention in residential aged care facilities.

Other studies have found that risk factors for falls among nursing home residents are similar to those for community dwellers [9–11]. The increased prevalence of a number of important falls risk factors among people within institutional settings is likely to contribute to the greater incidence of falls in this population. These are likely to include muscle weakness, gait and balance disorders [7, 12], poor vision, and dementia [13]. In addition, the increased prevalence of incontinence and anti-psychotic drug use within institutions probably means that these factors are of greater relative importance in these settings. The above literature has been recently reviewed by the UK National Institute of Clinical Excellence [14]. This group concluded that the key risk factors for falling in residential aged care facilities are a history of falls, gait deficit, balance deficit, visual impairment and cognitive impairment.

Two studies have shown that balance ability and ambulatory status are non-linearly related to falls in people living in residential aged care facilities. In a study involving 1228 residents, Thapa *et al.* [15] found that the incidence of injurious falls in those who could not walk was less than half that in those who could and that risk factors for falls differed between these groups. The strongest risk factor in the ambulatory residents was the use of psychotropic drugs, whereas the risk factors for falls in the non-ambulatory group were not being bed-bound and having the capacity for independent transfers.

In a prospective cohort study involving 1000 people aged 65 to 103 years living in residential aged care facilities, we also found a non-linear pattern

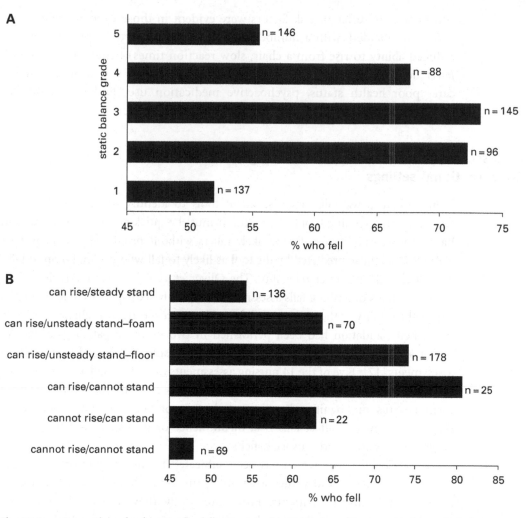

Fig. 15.1   Proportion of subjects who fell categorized by A: their performance in the static balance test, and B: ability to rise from a chair and stand unaided.

between balance and falls [16]. Fall rates were highest in those with fair standing balance, intermediate in those with the best standing balance and lowest in those with the worst standing balance (Figure 15.1A). This non-linear pattern was even more striking when subjects were categorized according to their standing balance and ability to rise from a chair (Figure 15.1B). Using this dual classification, fall rates were highest in those who could rise from a chair but could not stand unaided (81%), and lowest in those who could neither rise from a chair nor stand unaided (48%). In residents who could stand unaided, falls risk factors included increased age, male gender, higher care classifications, incontinence, psychoactive medication use, previous falls and slow reaction times. In contrast, quite different risk factors were evident in those residents who could not stand unaided, with a number of known fall risk factors (previous stroke, reduced ability to rise from a chair, slow reaction times) being associated with *fewer* falls. In this group, risk factors were intermediate versus nursing home care, poor health status, psychoactive medication use, Parkinson's disease, previous falls and being able to get out of a chair.

Assessment tools to identify those at high risk of falls in institutional settings

Many hospitals use falls risk assessment tools to identify those at high risk of falling. For a screening tool to be useful, it must be quick and easy to administer, have a proven ability to identify likely fallers without providing too many false positives (i.e. those predicted by the tool as likely to fall who do not go on to fall), as well as high interrater reliability. The Oliver *et al.* [6] systematic review identified 47 papers describing falls assessment tools. Only six papers were identified in which the validity of the screening tools had been prospectively evaluated and only two where validation had been performed in two or more patient cohorts. An earlier systematic review identified 14 nursing assessment tools and six functional assessments [17]. Five of the 14 nursing assessments identified had a sensitivity and specificity of above 70%. Risk factors commonly assessed by these tools included mental status or cognitive impairment, history of falls, mobility impairment, diagnoses known to affect falls risk, incontinence or difficulties toileting, use of culprit medications and sensory deficits.

To develop the tool which has been subjected to the most rigorous evaluation, Oliver *et al.* [18] identified a set of key predictors in an initial case-control study of 232 hospital patients. From this study they developed STRATIFY (St Thomas's risk assessment tool in falling elderly inpatients) which involves assessment of: (i) whether falls are the presenting complaint; (ii) transfer and mobility skills; (iii) whether the patient is agitated; (iv) the need for frequent toileting; or (v) visual impairment. This tool was then trialled in two large cohort studies (of 1217 and 331 patients), and found to have good sensitivity (ability to correctly identify people as fallers) and a good specificity (ability to correctly identify people as non-fallers). These findings indicate that simple, quick to administer assessment items are useful in identifying older persons at risk of falling while in hospital. However, subsequent validation in different settings yielded mixed results [19, 20].

Within residential aged care facilities, more extensive screening for falls risk is possible as the residents are there for longer periods of time than hospital inpatients. A useful screening tool has been developed by the Centre for

Education and Research on Ageing [21]. Assessment methods and manage-ment options are outlined for the following categories: medications, acute illness, mental state, ongoing medical conditions, history of falls, poor balance, use of walking aids, bowel or bladder problems, visual problems, hearing problems, foot problems, and footwear. Other physiological risk factors (such as reduced muscle strength) outlined in Part I of this book are also likely to be important.

Strategies for falls prevention in institutions

Identification of those at high risk of falls is relatively easy compared to the tailoring of appropriate intervention programmes to address this risk. Without such action falls risk screening tools are of little use. However, two recent RCTs in hospital aged care/rehabilitation settings [38, 39] and three RCTs in nursing home settings [22–24] have found that multi-faceted intervention programmes based on the results of falls risk assessment tools can reduce fall rates. A further nursing home trial found that falls could be reduced [25] and functional status improved [26] with regular functionally relevant activity and continence care. Another trial found that a physical therapy intervention improved mobility and reduced assis-tive device use, but did not reduce falls [27].

Strategies which have been used to minimize falls in hospitals and residential aged care facilities are summarized in Box 15.1.

Box 15.1 A comprehensive approach to preventing falls and fall injury.

(1) Use a screening protocol to identify high-risk patients

(2) Address the risk factors directly if possible
- Provide treatment of medical conditions that give rise to acute confusional states
- Provide treatment/therapy for agitation
- Provide treatment for co-morbidity where possible
- Monitor and attempt to remove or reduce dose of psychoactive drugs
- Initiate on-line prescribing systems to prevent adverse drug interactions
- Initiate physiotherapy programmes that include specific muscle strengthening exercises, gait and balance training
- Provide general exercise opportunities to prevent deterioration in motor function
- Provide regular supervised walking for those unsafe to walk independently
- Provide suitable walking aids
- Ensure safe shoes and clothing are worn
- Maximize vision with appropriate spectacles
- Provide occupational therapy training programmes to maximize safety and independence in functional tasks
- Initiate diversionary activities to prevent wandering

(3) Monitor patients
- Ensure regular checks of patients to see if assistance is required
- Ensure regular toileting [70] – especially if bladder or bowel control problems or medications with a diuretic or laxative effect
- Move high-risk patients to areas of the ward where they can be easily seen by nursing and other staff. Consider re-design of patient areas
- Use 'sitters' (family members or other volunteers) to supervise the patient [71]
- Consider electronic surveillance systems

(4) Implement environmental interventions
- Provide optimal lighting
- Remove or modify obstacle hazards or hazardous floor covering
- Ensure regular maintenance of wheelchairs and other equipment
- Minimize water and other spills on floors
- Install grab rails in bathroom and toilet areas
- Ensure toilet seats are of appropriate height
- Provide appropriate height chairs
- Provide easy access to call bells, light switches and personal effects
- Provide toileting aids (urine bottles/bedside commodes/bedpans)
- Provide other equipment (long-handle reachers, etc.)
- Locate at-risk patients near bathrooms and dining rooms
- Provide safe walking areas for people
- Consider use of restraints

(5) Increase awareness of falls risk
- Inform patients, relatives and staff of increased risk
- Consider method of quick identification of high-risk patients, e.g. coloured bracelet, code on patient file
- Initiate and repeat educational programmes for staff
- Ensure high level of monitoring on initial days of hospital stay (staff/relatives)

(6) Reduce fall injury
- Implement hip protector programme for very high-risk patients (e.g. those with delirium, agitation, confusion and multiple risk factors)
- Consider shock-absorbing floor surfaces
- Consider low-height beds

(7) Discharge planning
- Undertake full assessment of functional abilities prior to discharge
- Arrange appropriate assistance from carers and community services
- Arrange for ongoing physiotherapy, community exercise, home assessment and modification, and aged care team involvement as appropriate

(8) Post-fall assessment
- Document circumstances and investigate causes for each fall and intervene as appropriate
- Review environmental factors
- Review physical factors
- Perform functional assessment

Many of these strategies have recently been evaluated and incorporated into best practice guidelines on preventing falls and harm from falls in older people in hospitals and residential aged care facilities by the Australian Council for Safety and Quality in Health Care (www.powmri.edu.au/fallsnetwork) [28]. Recommendations from these guidelines are summarized in Box 15.2 and the results of RCTs evaluating falls prevention in institutional settings are discussed in the following section. The strength of each recommendation is based on the level of evidence from published studies using the following key.

- Level I: evidence obtained from a systematic review of all relevant randomized controlled trials (includes Cochrane reviews, other systematic reviews and meta-analyses).
- Level II: evidence obtained from at least one properly designed, randomized controlled trial.
- Level III: evidence obtained from well-designed controlled trials without randomization; from well-designed cohort or case-controlled analytic studies preferably from more than one centre or research group; or from multiple time series with or without the intervention.
- Level IV: opinion of respected authorities, based on clinical experience, descriptive studies or reports of expert committees.

- A: based directly on Level I evidence.
- B: based directly on Level II evidence or extrapolated recommendation from Level I evidence.
- C: based directly on Level III evidence or extrapolated recommendation from Level I or II evidence.
- D: based directly on Level IV evidence or extrapolated recommendation from Level I, II or III evidence.

Box 15.2 Summary of recommendations from the Australian Council for Safety and Quality in Health Care best practice guidelines on preventing falls and harm from falls in older people in hospitals and residential aged care facilities [28].

- A multi-faceted approach to the prevention of falls should be considered as part of routine care for all older people in hospitals and residential aged care facilities **(II-C)**.

- As part of a multi-component programme, conduct a systematic and comprehensive multidisciplinary falls risk assessment to inform the development of an individualized plan of care to prevent falls **(II-B)**.

- Develop and implement a targeted and individualized falls prevention plan of care based on the findings of a falls screen or assessment **(II-B)**.

- As part of a multifactorial falls prevention programme, identify balance, mobility and strength problems then tailor an individual programme to address these in hospital, post-hospital and residential aged care settings **(II-B)**.

- Managing the symptoms of cognitive impairment by addressing agitation, wandering and impulsive behaviour is necessary. When an older person presents with cognitive impairment, it is important that strategies are included to prevent the risk of delirium. It is essential to confirm that any disruptive behaviour is not due to acute delirium or delirium superimposed on dementia. Multi-component intervention to prevent delirium may provide an effective strategy for reducing falls in older patients. Provide supervision and assistance to ensure that patients/ residents with delirium, who are not capable of standing and walking safely, receive help with all transfers **(IV-D)**.

- Identify, assess and introduce a management plan for people with incontinence or who are at risk of becoming incontinent **(III-D)**.

- Screen older people for ill-fitting or inappropriate footwear, and give education and information about footwear features that may reduce fall risk (i.e. the use of slippers should be discouraged) **(III-C)**.

- Medications related to falls needs to be reviewed and appropriately modified as a component of a multifactorial approach to reducing the risk of falls in older people **(II-B)**.

- Attention to visual function screening and referral for visual function assessment and management should be included as part of a multi-faceted falls prevention programme **(II-C)**.

- Undertake annual eye examinations to reduce the incidence of visual impairment, which is associated with an increased risk of falls. Advise people who have had falls involving environmental obstacles (e.g. such as stairs and curbs) to use distance glasses when walking **(III-D)**.

- Environmental modifications should be included in multifactorial, multidisciplinary falls prevention interventions **(II-B)**.

- People considered to be at higher risk of falling should be assessed by an occupational therapist for specific environmental/equipment needs and training to maximize safety **(II-C)**.

- Alternatives to restraint should be considered and trialled for people with cognitive impairment. Restraint should be considered the last option for people who are at risk of falling **(III-C)**.

- Hip protector use should be considered for people living in residential aged care facilities with a high risk of hip fracture (defined as having limited independent mobility, a history of falls and osteoporosis). There needs to be commitment from the facility to introduce training for staff and continuing support for the use of hip protectors **(I-D)**.

- Hip protector use should be considered for patients in sub-acute hospital wards who are at high risk of falls (defined as having limited independent mobility, or confusion with agitation). There needs to be commitment from the facility to introduce training for staff and continuing support for the use of hip protectors **(III-D)**.

- Older people (in hospitals) who are at high risk of hip fracture (defined as greater than 80 years of age with a history of falls and/or osteoporosis), and who believe that they will be able to use hip protectors and see no barriers to their use, should be offered hip protectors **(III-D)**.

- Vitamin D and calcium supplementation should be considered as a routine management strategy as it appears to significantly reduce the risk of falls among ambulatory or institutionalized older people **(I-A)**.

- To decrease subsequent fracture rates, appropriate treatment with bisphosphonates should be undertaken for people who have previously sustained a fracture and who have osteoporosis **(II-B)**.

- Hospitals should establish protocols that increase osteoporosis treatment rates in people who have sustained their first osteoporotic fracture **(IV-D)**.

- As part of a multi-component falls prevention programme, post-fall assessment should be completed on all older people who fall whilst in hospital or residential aged care facilities **(III-C)**.

Risk factor modification

Where possible, risk factors, such as confusion, agitation, co-morbidity, psychoactive medication use, adverse drug interactions, reduced muscle strength, poor balance and poor vision, should be investigated and addressed. This needs to be done in conjunction with the patient's medical practitioner, and may involve referral to other professionals and appropriate intervention, as outlined in Chapter 12. There is evidence from one RCT that more intensive physiotherapy and occupational therapy intervention for those in nursing homes leads to improved functional abilities, and a resultant saving of nursing staff time [29].

Monitoring patients

Many falls in hospitals and residential care settings occur while the older person is attempting to attend to a basic need, such as fetching a drink or using the bathroom or toilet. The older person may select to undertake a task independently and underestimate the risk associated with the specific task given existing functional limitations. The addition of inadequate staffing levels or the use of agency support staff with little or no knowledge of individual patients serves only to compound the problems. Electronic surveillance systems may be of use but require further evaluation. These include video cameras, position sensors on beds, chairs or on an individual's lower limbs to alert staff when a potential faller moves into an upright position [30, 31] and an alarm which is triggered when a person goes beyond a certain point [5]. More sophisticated 'smart room' systems are being developed which collect information on various aspects of movement and the person's clinical status, and notify appropriate people if necessary [32].

Environmental interventions

Within hospitals and long term care institutions, there should be the potential to minimize environmental hazards as outlined in Chapter 8. Attention should also be given to the way in which each individual patient or resident interacts with the environment. For example, a person with limited mobility needs to have easy access to personal effects (tissues, books, drinks) so they do not attempt to get up to fetch them, or reach for them in an unsafe manner. Similarly, a call bell should always be in easy reach of the person. This enables patients to call for assistance for completing daily tasks and to alert staff quickly if they get into any difficulties. For those who are not able to move around their room independently, yet have the cognitive and physical abilities to carry out some self-care tasks, toilet aids should be located within easy reach (e.g. urine bottles for men, bedpans or bed side commodes for women). In this way independence can be safely enhanced. Chairs should be height-adjustable so they can be set at a height from which it is easy for the person to stand up, as it is more difficult to stand up from a lower chair due to the additional muscle force required [33]. Those who can carry out daily tasks independently may benefit from an occupational therapy assessment and the provision of additional equipment, such as long-handled reachers for picking dropped objects up off the floor.

Safety can be maximized with careful consideration of the optimal location for individual patients/residents. For example, those with difficulty walking may benefit from being closer to bathrooms and dining rooms.

While a number of the above strategies prevent older people from moving unsafely, care must be taken that people are not unnecessarily restricted from standing up and walking. This will contribute to greater losses of strength, balance and function, which in turn can lead to an increased risk of falls. Instead, regular supervised walking and exercise programmes should be undertaken. For those who 'wander', pleasant but safe walking areas should be provided.

Among those at very high risk of falling the use of restraints may be considered. The issue of restraints in institutional settings is a complicated and controversial one, and is discussed in Chapter 13.

Increasing awareness of falls risk

Education is a crucial part of any falls prevention programme [21, 22]. Patients/residents, family members and staff should be informed if an individual is at an increased risk of falls, and the particular activities that they should avoid attempting unassisted or unsupervised. Systems are required to ensure that specific patient information is conveyed from each nursing shift to the next and that no lapses in vigilance occur during staff changeovers [7]. Education sessions should also be held regularly due to staff and resident changes. An information booklet may also be useful for patients [34].

Reducing fall injury

Even the most conscientious application of a falls prevention programme will not totally eradicate falls, particularly among very high-risk individuals. Therefore, as outlined in Box 15.1, attention must also be given to the prevention of injury following a fall.

Discharge planning

Programmes to prevent falls among hospital inpatients should not cease as soon as the person leaves the hospital. Effective discharge planning has a role to play in minimizing the risk of falls soon after the return home. This is vital as several studies have shown that people recently discharged from hospital are at an increased risk of falling. For example, Forster and Young [35] found that 73% of stroke patients fell in the six months after discharge from hospital. Similarly, Mahoney et al. [36] found that 14% of 214 older patients fell in the first month after returning home from a period of hospitalization for a medical condition.

Assessments of a person's functional abilities and risk of falling should be carried out prior to discharge from hospital. The person should not leave the hospital until it is clear that they are able to safely manage essential self-care and household tasks, or assistance with these tasks has been arranged. An occupational therapy home visit may be necessary to establish safety at home and has been shown to reduce falls rate among past fallers who have recently been in hospital [37]. Short periods of intensive rehabilitation should be considered for those recovering from major illness or surgery. Such a rehabilitation programme should aim to maximize the person's physical ability and thus independence.

Post-fall assessment

Is it important that systems be put in place for the investigation of all falls that do occur [7]. Any environmental hazards associated with the fall should be identified and acted on as appropriate. A physical examination of the faller may identify additional intrinsic risk factors. A review of the person's functional abilities and the interaction between these and the environment will also assist in identification of modifiable risk factors.

Research evaluating strategies for falls prevention in institutions

Hospitals

Two recent RCTs have evaluated the effects of multi-faceted falls prevention programmes in hospital settings. Haines *et al.* [38] developed a targeted, multiple intervention falls prevention programme and evaluated this in a RCT among 626 patients of three sub-acute wards in Melbourne, Australia. Interventions included a falls risk alert card with information brochure, an exercise programme, an education programme and hip protectors. Participants in the intervention group experienced 30% fewer falls than participants in the control group. This difference was significant (Peto log rank test $p = 0.045$) and was most obvious after 45 days of observation. The results of this study are encouraging but as many patients will leave hospitals prior to 45 days, some caution is required in drawing conclusions for other settings.

Encouraging findings regarding the effectiveness of interventions for preventing falls in hospitals have also been reported by Healy *et al.* [39], who conducted a cluster RCT in matched pairs of eight aged care wards and associated community units of a district general hospital in northern England. The intervention involved a pre-printed care plan for patients identified as at risk of falling with targeted interventions addressing eyesight, medication, blood pressure, urine test results, mobility, bedrail risk/benefit assessment, footwear, bed height, simple environmental factors, patients' position in the ward and a nurse call bell being within reach. They found a reduction of falls on the intervention wards but not control wards, with a significant between-group difference (relative risk = 0.71, 95% CI = 0.55–0.90).

In a recent non-randomized controlled trial on three similar aged care wards, Vassallo *et al.* [40] evaluated a falls prevention programme involving a multi-disciplinary team who met weekly specifically to discuss patients' falls risk and formulate a targeted plan. Patients at risk were identified using wristbands; risk factors were corrected or environmental changes made to enhance safety. Control wards had proportionally more fallers (20.2% vs. 14.2%, $p = 0.033$), patients sustaining injury (8.2% vs. 4%, $p = 0.025$) and total number of falls

(170 vs. 72, $p = 0.045$). However, these results did not remain significant after controlling for differing length of stay. Many multi-faceted programmes to prevent falls in hospitals have been evaluated in before/after studies. Most [5, 41–45] but not all [46, 47] of these studies have found a reduction in falls after the intervention period.

Several small RCTs have looked at single interventions to prevent falls in hospitals. Mayo et al. [48] found that an identification bracelet worn by those identified as being at high risk of falling was not effective in preventing falls. In a RCT among 54 patients in an aged care rehabilitation ward, Donald et al. [49] found a trend for fewer falls occurring on vinyl floors than on carpeted floors, and some additional benefits from leg strengthening exercises in addition to conventional physiotherapy. Tideiksaar et al. [50] trialled a bed alarm system in a RCT among 70 patients at high risk of falling. The device involved a sensor strip under the bedclothes, which alerted nursing staff to a patient's attempt to get out of bed, thus enabling them to provide assistance. Although not statistically significant, fewer falls occurred in the intervention group. These interventions all need further investigation with larger samples.

Before/after or historical control studies have also been conducted to assess the effects of single intervention strategies. These studies have reported reductions in repeat falls, with a policy of taking standing and lying blood pressure after a fall in a psychiatric hospital [51]. Also a reduction in falls with a thigh-position device which alerts staff when a person attempts to get out of bed or stand up [30, 31].

While it is unclear whether the provision of exercise as a single intervention affects falls in hospital patients, a recent RCT [52] found that functional ability could be improved with an exercise programme among 300 people with non-disabling medical and surgical diagnoses who were admitted to an acute care hospital.

As with any healthcare intervention the effect of falls prevention programmes is difficult to evaluate in a non-controlled study. It is difficult to separate the effects of the falls prevention programme from other changes in healthcare systems and community-wide falls prevention programmes. However, it will usually not be possible or desirable to conduct a RCT to evaluate the effects of a single intervention programme in each setting. Once elements of effective programmes have been determined in randomized studies, a quality improvement model to implement these strategies locally is appropriate. The recent publication of the successful large RCTs of falls prevention programmes in hospitals [38, 39] provides an initial body of evidence on which to base local programmes.

Data collection is a key issue in the design of studies to evaluate falls prevention programmes. Falls monitoring relies on incident forms being completed rigorously, but this may not always occur – one recent study found that incident forms were only completed for an average of 60% of falls [46]. Another issue is that an increased awareness of falls can accompany the introduction of a falls prevention programme. This may lead to a greater rigour in completing incident forms and may increase the rate of reported falls, confounding the effects of the intervention strategy.

Residential aged care

In residential aged care there have been several RCTs investigating falls prevention programmes. Three recent RCTs have found that *multi-faceted programmes* have the potential to decrease falls. Jensen *et al.* [22] conducted a cluster RCT among 439 residents of nine residential care facilities in Sweden. An 11-week multidisciplinary programme of general and resident-specific tailored strategies was found to significantly reduce falls during a 34-week follow-up period (adjusted incidence rate ratio = 0.60, 95% CI = 0.50–0.73). This programme involved educating staff, modifying the environment, implementing exercise programmes, supplying and repairing aids, reviewing drug regimens, providing hip protectors, having post-fall problem-solving conferences, and guiding staff.

Becker *et al.* [23] conducted a cluster RCT among 981 long-stay residents of six nursing homes and found a markedly lower incidence density ratio of falls in the intervention group compared with the control group over a 12 month period (relative risk = 0.55, 95% CI = 0.41–0.73). A total of 52% of the control group were fallers compared with 37% of the intervention group (relative risk = 0.75, 95% CI = 0.57–0.98). The intervention involved staff training and feedback, information provision and education for residents, environmental adaptations, exercise (balance exercises and progressive resistance training with ankle weights and dumbbells), and hip protectors. Interestingly, intervention effects were not apparent before six months and the authors suggested that it may have taken this long for improvement in the mediating variables (physical performance, staff adherence and environmental adaptations) to take effect.

In an earlier cluster RCT of multi-faceted programmes in residential aged care, Ray *et al.* [24] studied 482 residents who had previously fallen. Seven pairs of nursing homes were randomized to receive no intervention or the intervention programme, which involved structured individual assessment (of environmental safety, wheelchair use, psychotropic drug use, and transfers and ambulation) by medical, nursing and occupational therapy professionals. At post-test there was a mean reduction of 19% in the proportion of recurrent fallers in the intervention homes. Greater effects were evident for homes with a higher compliance with recommendations and for residents with three or more previous falls.

However, another recent RCT did not find such positive results. Kerse *et al.* [53] reported an increased falls rate following a trial that involved residential care staff, used existing resources and implemented systematic individualized fall risk management for all residents, using a falls risk assessment tool, high-risk logo and strategies to address identified risks (incident rate ratio = 1.34, 95% CI = 1.06–1.72). This intervention was less intensive than the three other RCTs conducted in residential care settings and the authors suggested that low intensity interventions may be worse than usual care [53]. In the only RCT of a comprehensive post-fall assessment by a nurse practitioner with physician referral, Rubenstein *et al.* [54] found that while this approach reduced hospitalizations and hospital stays, it did not significantly reduce the rate of subsequent falls.

People with *impaired cognition* comprise a large percentage of people residing in residential care facilities. Unfortunately, the role and optimal design of a falls prevention programme for this group is unclear. In a pre-planned sub-group analysis of data from the Jensen *et al.* [22] study described above, the intervention was only effective in residents with a higher level of cognition (Mini-mental State Examination Score of > 18) [55]. In a RCT among 25 previous fallers with dementia, Buettner [56] described an interesting programme for people with dementia living in residential aged care. This programme targeted times of day and locations in which falls were observed to occur. It involved early morning walking groups, exercise aimed at improving functional abilities in the mid-afternoon and relaxation sessions using a sensory air flow mat in the evenings. The authors reported a marked reduction in falls following two months of the programme. Unfortunately the groups were not well matched at baseline and statistical analyses were not presented.

Vitamin D supplementation appears to have an important role in preventing falls in residential care facilities. Vitamin D deficiency is common in this setting, even in countries with high levels of sunlight. A recent meta-analysis found that vitamin D supplementation reduces the risk of falls among institutionalized older people with stable health by more than 20% [57]. There may be added benefits of calcium supplementation. A landmark study has shown that vitamin D plus calcium supplementation taken daily for three years by frail older people in residential aged care facilities or sheltered accommodation could significantly reduce the incidence of hip fracture [58].

As discussed in Chapter 13, early studies [59] indicated that *hip protectors* may have a role to play in injury prevention in residential aged care settings. More recent studies [60] have not found such positive results, primarily due to compliance problems [61].

Few large scale RCTs have investigated the effects on falls of *exercise* as a single intervention in residential aged care. Schnelle *et al.* [25, 26] conducted an interesting RCT among 190 nursing home residents. Intervention participants were seen by a research assistant up to four times a day for eight months, and were given a continence prompt, a supervised walk, asked to sit-to-stand eight times and encouraged to take on fluids. Additional upper-limb resistance training was provided at tailored intensity, walking distance was gradually increased if possible and sit-to-stand exercise encouraged with minimal use of upper limbs for support. This programme resulted in improved or maintained functional abilities among exercise subjects, while the abilities of control subjects deteriorated (between-group differences for 14 of 15 outcome measures). The control group also had an increased incidence of falls from baseline to follow-up while the intervention group remained stable (OR $\pm$, standard error $= 0.46 \pm 0.18$).

Mulrow *et al.* [27] analysed the effect of one-to-one physiotherapy compared to controls in 194 people living in nursing homes. The programme consisted of resistance, balance, functional task training, endurance and flexibility exercises, and took place three times a week for four months. The programme did enhance mobility and reduce assistive device use but did not reduce falls in a six month period [27].

There have been several other RCTs that have evaluated the effect of exercise on falls in residential aged care settings, but were probably too small to detect effects if they were present. In a RCT among 110 residents of two senior housing communities with a variety of living arrangements, Nowalk *et al.* [62] compared fall rates among three groups: a resistance and endurance training group; a Tai Chi group; and a falling modulation (control) group. Over the two year trial period, adherence was only 40% and was higher in the resistance and endurance training group. No differences in fall rates among the three groups were found. In another small RCT ($n = 133$) among nursing home residents, McMurdo *et al.* [63] found no significant differences between fall rates in exercise and control groups in the six month period after completing a seated exercise programme as well as a risk-factor modification programme.

Several RCTs have indicated that risk factors for falling among residents of aged care facilities can be improved with training. In a systematic review of 16 RCTs, Rydwik *et al.* [64] concluded that there is strong evidence for a positive effect of physical training on muscle strength and mobility, moderate evidence for an effect on range of motion, and inconsistent evidence regarding gait, activities of daily living, balance and endurance. Schoenfelder and Rubenstein [65] found that a three-month ankle-strengthening and walking programme led to balance and fear of falling levels being maintained or improved for the exercise group in comparison to the control group. Although limited by very small subject numbers and a lack of between-group comparisons, two other RCTs have shown that physical training can improve functional ability in residents of aged care facilities [66, 67]. For more discussion of exercise prescription principles and results of RCTs evaluating the effect of exercise on falls and functional abilities, please refer to Chapters 10 and 11.

Some additonal information on the potential role of exercise in residential aged care can be gleaned from recent studies in retirement village settings among transitionally frail older people, as discussed in Chapter 10. Our group [68] conducted a cluster RCT among 551 residents of 20 retirement villages that compared weight-bearing group exercise with control activities of flexibility and relaxation exercises, and no intervention. The exercise classes were held twice weekly by exercise instructors and involved aerobic exercise, strengthening exercises, as well as activities for balance, hand-eye and foot-eye coordination, and flexibility. After adjusting for age and sex, there were 22% fewer falls during the 12 month trial in the exercise group compared with the combined controls (incidence rate ratio $= 0.78$, 95% CI$=0.62$–0.99). In those who had fallen in the previous year there was a stronger effect (incidence rate ratio $= 0.69$, 95% CI$=0.48$–0.99). In a cluster RCT, Wolf et al. [69] compared a twice-weekly Tai Chi programme with a wellness education programme in 311 residents aged 70–9 from 20 congregate living facilities (retirement villages). To be eligible for the study, subjects had to be assessed as 'transitioning to frailty' and to have fallen at least once in the past year. Following 48 weeks of intervention, there was a trend to a reduction in falls in the intervention group compared with the control group, but this did not reach statistical significance (relative risk $= 0.75$, 95% CI$=0.52$–1.08). The authors reported that over the intervention period, 48% of subjects in the Tai Chi group and 60% of subjects in the wellness education group fell at least once.

It is important to remember the non-linear pattern of falls seen most noticeably in the residential and nursing home care population, and to recognize the limited benefits of considering falls in isolation in clinical trials. Many intervention programmes in these settings promote activity, independence and quality of life, and with this comes an inevitable increased exposure to risk of falls. One must weigh up the outcome of increased exposure to risk and falls against the benefits of improved functional performance, both from the individual patient's perspective and the level of care required for these individuals.

Conclusion

Many older people within hospitals and aged care facilities are at an increased risk of falling. There is now good evidence that a multidisciplinary, multifactorial assessment and intervention programme can be effective in reducing the risk of falls in nursing homes. The findings of the RCTs completed to date suggest that interventions may need to be in place six months before benefits are seen and low intensity interventions may be worse than usual care. Vitamin D supplementation appears to be an effective means of preventing falls in nursing homes. In terms of other single intervention strategies, there is insufficient evidence that exercise can prevent falls in residential care, and problems related to compliance preclude hip protectors from being an effective fall injury prevention strategy. Studies are yet to demonstrate that falls interventions can be effective in older people with cognitive impairment living in residential care. Initial findings indicate that multidisciplinary approaches can prevent falls in hospital patients. While many of the individual strategies for preventing falls outlined above are common sense, most have not been rigorously tested for their effectiveness and cost-effectiveness in research trials. The implementation of these strategies in institutional settings, therefore, requires further evaluation.

REFERENCES

1. N. E. Mayo, N. Korner-Bitensky, R. Becker & P. Georges, Predicting falls among patients in a rehabilitation hospital. *American Journal of Physical Medicine and Rehabilitation*, **68**(3) (1989), 139–46.

2. A. Dromerick & M. Reding, Medical and neurological complications during inpatient stroke rehabilitation. *Stroke*, **25**(2) (1994), 358–61.

3. L. Nyberg & Y. Gustafson, Patient falls in stroke rehabilitation. A challenge to rehabilitation strategies. *Stroke*, **26**(5) (1995), 838–42.

4. D. A. Evans, B. Hodgkinson, L. Lambert, J. Wood & I. Kowanko, *Falls in Acute Hospitals: a Systematic Review* (Adelaide: The Joanna Briggs Institute for Evidence Based Nursing and Midwifery, 1998).

5. M. Gowdy & S. Godfrey, Using tools to assess and prevent inpatient falls. *Joint Commission Journal on Quality and Safety*, **29**(7) (2003), 363–8.

6. D. Oliver, F. Daly, F. C. Martin & M. E. T. McMurdo, Risk factors and risk assessment tools for falls in hospital in-patients: a systematic review. *Age and Ageing*, **33** (2004), 122–30.

7. L. Z. Rubenstein, K. R. Josephson & D. Osterweil, Falls and fall prevention in the nursing home. *Clinics in Geriatric Medicine*, **12**(4) (1996), 881–902.

8. D. K. Kiely, D. P. Kiel, A. B. Burrows & L. A. Lipsitz, Identifying nursing home residents at risk for falling. *Journal of the American Geriatrics Society*, **46**(5) (1998), 551–5.

9. L. A. Lipsitz, P. V. Jonsson, M. M. Kelley & J. S. Koestner, Causes and correlates of recurrent falls in ambulatory frail elderly. *Journal of Gerontology*, **46**(4) (1991), M114–22.

10. H. Luukinen, K. Koski, P. Laippala & S. L. Kivela, Risk factors for recurrent falls in the elderly in long-term institutional care. *Public Health*, **109**(1) (1995), 57–65.

11. P. B. Thapa, P. Gideon, R. L. Fought & W. A. Ray, Psychotropic drugs and risk of recurrent falls in ambulatory nursing home residents. *American Journal of Epidemiology*, **142**(2) (1995), 202–11.

12. L. Z. Rubenstein, K. R. Josephson & A. S. Robbins, Falls in the nursing home. *Annals of Internal Medicine*, **121**(6) (1994), 442–51.

13. P. O. Jantti, V. I. Pyykko & A. L. Hervonen, Falls among elderly nursing home residents. *Public Health*, **107**(2) (1993), 89–96.

14. National Institute for Clinical Excellence, *Clinical Practice Guideline for the Assessment and Prevention of Falls in Older People* (London: National Institute for Clinical Excellence, 2004).

15. P. B. Thapa, K. G. Brockman, P. Gideon, R. L. Fought & W. A. Ray, Injurious falls in nonambulatory nursing home residents: a comparative study of circumstances, incidence, and risk factors. *Journal of the American Geriatrics Society*, **44**(3) (1996), 273–8.

16. S. R. Lord, L. M. March, I. D. Cameron *et al.*, Differing risk factors for falls in nursing home and intermediate-care residents who can and cannot stand unaided. *Journal of the American Geriatrics Society*, **51**(11) (2003), 1645–50.

17. K. L. Perell, A. Nelson, R. L. Goldman *et al.*, Fall risk assessment measures: an analytic review. *Journals of Gerontology. Series A, Biological Sciences and Medical Sciences*, **56**(12) (2001), M761–6.

18. D. Oliver, M. Britton, P. Seed, F. C. Martin & A. H. Hopper, Development and evaluation of evidence based risk assessment tool (STRATIFY) to predict which elderly inpatients will fall: case-control and cohort studies. *British Medical Journal*, **315**(7115) (1997), 1049–53.

19. E. Coker & D. Oliver, Evaluation of the STRATIFY falls prediction tool on a geriatric unit. *Outcomes Management*, **7** (2003), 8–17.

20. A. Papaioannou, W. Parkinson, R. Cook *et al.*, Prediction of falls using a risk assessment tool in the acute care setting. *Biomed Central Medicine*, **2**(1) (2004), 1.

21. C. Shanley, *Putting Your Best Foot Forward: Preventing and Managing Falls in Aged Care Facilities* (Sydney: The Centre for Education and Research on Ageing (CERA), 1998).

22. J. Jensen, L. Lundin-Olsson, L. Nyberg & Y. Gustafson, Fall and injury prevention in older people living in residential care facilities: a cluster randomized trial. *Annals of Internal Medicine*, **136**(10) (2002), 733–41.

23. C. Becker, M. Kron, U. Lindemann *et al.*, Effectiveness of a multifaceted intervention on falls in nursing home residents. *Journal of the American Geriatrics Society*, **51** (2003), 306–13.

24. W. A. Ray, J. A. Taylor, K. G. Meador *et al.*, A randomized trial of a consultation service to reduce falls in nursing homes. *JAMA: Journal of the American Medical Association*, **278**(7) (1997), 557–62.

25. J. F. Schnelle, K. Kapur, C. Alessi *et al.*, Does an exercise and incontinence intervention save healthcare costs in a nursing home population? *Journal of the American Geriatrics Society*, **51**(2) (2003), 161–8.

26. J. F. Schnelle, C. A. Alessi, S. F. Simmons *et al.*, Translating clinical research into practice: a randomized controlled trial of exercise and incontinence care with nursing home residents. *Journal of the American Geriatrics Society*, **50**(9) (2002), 1476–83.

27. C. D. Mulrow, M. B. Gerety, D. Kanten *et al.*, A randomized trial of physical rehabilitation for very frail nursing home residents. *JAMA: Journal of the American Medical Association*, **271**(7) (1994), 519–24.

28. Australian Council for Safety and Quality in Health Care, *Preventing Falls and Harm from Falls in Older People. Best Practice Guidelines for Australian Hospitals and Residential Aged Care Facilities.* (Canberra: Australian Council for Safety and Quality in Health Care, 2005).

29. B. Przybylski, E. Dumont, M. Watkins *et al.*, Outcomes of enhanced physical and occupational therapy service in a nursing home setting. *Archives of Physical Medicine and Rehabilitation*, **77**(6) (1996), 554–61.

30. B. Widder, A new device to decrease falls. *Geriatric Nursing – American Journal of Care for the Aging*, **6**(5) (1985), 287–8.

31. K. E. Kelly, C. L. Phillips, K. C. Cain, N. L. Polissar & P. B. Kelly, Evaluation of a nonintrusive monitor to reduce falls in nursing home patients. *Journal of the American Medical Directors Association*, **3**(6) (2002), 377–82.

32. V. Rialle, N. Lauvernay, A. Franco, J. F. Piquard & P. Couturier, A smart room for hospitalised elderly people: essay of modelling and first steps of an experiment. *Technology and Health Care*, **7**(5) (1999), 343–57.

33. U. Arborelius, P. Wretenberg & F. Lindberg, The effects of armrests and high seat heights on lower-limb joint load and muscular activity during sitting and rising. *Ergonomics*, **35** (1992), 1377–91.

34. H. Buri, A group programme to prevent falls in elderly hospital patients. *British Journal of Therapy and Rehabilitation*, **4**(10) (1997), 550.

35. A. Forster & J. Young, Incidence and consequences of falls due to stroke: a systematic inquiry. *British Medical Journal*, **311**(6997) (1995), 83–6.

36. J. Mahoney, M. Sager, N. C. Dunham & J. Johnson, Risk of falls after hospital discharge. *Journal of the American Geriatrics Society*, **42**(3) (1994), 269–74.

37. R. G. Cumming, M. Thomas, G. Szonyi *et al.*, Home visits by an occupational therapist for assessment and modification of environmental hazards: a randomized trial of falls prevention. *Journal of the American Geriatrics Society*, **47**(12) (1999), 1397–402.

38. T. P. Haines, K. L. Bennell, R. H. Osborne & K. D. Hill, Effectiveness of targeted falls prevention programme in subacute hospital setting: randomised controlled trial. *British Medical Journal*, **328** (2004), 676.

39. F. Healey, A. Monro, A. Cockram, V. Adams & D. Heseltine, Using targeted risk factor reduction to prevent falls in older in-patients: a randomised controlled trial. *Age and Ageing*, **33**(4) (2004), 390–5.

40. M. Vassallo, R. Vignaraja, J. C. Sharma *et al.*, The effect of changing practice on fall prevention in a rehabilitative hospital: the Hospital Injury Prevention Study. *Journal of the American Geriatrics Society*, **52**(3) (2004), 335–9.

41. A. Ward, L. Candela & J. Mahoney, Developing a unit-specific falls reduction program. *Journal for Healthcare Quality*, **26**(2) (2004), 36–40.

42. V. Kilpack, J. Boehm, N. Smith & B. Mudge, Using research-based interventions to decrease patient falls. *Applied Nursing Research*, **4**(2) (1991), 50–6.

43. E. Barry, M. Laffoy, E. Matthews & D. Carey, Preventing accidental falls among older people in long stay units. *Irish Medical Journal,* **94**(6) (2001), 172, 174–6.

44. P. K. Lieu, N. K. Ismail, P. W. Choo *et al.,* Prevention of falls in a geriatric ward. *Annals of the Academy of Medicine, Singapore,* **26**(3) (1997), 266–70.

45. A. Mitchell & N. Jones, Striving to prevent falls in an acute care setting – action to enhance quality. *Journal of Clinical Nursing,* **5**(4) (1996), 213–20.

46. A. Semin-Goossens, J. M. van der Helm & P. M. Bossuyt, A failed model-based attempt to implement an evidence-based nursing guideline for fall prevention. *Journal of Nursing Care Quality,* **18**(3) (2003), 217–25.

47. A. J. Lane, Evaluation of the fall prevention program in an acute care setting. *Orthopaedic Nursing,* **18**(6) (1999), 37–43.

48. N. E. Mayo, L. Gloutney & A. R. Levy, A randomized trial of identification bracelets to prevent falls among patients in a rehabilitation hospital. *Archives of Physical Medicine and Rehabilitation,* **75**(12) (1994), 1302–8.

49. I. P. Donald, K. Pitt, E. Armstrong & H. Shuttleworth, Preventing falls on an elderly care rehabilitation ward. *Clinical Rehabilitation,* **14**(2) (2000), 178–85.

50. R. Tideiksaar, C. F. Feiner & J. Maby, Falls prevention: the efficacy of a bed alarm system in an acute-care setting. *Mount Sinai Journal of Medicine,* **60**(6) (1993), 522–7.

51. C. Murdock, R. Goldney, L. Fisher, P. Kent & S. Walmsley, A reduction in repeat falls in a private psychiatric hospital. *Australian and New Zealand Journal of Mental Health Nursing,* **7**(3) (1998), 111–5.

52. H. Siebens, H. Aronow, D. Edwards & Z. Ghasemi, A randomized controlled trial of exercise to improve outcomes of acute hospitalization in older adults. *Journal of the American Geriatrics Society,* **48**(12) (2000), 1545–52.

53. N. Kerse, M. Butler, E. Robinson & M. Todd, Fall prevention in residential care: a cluster, randomized, controlled trial. *Journal of the American Geriatrics Society,* **52**(4) (2004), 524–31.

54. L. Z. Rubenstein, A. S. Robbins, K. R. Josephson, B. L. Schulman & D. Osterweil, The value of assessing falls in an elderly population. A randomized clinical trial. *Annals of Internal Medicine,* **113**(4) (1990), 308–16.

55. J. Jensen, L. Nyberg, Y. Gustafson & L. Lundin-Olsson, Fall and injury prevention in residential care – effects in residents with higher and lower levels of cognition. *Journal of the American Geriatrics Society,* **51**(5) (2003), 627–35.

56. L. L. Buettner, Focus on caregiving. Falls prevention in dementia populations: following a trial program of recreation therapy, falls were reduced by 164 percent. *Provider,* **28**(2) (2002), 41–3.

57. H. Bischoff-Ferrari, B. Dawson-Hughes, W. Willett *et al.,* Effect of Vitamin D on falls: a meta-analysis. *JAMA: Journal of the American Medical Association,* **291** (2004), 1999–2006.

58. M. C. Chapuy, M. E. Arlot, F. Duboeuf *et al.,* Vitamin D_3 and calcium to prevent hip fractures in the elderly women. *New England Journal of Medicine,* **327**(23) (1992), 1637–42.

59. J. B. Lauritzen, M. M. Petersen & B. Lund, Effect of external hip protectors on hip fractures. *The Lancet,* **341**(8836) (1993), 11–3.

60. P. O'Halloran, G. Cran, T. Beringer *et al.*, A cluster randomised controlled trial to evaluate a policy of making hip protectors available to residents of nursing homes. *Age and Ageing*, **33**(6) (2004), 582–8.

61. M. Parker, W. J. Gillespie & L. D. Gillespie, *Hip Protectors for Preventing Hip Fractures in Older People*. Cochrane Database of Systematic Reviews (3) (2005), CD0001255.

62. M. P. Nowalk, J. M. Prendergast, C. M. Bayles, F. J. D'Amico & G. C. Colvin, A randomized trial of exercise programs among older individuals living in two long-term care facilities: the FallsFREE program. *Journal of the American Geriatrics Society*, **49**(7) (2001), 859–65.

63. M. E. McMurdo, A. M. Millar & F. Daly, A randomized controlled trial of fall prevention strategies in old peoples' homes. *Gerontology*, **46**(2) (2000), 83–7.

64. E. Rydwik, K. Frandin & G. Akner, Effects of physical training on physical performance in institutionalised elderly patients (70 +) with multiple diagnoses. *Age and Ageing*, **33**(1) (2004), 13–23.

65. D. P. Schoenfelder & L. M. Rubenstein, An exercise program to improve fall-related outcomes in elderly nursing home residents. *Applied Nursing Research*, **17**(1) (2004), 21–31.

66. C. Toulotte, C. Fabre, B. Dangremont, G. Lensel & A. Thevenon, Effects of physical training on the physical capacity of frail, demented patients with a history of falling: a randomised controlled trial. *Age and Ageing*, **32**(1) (2003), 67–73.

67. D. P. Schoenfelder, A fall prevention program for elderly individuals. Exercise in long-term care settings. *Journal of Gerontological Nursing*, **26**(3) (2000), 43–51.

68. S. R. Lord, S. Castell, J. Corcoran *et al.*, The effect of group exercise on physical functioning and falls in frail older people living in retirement villages: a randomized, controlled trial. *Journal of the American Geriatrics Society*, **51**(12) (2003), 1685–92.

69. S. L. Wolf, R. W. Sattin, M. Kutner *et al.*, Intense tai chi exercise training and fall occurrences in older, transitionally frail adults: a randomized, controlled trial. *Journal of the American Geriatrics Society*, **51**(12) (2003), 1693–701.

70. A. Bakarich, V. McMillan & R. Prosser, The effect of a nursing intervention on the incidence of older patient falls. *Australian Journal of Advanced Nursing*, **15**(1) (1997), 26–31.

71. D. J. Boswell, J. Ramsey, M. A. Smith & B. Wagers, The cost-effectiveness of a patient-sitter program in an acute care hospital: a test of the impact of sitters on the incidence of falls and patient satisfaction. *Quality Management in Health Care*, **10**(1) (2001), 10–6.

16

A physiological profile approach to falls risk assessment and prevention

As outlined in Chapter 6, research studies have identified a broad range of medical conditions which contribute to falls risk. These include chronic and degenerative diseases, such as stroke [1–5], Parkinson's disease [6–8], arthritis [9], foot problems [10], cognitive impairment [1, 11, 12], peripheral neuropathy and diabetes [13, 14], cataracts [15] and vestibular disorders [16, 17]. However, attributing a degree of falls risk to a specific medical diagnosis is often problematic because the severity of these conditions varies considerably among individuals. Furthermore, impairments in sensorimotor function and balance associated with increased age, inactivity, medication use or minor pathology, may be evident in older people without diagnosed medical conditions.

To address this issue, we have devised a Physiological Profile Assessment (PPA) for assessing falls risk that involves quantitative assessment of sensorimotor and balance abilities. Physiological factors that are the important contributors to stability are shown in Figure 16.1. Functioning in each of these factors declines with age [18] and impairments in each factor increases the risk of falling [19–22]. A marked deficit in any one of these factors may be sufficient to predispose an older person to fall; however, a combination of mild or moderate impairments across physiological domains also may increase the risk of falling. By assessing an individual's physiological abilities, impairments in one or more physiological domains can be identified and cumulative falls risk can be determined.

In many cases the postural effects of medical conditions, whether diagnosed or not, will be manifest in one or more of the PPA tests. For example, poor vision is likely to be the prime impairment and risk factor for falls in older people with cataracts or macular degeneration. Similarly, poor peripheral sensation is likely to be a major falls risk factor for people with diabetic neuropathy and muscle weakness the main risk factor for people with prior poliomyelitis. Finally, older people following a stroke, with limiting arthritis or multiple pathologies may have several impairments, including poor peripheral sensation, muscle weakness, slowed reaction time and poor balance.

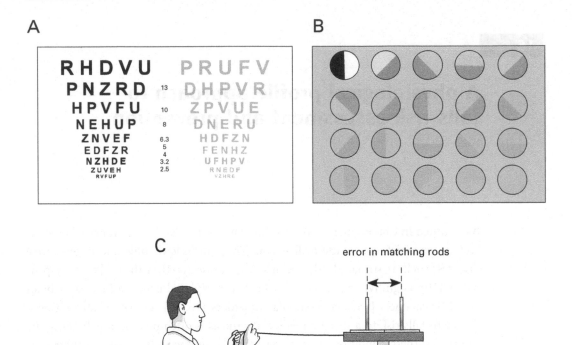

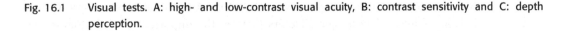

Fig. 16.1   Visual tests. A: high- and low-contrast visual acuity, B: contrast sensitivity and C: depth perception.

This chapter outlines the nature and elements of the PPA and describes how it can be used for assessing falls risk, tailoring a falls prevention programme and evaluating the effectiveness of intervention in both the research and clinical settings.

The PPA components

The PPA involves the measurement of sensorimotor and balance abilities with simple quantitative tests. Using population norms, impairments in specific physiological domains and an individual's overall falls risk can be identified [23]. The PPA has two versions: a comprehensive version and a screening version. The two versions provide the same falls risk score. However, the comprehensive version provides additional information on a broad range of physiological measures that provide insight into each subject's impairments, including complementary assessments of vision and peripheral sensation, measurements of strength in multiple lower-extremity muscle groups, and assessments of balance under a series of increasingly challenging conditions. Thus the comprehensive version is suitable for research settings and in clinical settings, where the outcome of the more detailed assessment may alter subsequent treatment or referral patterns. It takes an hour per person to complete.

The screening version takes 15–20 minutes to administer, and is suitable for settings in which time constraints are an issue and where the PPA forms only part of a broader medical examination. The screening version contains five tests: vision (edge-contrast sensitivity), peripheral sensation (proprioception), lower-extremity strength (knee extension strength), reaction time using a finger press as the response, and body sway (sway when standing on the medium-density foam rubber mat). We identified these five items from discriminant function analyses as being the most important for discriminating between fallers and non-fallers in prospective studies [19, 20].

Rationale for test selection

In order for the PPA to be practical in a clinical setting, the tests have been selected to meet the following criteria:

(1) *Short administration time.* To test the many domains important in balance control in one session, it is important that each test item take only a few minutes to administer. Quick administration time also aids participation and avoids fatigue in frail older people.

(2) *Simple to administer.* As with all tests of physical functioning, the PPA needs to be administered in a standardized, rigorous way. Each test has been designed in an effort to facilitate test administration. Only one day of training is required for allied healthcare personnel to be proficient in test administration and use of the computer programme.

(3) *Feasible for older people to undertake.* The selected tests need to be non-invasive, not require excessive effort, or cause pain or discomfort. However, the tests need to be challenging so as to discriminate between older people with and without sensorimotor and balance impairments, with minimal ceiling and floor effects.

(4) *Valid and reliable measurements.* The measurements obtained with the test must have high criterion validity; that is, they must be able to predict falling in older people. The test's items also need to have good inter-rater and test-retest reliability [23].

(5) *'Low-tech' and robust.* If the tests are to be used successfully in large community studies and assessment clinics they need to be 'low-tech' and robust.

(6) *Transportability.* A compact, lightweight test battery enables testing in a variety of physical settings. Thus, assessment can be done in community settings, retirement villages and healthcare institutions. Such transportability

improves participation and adherence, because the clinic can be brought to the target population of older frail people, rather than requiring them to attend a fixed-location laboratory. One person can carry each equipment item and all equipment can fit into a car for transportation.

(7) *Quantitative measurements.* Finally, all tests provide continuously scored measurements, that is, quantitative rather than discrete or graded scores. This enables the test scores to be analysed with univariate and multivariate parametric statistics, such as analysis of variance, correlation and regression techniques, and discriminant analysis.

The PPA tests

The PPA tests for the comprehensive version are described in Table 16.1 and are illustrated in Figures 16.1, 16.2, 16.3, 16.4, 16.5 and 16.6. At present, the PPA does not contain a test of vestibular function. Our group have previously used Fukuda's vestibular x-writing and stepping tests [24, 25] to assess this domain [19, 20]. However, we found that poor performances in these tests were not related to either poor balance, [26] or falls [19] and that measurements obtained with these tests have low test-retest reliability [26]. We are currently evaluating more direct screening tests of vestibular functioning for subsequent versions of the PPA.

The web-based normative database and assessment report programme

For both the comprehensive and screening versions, a web-based computer software programme (www.powmri.edu.au/FBRG/calculator.htm) has been developed to compare an individual's performance in the PPA tests in relation to a normative database compiled from the large population studies[1] [18–21]. This programme produces a falls risk assessment report for each individual that includes the following components:

(1) A graph indicating an individual's overall falls risk score.
(2) A profile of the individual's test performances. This profile allows a quick identification of physiological strengths and impairments.
(3) A table indicating the individual's test performances in relation to age- and sex-matched norms.
(4) A written report that makes recommendations for improving functional performances or compensating for impairments identified.

Figures 16.7 and 16.8 and Table 16.2 present the report components for a 79-year-old woman who underwent the comprehensive version of the PPA. Figure 16.7 shows her falls risk score – a single index score derived from

---

[1] The PPA equipment and computer programme are commercially available. Further information can be obtained from the Prince of Wales Medical Research Institute at FallScreen@unsw.edu.au or www.powmri.edu.au/FBRG/.

Table 16.1 The Physiological Profile Assessment (PPA) tests

Test	Test description
High- and low-contrast visual acuity	Visual acuity is measured using a letter chart with high- and low-contrast (10%) letters. Acuity is assessed binocularly with subjects wearing their distance glasses (if applicable) at a test distance of 3 m and measured in terms of the minimum angle resolvable in minutes of arc.
Contrast sensitivity	Edge-contrast sensitivity is assessed using the Melbourne Edge Test [27]. The chart has 15 circular 25-mm-diameter patches containing edges with reducing contrast, with variable orientation as the identifying feature. The test uses a four-alternative forced-choice method of presentation. The edges are presented in the orientations: horizontal, vertical, 45 degrees left and 45 degrees right. A key card containing the four possible edge angles is provided for subject instruction. The lowest contrast patch correctly identified is recorded as the subject's contrast sensitivity in decibel units, where $1 \, dB = 10 \log_{10}$ contrast.
Depth perception	Depth perception is measured with a Howard-Dohlman apparatus. [28]. This test presents two vertical rods, the objective being to align these rods side-by-side. The subject is seated 3 m away and pulls on the cord to move the right rod while the left rod remains fixed. Any discrepancies in the position of the rods are measured in millimetres.
Tactile sensitivity	Tactile sensitivity is measured with a pressure aesthesiometer. This instrument contains eight nylon filaments of equal length, but varying in diameter. The force (in grams) required to bend each filament is calibrated and ranges from 0.0045 g to 447 g. The filaments are applied to the centre of the lateral malleolus of the ankle using a staircase method. The touch threshold is determined from the finest filament the subject can detect.
Vibration sense	Vibration sense is measured using an electronic device that generates a 200-Hz vibration of varying intensity. The vibration is applied to the tibial tuberosity via a 1-cm-diameter rubber button. A staircase method is used to determine vibration thresholds which are measured in microns of motion perpendicular to the body surface.
Proprioception	Proprioception is assessed using a lower-limb matching task. In this test, subjects are seated with their eyes closed and are asked to align their lower limbs simultaneously on either side of a vertical clear acrylic sheet ($60 \times 60 \times 1$ cm) inscribed with a protractor and placed between the legs. Any difference in aligning the lower limbs (indicated by disparities in matching the great toes on either side of the acrylic sheet) is measured in degrees. After two practise trials, an average of five experimental trials is recorded.
Lower-limb strength	The strength of three leg muscle groups (knee extensors and flexors, ankle dorsiflexors) is measured isometrically while subjects are seated. Testing the

Table 16.1 (*cont.*)

Test	Test Description
	knee extensor and flexor muscles is performed using a spring gauge attached to the subject's leg using a webbing strap with a Velcro fastener. The strength of the knee extensor and flexor muscles is measured with the subject sitting in a tall chair with a strap around the leg 10 cm above the ankle joint, and the hip and knee joint angles positioned at 90 degrees. In three trials per muscle group, the subject attempts to pull against the strap assembly with maximal force for two to three seconds and the greatest force for each muscle group is recorded. The testing of ankle dorsiflexion strength is undertaken using a footplate attached to a spring gauge. While the subject is sitting in a tall chair, the foot is secured to the footplate using a webbing strap with a Velcro fastener, with the angle of the knee at 110 degrees. In three trials, the subject attempts maximal dorsiflexion of the ankle and the greatest force (in kilograms) is recorded.
Reaction time	Reaction time is assessed in milliseconds using a handheld electronic timer and a light as the stimulus, and depression of a switch by the finger and the foot as the responses. The light stimulus is located adjacent to the response switches and is bright (i.e. supra-threshold) to ensure that the tests are not influenced by the subject's visual acuity. The timer has a built-in variable delay of one to five seconds to remove any cues that could be gained from the test administrator commencing each trial by pressing the 'start' button. Five practise trials are undertaken, followed by ten experimental trials.
Postural sway	Postural sway is measured using a sway-meter that measures displacements of the body at waist level. The device consists of a 40-cm-long rod with a vertically mounted pen at its end. The rod is attached to the subject by a firm belt and extends posteriorly. As the subject attempts to stand as still as possible for 30 seconds, the pen records the subject's sway on a sheet of millimetre graph paper fastened to the top of an adjustable-height table. Testing is performed, with eyes open and closed, on a firm surface and on a medium-density foam rubber mat (15 cm thick). Total sway (number of square millimetre squares traversed by the pen) and antero-posterior and medio-lateral sway are recorded for the four tests.
Maximal balance range	In the maximal balance range test subjects are asked to lean forward from the ankles without moving the feet, as far as possible, i.e. to the point where they can just retain balance. Subjects are then asked to lean back as far as possible. In this test the sway-meter is attached to the subject at waist level with the rod extending anteriorly. A pen attached to the end of the rod records the anterior and posterior movements of the pen on a sheet of graph paper that is fastened to the top of an adjustable-height table. The subject, who can see the pen, has three attempts at the test. The score recorded is the maximal anterio-posterior excursion of the pen recorded during the three trials.

Table 16.1 (*cont.*)

Test	Test Description
Coordinated stability	As with the maximal balance range test, the sway-meter is attached to the subject at waist level with the rod extending anteriorly. The subject is then asked to adjust balance by bending or rotating the body without moving the feet, so that the pen on the end of the rod follows and remains within a convoluted track that is marked on a sheet of paper attached to the top of an adjustable-height table. To complete the test without errors, the pen has to remain within the track, which is 1.5 cm wide, and adjust the position of the pen 29 cm laterally and 18 cm in the anterio-posterior plane. A total error score is calculated by summing the number of occasions the pen on the sway-meter fails to stay within the path. Where subjects fail to negotiate an outside corner (because they cannot adjust their centre of gravity sufficiently), five error points are accrued. Subjects attempt the test twice, with the better trial taken as the test result.

discriminant function analysis using the data from the population studies [19–21] The falls risk score is comprised of weighted scores of independent risk factors (i.e. visual contrast sensitivity, lower-extremity proprioception, knee extension strength, reaction time and sway on the foam rubber mat). The graph presents the falls risk score in relation to age and categorizes falls risk into grades ranging from very low to very marked.

Figure 16.8 shows the subject's test performance profile graph. This graph presents the test results in standardized (*z*) scores form, again using the reference data from the population studies. Thus, a score of zero indicates average performance for people aged 60 years and over, positive scores indicate above-average performances, and negative scores indicate below-average performances. Each unit represents one standard deviation. Because the scores have been standardized, the test results can be compared with each other to determine relative performances.

Table 16.2 shows the subject's test scores presented in a tabular format to complement the test performance profile graph. For each individual, reference ranges for each test are provided for: (i) sex-matched young people without known pathology or impairments; and (ii) age- and sex-matched people.

Finally, the computer programme compiles a written report for each subject. An example is presented in Figure 16.9. It summarizes the findings, highlights below-average performances and makes individual recommendations for reducing the risk for falls. In a clinical setting, the reports can be produced immediately following the assessment. This allows the therapist and the patient to examine and discuss the results of the tests together and for the patient to take away the report as a record of the assessment.

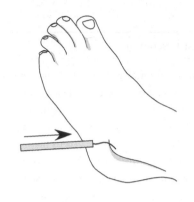

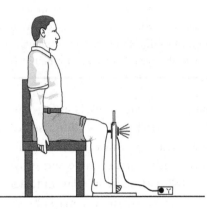

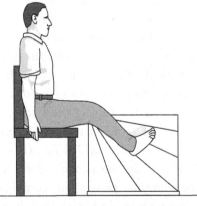

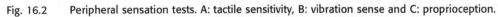

Fig. 16.2   Peripheral sensation tests. A: tactile sensitivity, B: vibration sense and C: proprioception.

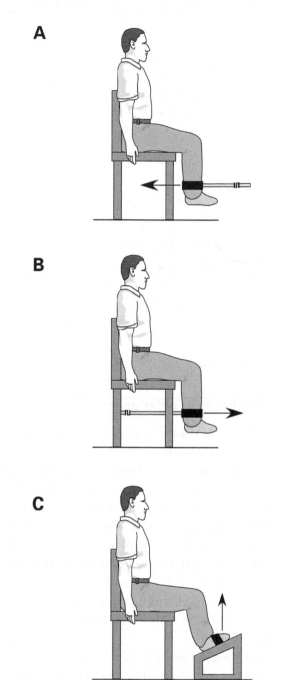

Fig. 16.3   Muscle strength tests. A: knee flexion, B: knee extension and C: ankle dorsiflexion.

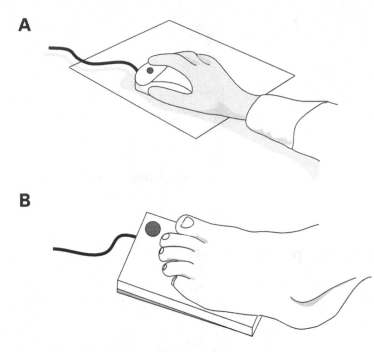

Fig. 16.4   Reaction time tests. A: hand, B: foot.

The PPA as a predictor of falls in older people

We have conducted a series of studies to evaluate the ability of the PPA tests to discriminate between elderly fallers and non-fallers [19–22, 29–31]. In a one-year prospective study of 95 residents at an intermediate care hostel, aged 59 to 97 years, the PPA measurements were used to correctly classify subjects into a multiple falls group (two or more falls) or a non-multiple falls group (no falls or one fall) with an accuracy of 79% [19]. This categorization of falls status was used because it has frequently been found that multiple falls within a year are more likely to indicate physiological impairments and chronic conditions than does a single fall [3, 15]. In a subsequent study of intermediate care residents we found that the discrimination between faller and non-faller groups could be increased to 86% with the addition of a validated assessment of cognitive functioning [29].

The PPA also has good predictive ability in community-dwelling populations. In a one-year prospective study involving 414 community-dwelling women aged 65 to 99 years, the PPA measurements correctly classified subjects into a multiple falls group or a non-multiple falls group with 75% accuracy [20]. The largest study using the PPA was a cross-sectional investigation of 1762 community-dwelling people aged 60 to 100 years. Subjects with a history of falls

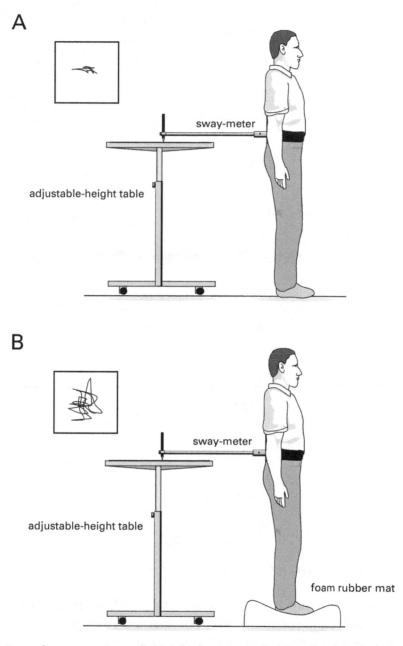

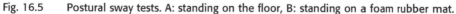

Fig. 16.5   Postural sway tests. A: standing on the floor, B: standing on a foam rubber mat.

exhibited reduced knee extension strength, poorer tactile sensitivity and greater sway (independently of age) than those without a history of falls [21]. The PPA test measures have also been found to discriminate between older community-dwelling people with and without a history of injurious falls [30].

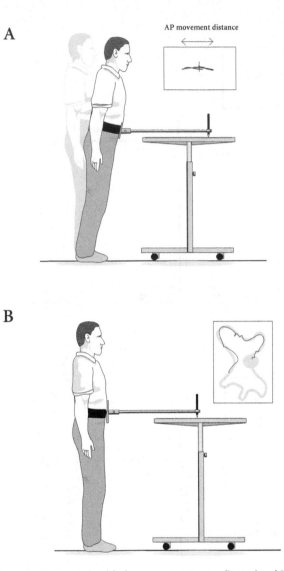

Fig. 16.6   Leaning balance tests. A: maximal balance range, B: coordinated stability.

In recent studies, we have enhanced the PPA by adding additional measures of vision (depth perception) [22] and leaning balance [31] to the assessment to include these complementary physiological domains.

Examples of the PPA in clinical groups

We have used the PPA in studies of clinical groups who have an increased risk of falling, including people with diabetes mellitus [32], lower limb osteoarthritis

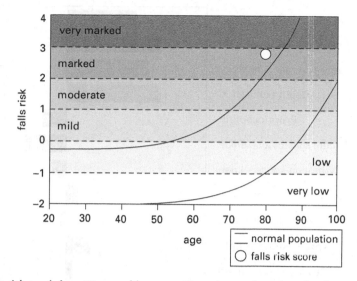

Fig. 16.7   Falls risk graph for a 79-year-old woman. Normal range based on data for a randomly selected sample of 2312 community-dwelling people aged 20 to 99 years.

[9] and a history of poliomyelitis [33]. Figures 16.10, 16.11, 16.12, 16.13 and 16.14, respectively show typical examples of the z-score output for: a young person (age 27 years) without known pathology or impairments; a person with age-related macular degeneration (age 82 years); a person with diabetes mellitus (age 67 years); a person with lower limb osteoarthritis (age 76 years); and a person with a history of poliomyelitis (age 51 years).

As expected, the older person with macular degeneration performed poorly in each of the visual tests. She also demonstrated impaired balance, particularly in the postural sway test with eyes open on the foam rubber mat. Our research group has previously found that although vision is not critical for the maintenance of stability when standing on a firm surface, standing on a compliant surface relies more strongly on visual input because proprioceptive input from the feet and ankles is reduced [18, 26, 34]. In this situation, visual acuity and stereopsis play an important role in stabilizing balance [34]. This finding indicates that people with macular degeneration are at risk for falling, not only because of a reduced ability to perceive hazards in the environment but also because of impaired balance. Older people with this condition are likely to be at particular risk when standing or walking in challenging environmental conditions, such as on uneven or compliant surfaces.

The older person with diabetes mellitus scored poorly on tests of peripheral sensation, which reflects the presence of diabetic peripheral neuropathy. This finding is consistent with the results from a previous study conducted by our group [32] comparing 25 people with diabetes mellitus with 40 age-matched

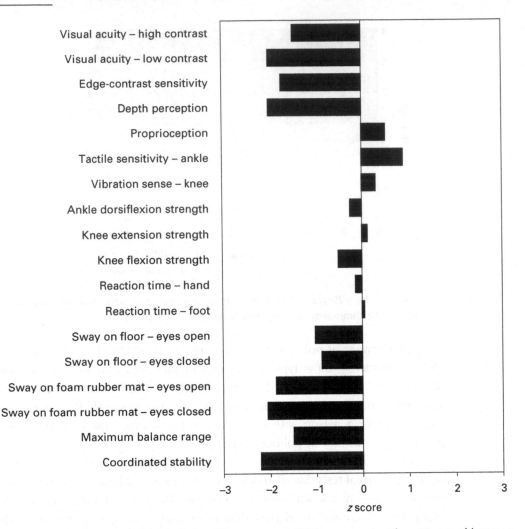

Fig. 16.8   Comprehensive Physiological Profile Assessment (PPA) z-score output for a 79-year-old woman.

control subjects. Despite exhibiting above-average lower-extremity muscle strength, this subject performed poorly on the postural sway tests, most notably (in relative terms) in the unchallenged standing on floor conditions. This finding is consistent with research showing that peripheral sensation is the most important contributor to postural stability in quiet standing [18, 26] and provides insight into why patients with diabetes have an increased risk for falls [13].

The older person with lower-limb osteoarthritis scored poorly on tests of knee and ankle muscle strength, lower-limb proprioception, postural sway and leaning balance, but was comparable to aged-matched peers without arthritis in the tests of vision, tactile sensitivity and reaction time. This finding is consistent

Table 16.2 Table of individual test performance for a 79-year-old woman in relation to reference ranges for: (i) sex-matched young subjects without known pathology or impairments; and (ii) age- and sex-matched subjects

Test	Score	Young normal	Age-matched[a]
Vision			
Visual acuity – high contrast (mar)	2.5[b]	0.54–0.82	0.83–1.58
Visual acuity – low contrast (mar)	6[b]	0.76–1.05	1.32–2.65
Edge-contrast sensitivity (dB)	13[b]	23–24	20–24
Depth perception (cm error)	5.2	0.0–2.0	0.8–8.3
Sensation			
Tactile sensitivity – ankle ($\log_{10}$ 0.1 mg)	3.7	3.22–4.08	3.61–4.31
Vibration sense – knee (microns)	15.5	2–5	7–34
Proprioception (degrees error)	1	0.2–1.4	0.4–2.4
Muscle strength			
Ankle dorsiflexion (kg)	7	10–15	6–10.5
Knee extension (kg)	21	35–58	15–29
Knee flexion (kg)	10	22–29	7–34
Reaction time			
Hand (ms)	251	182–236	197–267
Foot (ms)	278	213–273	230–305
Balance			
Sway on floor – eyes open (mm)	120[b]	35–70	40–100
Sway on floor – eyes closed (mm)	158	55–95	50–160
Sway on foam rubber mat – eyes open (mm)	286[b]	60–110	65–163
Sway on foam rubber mat – eyes closed (mm)	581[b]	70–185	108–285
Maximal balance range (mm)	140	198–252	132–198
Coordinated stability (errors)	15[b]	0–3	1–12

[a] Women aged 75–79 years
[b] Worse than average age-matched
    mar = minimum angle resolvable

with the results from a study by our group comparing 283 older people with lower-limb arthritis with 401 age-matched control subjects [9]. The arthritis groups suffered significantly more falls and falls injuries than the non-arthritis group in this study.

The person with a history of poliomyelitis performed poorly on the tests of lower-extremity strength, proprioception and postural sway on a foam rubber mat, but exhibited above-average vision and average tactile sensation and vibration sense. A case-control study of 40 people with a history of poliomyelitis

21st June, 2005

Mrs Jane Smith
1 Australia St
Sydney, New South Wales 2000

Dear Mrs Smith,

Please find attached the report regarding your falls risk assessment at the Prince of Wales Medical Research Institute on 21st June 2005. These test results indicate that you have an increased risk of falling.

You performed well in the important tests of visual field dependence, proprioception and tactile sensitivity. In some areas, however, you were below average for your age group, so the following recommendations may be of help to you.

One or more of your vision tests were below average. Reduced vision can increase the risk of a trip over an unseen object in the environment such as steps, gutters and footpath cracks and raised edges. It is recommended that you see an eye specialist for an assessment if you have not done so in the past year. You may also benefit from wearing a single lens pair of glasses, especially when outside. It is recommended that you do not wear bifocal or multifocal spectacles, as the lower sections of these spectacles blur items at critical distances on the ground and this can lead to trips. Wearing a hat outside also improves vision by reducing glare substantially.

Your sway scores were high indicating reduced balance control. There are certain situations where you should take particular care: when walking on soft or uneven surfaces such as thick carpets and soft or rough ground. You may also be at risk of losing balance in dim or unlit areas, so avoid such areas where possible and make sure you turn the light on before walking in the house at night. Exercises can improve strength, coordination and balance. It is recommended that you increase your current level of physical activity, with a program of planned walks 3 times a week and a complementary program of group or home-based exercises. However, you should be assessed by your general practitioner prior to undertaking any exercise program. The attached home exercises could benefit you in this area. Finally, it is recommended that you wear shoes with low heels and firm rubber soles. These are best for balance.

For inquiries regarding this report, please contact the Falls and Balance Research Group at the Prince of Wales Medical Research Institute on 9999-9999.

Yours sincerely,

Dr Anthony Jones

Fig. 16.9   Written report summarizing the physiological profile approach findings (NB the name Jane Smith is a pseudonym).

(aged 28 to 71 years) and 38 age-matched control subjects confirmed that people with a history of poliomyelitis represent a clinical group with lower-limb weakness, but in whom most other physiological factors associated with balance are similar to those in the general community [33]. Consistent with previous studies of older people [18, 26, 34], reduced muscle strength impairs standing balance when subjects stand on a compliant surface.

Use of the PPA in falls prevention trials

The individual PPA strength, speed and balance tests have been used to assess the effectiveness of falls prevention strategies [31, 35–38]. By including these measures in randomized controlled trials, it is possible to elucidate the

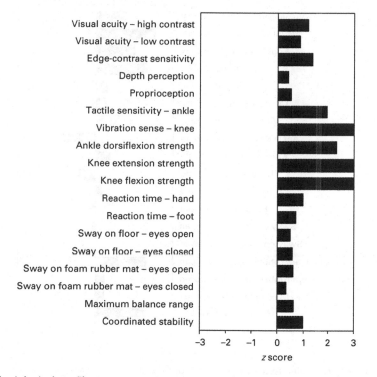

Fig. 16.10   Physiological Profile Assessment z-score output for a young adult (age 27 years), falls risk score = 0.87.

mechanisms by which interventions may prevent falls. The findings of the completed randomized controlled trials indicate that exercise programmes that improve balance in populations with strength and balance impairments are the most effective group exercise interventions for preventing falls [36, 37].

The PPA falls risk score has also been used as an outcome measure in randomized controlled trials [39, 40]. The first of these compared the effectiveness of group resistance and agility training programmes in reducing falls risk in community-dwelling older women with low bone mass. At the end of the 25-week trial, the PPA falls risk scores were reduced by 57% and 48% in the resistance and agility training groups, respectively, but by only 20% in a control group that undertook stretching exercises. In both the resistance and agility groups, the reduction in falls risk was mediated primarily by improved postural stability, where sway was reduced by 31% and 29% respectively. Based on the PPA normative data, these changes represented a reduction in the risk of falling over 12 months from over 80% to 50%–55%.

The second randomized controlled trial was conducted to determine whether tailored interventions, identified by the comprehensive PPA could reduce falls

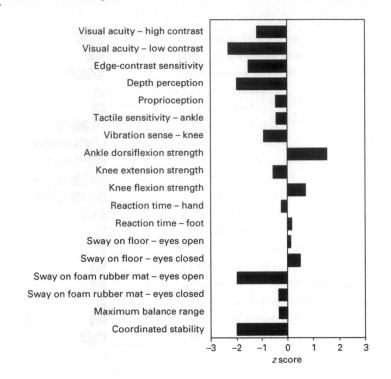

Fig. 16.11   Physiological Profile Assessment z-score output for person with macular degeneration (age 82 years), falls risk score = 1.55.

risk by maximising vision, muscle strength, coordination and balance in 620 community-dwelling people aged 75 years and over [40]. The participants underwent the PPA at baseline and at the mid-point of the trial. At retest, the subjects who undertook the exercise intervention showed significant improvements in knee flexion strength and sit-to-stand times compared to the controls. Similarly, subjects who underwent the visual interventions (referral to an eye care specialist) showed significant improvements in visual acuity and contrast sensitivity. Overall, PPA falls risk scores decreased significantly in the intervention group, but the interventions were not sufficiently targeted to those at increased risk of falls. The intervention appeared to have had the greatest effect (although still not significant) in those with PPA falls risk scores ≥ 2, i.e. in those with an increased risk of falls – relative risk = 0.76, 95% CI = 0.53–1.09.

Use of the PPA in falls clinics

The PPA has now been incorporated into falls clinics. In one UK falls service, the PPA has been used in association with the Timed Up and Go Test (TUGT) to provide an evidence-based approach for assessment and management of older

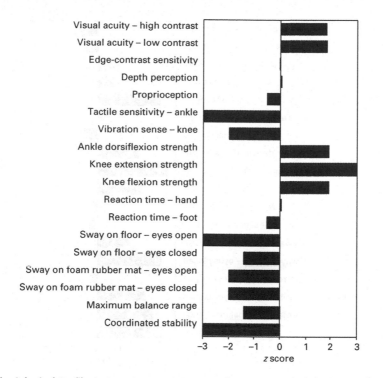

Fig. 16.12   Physiological Profile Assessment z-score output for person with diabetic peripheral neuropathy (age 67 years), falls risk score = 1.55.

people at risk of falls related predominantly to postural instability [41]. Initially the TUGT [42] is used as a screening test to identify those at increased risk of falling (i.e. those who take more than 15 seconds to complete the test). The screening version PPA is then administered to quantify the risk and provide direction for tailored intervention. The Otago strength and balance training programme is prescribed for those with impairments in knee extension strength, reaction time and/or postural sway [43]. A vision management plan encompassing correction of refractive errors with prescription spectacles and cataract surgery, and limiting the use of multifocal and bifocal spectacles [44], is put in place for those with impaired contrast sensitivity. Information regarding how reduced lower limb proprioception can impair balance is given to those with proprioceptive loss. This advice includes recommendations regarding wearing shoes with low heels and firm rubber soles, and using a walking stick or cane to supplement sensory input [45, 46]. Investigation of the causes of peripheral neuropathy in this group is also undertaken. Six-month follow-up of patients with repeat PPA testing has shown statistically significant improvements in an overall PPA score as well as those of strength, balance and reaction time [41].

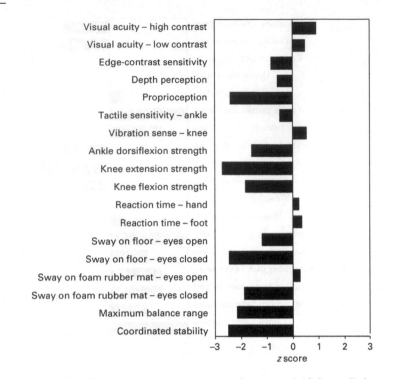

Fig. 16.13   Physiological Profile Assessment z-score output for person with lower-limb osteoarthritis (age 76 years), falls risk score = 1.50.

Clinicians at another falls clinic based in an acute hospital in Sydney have evaluated their interventions using the PPA [47]. A total of 142 patients were assessed with the screening version PPA at initial assessment. They then received medical care and recommendations for home based exercise, visual examinations, appropriate footwear and gait aids, based on the assessment and PPA scores. The overall compliance rate for adopting the interventions was 72%. At a four-month follow-up assessment, there were significant improvements in quadriceps strength, reaction time, postural sway and the overall falls risk score. Falls rate in the period following the initial clinic visit (0.16 falls per patient-month) was significantly lower than in the 12 months prior to the clinic visit (0.32 falls per patient-month) – relative risk = 0.52, 95% CI = 0.33–0.71.

Due to the inherent limitations of service evaluations with regard to the necessity of providing optimal care for all patients, with consequent lack of outcome assessment blinding and controls, these findings cannot be compared to those reported by randomized controlled trials. However, unlike most randomized controlled trials, they represent real-life service settings, and the evidence to date suggests that the PPA is a clinically useful and feasible tool for assessment and evaluation of targeted interventions.

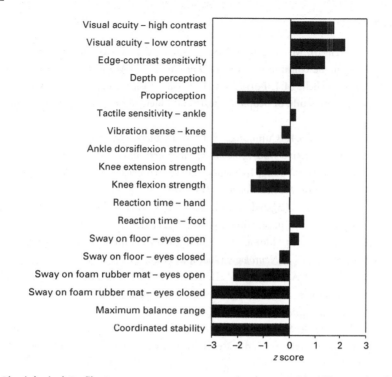

Fig. 16.14 Physiological Profile Assessment z-score output for person with a history of poliomyelitis (age 51 years), falls risk score = 1.75.

Conclusion

The Cochrane systematic review of interventions used to prevent falls in older people, concluded that protection against falling may be maximized by interventions that target multiple risk factors in individual patients. Also, that healthcare providers should consider screening of older people who are at risk for falls, followed by targeted interventions for deficit areas [48]. The PPA fulfils these criteria by using validated assessments and normative data from large scale studies to identify key physiological risk factors (impairments) that can be targeted with interventions.

A major strength of the PPA is that it uses a function-based and quantitative model, and thus provides a useful tool for falls risk factor identification and the evaluation of interventions aimed at maximizing physical functioning. We acknowledge that there are falls risk factors not measured by the PPA, including psychological factors, adverse effects of medications and postural effects of certain medical conditions, particularly cardiovascular disorders. Therefore, the PPA should be viewed as being able to complement and guide in the multidisciplinary assessment and management of older people who fall.

REFERENCES

1. M. E. Tinetti, M. Speechley & S. F. Ginter, Risk factors for falls among elderly persons living in the community. *New England Journal of Medicine*, **319** (1988), 1701–7.

2. A. J. Campbell, M. J. Borrie & G. F. Spears, Risk factors for falls in a community-based prospective study of people 70 years and older. *Journal of Gerontology*, **44** (1989), M112–17.

3. M. C. Nevitt, S. R. Cummings, S. Kidd, D. Black, Risk factors for recurrent nonsyncopal falls: a prospective study. *Journal of the American Geriatrics Society*, **261** (1989), 2663–8.

4. A. Forster & J. Young, Incidence and consequences of falls due to stroke: a systematic inquiry. *British Medical Journal*, **311** (1995), 83–6.

5. L. Jorgensen, T. Engstad & B. K. Jacobsen, Higher incidence of falls in long-term stroke survivors than in population controls. *Stroke*, **33** (2002), 542–7.

6. A. Schrag, Y. Ben-Shlomo & N. Quinn, How common are complications of Parkinson's disease? *Journal of Neurology*, (2002), 419–23.

7. B. H. Wood, J. A. Bilclough, A. Bowron & R. W. Walker, Incidence and prediction of falls in Parkinson's disease: a prospective multidisciplinary study. *Journal of Neurology, Neurosurgery and Psychiatry*, **72** (2002), 721–5.

8. A. Ashburn, E. Stack, R. M. Pickering & C. D. Ward, A community-dwelling sample of people with Parkinson's disease: characteristics of fallers and non-fallers. *Age and Ageing*, **30** (2001), 47–52.

9. D. Sturnieks, S. R. Lord, A. Tiedemann *et al.*, Physiological risk factors for falls in older people with lower limb arthritis. *Journal of Rheumatology*, **31** (2004), 2272–9.

10. H. B. Menz & S. R. Lord, The contribution of foot problems to mobility impairment and falls in community-dwelling older people. *Journal of the American Geriatrics Society*, **49** (2001), 1651–6.

11. P. T. M. van Dijk, O. G. R. M. Meulenberg, H. J. van del Sande & J. D. F. Habbema, Falls in dementia patients. *Gerontologist*, **33** (1993), 200–4.

12. F. E. Shaw, J. Bond, D. A. Richardson *et al.*, Multifactorial intervention after a fall in older people with cognitive impairment and dementia presenting to the accident and emergency department: randomised controlled trial. *British Medical Journal*, **326** (2003), 73–8.

13. J. Richardson, C. Ching & E. Hurvitz, The relationship between electromyographically documented peripheral neuropathy and falls. *Journal of the American Geriatrics Society*, **40** (1992), 1008–12.

14. A. V. Schwartz, T. A. Hillier, D. E. Sellmeyer *et al.*, Older women with diabetes have a higher risk of falls: a prospective study. *Diabetes Care*, **25** (2002), 1749–54.

15. R. Q. Ivers, R. G. Cumming, P. Mitchell *et al.*, Visual impairment and falls in older adults: the Blue Mountains Eye Study. *Journal of the American Geriatrics Society*, **46** (1998), 58–64.

16. S. L. Whitney, M. T. Hudak & G. F. Marchetti, The dynamic gait index relates to self-reported fall history in individuals with vestibular dysfunction. *Journal of Vestibular Research*, **10** (2000), 99–105.

17. S. J. Herdman, P. Blatt, M. C. Schubert & R. J. Tusa, Falls in patients with vestibular deficits. *American Journal of Otology*, **21** (2000), 847–51.

18. S. R. Lord & J. A. Ward, Age-associated differences in sensori-motor function and balance in community dwelling women. *Age and Ageing*, **23** (1994), 452–60.

19. S. R. Lord, R. D. Clark & I. W. Webster, Physiological factors associated with falls in an elderly population. *Journal of the American Geriatrics Society*, **39** (1991), 1194–200.

20. S. R. Lord, J. A. Ward, P. Williams & K. Anstey, Physiological factors associated with falls in older community-dwelling women. *Journal of the American Geriatrics Society*, **42** (1994), 1110–17.

21. S. R. Lord, P. N. Sambrook, C. Gilbert *et al.*, Postural stability, falls and fractures in the elderly: results from the Dubbo Osteoporosis Epidemiology Study. *Medical Journal of Australia*, **160** (1994), 684–5, 688–91.

22. S. R. Lord & J. Dayhew, Visual risk factors for falls in older people. *Journal of the American Geriatrics Society*, **49** (2001), 676–7.

23. S. R. Lord, H. B. Menz & A. Tiedemann, A physiological profile approach to falls risk assessment and prevention. *Physical Therapy*, **83** (2003), 237–252.

24. J. Kosoy, The oto-neurologic examination. *Acta Otolaryngologica*, **S343** (1977), 1–95.

25. T. Fukuda, The stepping test: two phases of the labyrinthine reflex. *Acta Otolaryngologica*, **50** (1959), 95–108.

26. S. R. Lord, R. D. Clark & I. W. Webster, Postural stability and associated physiological factors in a population of aged persons. *Journal of Gerontology*, **46** (1991), M69–76.

27. J. H. Verbaken & A. W. Johnston, Population norms for edge contrast sensitivity. *American Journal of Optometry and Physiological Optics*, **63** (1986), 724–732.

28. C. H. Graham, Visual space perception. In *Vision and Visual Perception*, ed. C. H. Graham (New York: John Wiley and Sons Inc., 1965), pp. 504–47.

29. S. R. Lord & R. D. Clark, Simple physiological and clinical tests for the accurate prediction of falling in older people. *Gerontology*, **42** (1996), 199–203.

30. S. R. Lord, D. McLean & G. Stathers, Physiological factors associated with injurious falls in older people living in the community. *Gerontology*, **38** (1992), 338–46.

31. S. R. Lord, J. A. Ward & P. Williams, The effect of exercise on dynamic stability in older women: a randomized controlled trial. *Archives of Physical Medicine and Rehabilitation*, **77** (1996), 232–6.

32. S. R. Lord, G. A. Caplan, R. Colagiuri *et al.*, Sensori-motor function in older persons with diabetes. *Diabetic Medicine*, **10** (1993), 614–18.

33. S. R. Lord, G. M. Allen, P. Williams & S. C. Gandevia, Risk of falling: predictors based on reduced strength in persons previously affected by polio. *Archives of Physical Medicine and Rehabilitation*, **83** (2001), 907–11.

34. S. R. Lord & H. B. Menz, Visual contributions to postural stability in older adults. *Gerontology*, **46** (2000), 306–10.

35. S. R. Lord, J. A. Ward, P. Williams & M. Strudwick, The effect of a 12-month exercise program on balance, strength, and falls in older women: a randomized controlled trial. *Journal of the American Geriatrics Society*, **43** (1995), 1198–206.

36. L. Day, B. Fildes, I. Gordon *et al.*, A randomised factorial trial of falls prevention among community-dwelling older people. *British Medical Journal*, **325** (2002), 128–31.

37. A. Barnett, B. Smith, S. R. Lord *et al.*, Community-based group exercise improves balance and reduces falls in at-risk older people: a randomised controlled trial. *Age and Ageing*, **32** (2003), 407–14.

38. S. R. Lord, S. Castell, J. Corcoran *et al.*, The effect of group exercise on physical functioning and falls in frail older people living in retirement villages: a randomised controlled trial. *Journal of the American Geriatrics Society*, **51** (2003), 1685–92.

39. T. Liu-Ambrose, K. M. Khan, J. J. Eng *et al.*, Both resistance and agility training reduce fall risk in 75–85 year old women with low bone mass: a six-month randomized controlled trial. *Journal of the American Geriatrics Society*, **52** (2004), 657–65.

40. S. R. Lord, A. Tiedemann, K. Chapman *et al.*, The effect of a tailored falls prevention program on fall risk and falls in older people: a randomised controlled trial. *Journal of the American Geriatrics Society*, **53** (2005), 1296–304.

41. J. C. Whitney, S. R. Lord & J. C. T. Close, Streamlining assessment and intervention in a falls clinic using the timed up and go and physiological profile assessments. *Age and Ageing*, **34** (2005), 567–71.

42. D. Podsiadlo & S. Richardson, The timed "up and go" a test of basic functional mobility for frail elderly persons. *Journal of the American Geriatrics Society*, **39** (1991), 142–8.

43. A. J. Campbell, M. C. Robertson, M. M. Gardner *et al.*, Randomised controlled trial of a general practice programme of home based exercise to prevent falls in elderly women. *British Medical Journal*, **315** (1997), 1065–9.

44. S. R. Lord, J. Dayhew & A. Howland, Multifocal glasses impair edge contrast sensitivity and depth perception and increase the risk of falls in older people. *Journal of the American Geriatrics Society*, **50** (2002), 1760–6.

45. J. J. Jeka, Light touch contact as a balance aid. *Physical Therapy*, **77** (1997), 476–87.

46. M. W. Rogers, D. L. Wardman, S. R. Lord & R. Fitzpatrick, Passive tactile input improves stability during standing. *Experimental Brain Research*, **136** (2001), 514–22.

47. T. Murrant, M. J. Haran, R. A. Carroll *et al.*, Experience from an outpatient multidisciplinary falls prevention clinic for older people. Manuscript in preparation.

48. L. D. Gillespie, W. J. Gillespie, M. C. Robertson *et al.*, Interventions for preventing falls in elderly people. *Cochrane Database of Systematic Reviews*, (4) (2003), CD000340.

17

Research into practice

Over the past decade, some 50 randomized controlled trials for the prevention of falls in older people have been published. These have built on epidemiological and risk factor studies from the last 30–40 years, and provide strong evidence that falls can be prevented. Despite remaining gaps in the literature, the published research findings can be used to guide the development and delivery of clinical services to prevent falls in older people.

However, one of the challenges for those implementing falls prevention services is how to interpret the findings from research publications that have studied diverse populations of older people and have employed a multiplicity of interventions. Further, older people who present to healthcare systems are often not representative of populations studied in research settings. Unlike specific diseases such as osteoporosis, for which there is a clear definition, an agreed diagnostic gold standard and a limited range of treatment options, falls present more difficult diagnostic and therapeutic dilemmas. The previous chapters have identified and discussed falls risk factors and have considered the evidence on a range of approaches to prevention. This chapter synthesizes this evidence and collates the information in a format that can be used to facilitate the translation of research findings into routine clinical practice.

Screening versus assessment

As yet there is no firm data to support a population-based approach to the prevention of falls, and as such there is a need to identify appropriate populations in order to effectively target interventions and resources. Screening permits the identification of high-risk populations based on known risk factors but does not necessarily provide sufficient information to allow for the tailoring of intervention. Age and history of falls are both good indicators of a high-risk population but neither risk factor is modifiable. The Timed Up and Go Test represents a validated screening tool used to identify at risk fallers, but the tool in itself does not give detailed information as to the underlying deficits contributing to overall risk. Assessment tools on the other hand should provide detailed information on the underlying deficits contributing to overall risk, and should be linked to intervention and/or evaluation. The Physiological Profile Assessment represents a validated risk assessment tool which can be easily linked to evidence-based approaches to intervention.

What intervention and in which population?

There is no single all-encompassing approach to the prevention of falls in older people. This is particularly true of community-dwelling populations where there is marked heterogeneity in physical and cognitive abilities. The challenge remains both to identify at-risk populations, and design appropriate interventions which are likely to prevent falls and fall-related injury.

Table 17.1. Successful prevention strategies by populations identified and type of intervention

Community dwelling populations	Emergency Department attendees
Single Interventions	*Single Interventions*
Wolf, 1996 [1]	Kenny, 2001 [18]
Campbell, 1999 [3]	
Campbell, 1997 [4]	*Multifaceted Interventions*
Buchner, 1997 [29]	Close, 1999 [19]
Cumming , 1999 [5]	Davison, 2005 [20]
Barnett, 2003 [2]	
Lord, 2003 [8]	**Hospital In-patients**
Robertson, 2001 [9]	*Single Interventions*-Nil
Means, 2005 [10]	*Multifaceted Interventions*
Harwood, 2005 [6]	Haines, 2004 [25]
Li, 2005 [7]	Healey, 2004 [26]
Skelton, 2005 [30]	
Campbell, 2005 [17]	**Care Home Residents**
	Single Interventions-Nil
Multifaceted Interventions	*Multifaceted Interventions*
Tinetti, 1994 [15]	Ray, 1997 [23]
Hornbrook, 1994 [13]	Jensen, 2002 [22]
Day, 2002 [12]	Becker, 2003 [21]
Clemson, 2004 [11]	
Nikolaus, 2003 [14]	
Wagner, 1994 [16]	

Table 17.1 highlights the existing literature of successful randomized controlled trials, categorizes studies by place of residence/presentation of participants and shows whether the intervention was single or multi-faceted in nature. Both single and multi-faceted approaches to prevention have been shown to be effective in community-dwelling populations, whereas prevention in residential care homes and hospitals has only been successful when a multi-faceted approach has been taken. This suggests that caution is required in extrapolating research findings from one population and/or setting to another.

Community-based populations

Much of the research evidence relates to community-dwelling populations, and as indicated, both single [1–10] and multi-faceted [11–16] approaches to prevention have been shown to be effective. The majority of older people live in their own homes and this population has the greatest heterogeneity. This is reflected in falls prevention studies conducted to date which have included study samples ranging from representative samples of older people recruited from the electoral roll [12] to high-risk individuals with predetermined risk factors [15]. Table 17.2 (a and b) summarizes the successful randomized controlled trials in community-dwelling populations.

Exercise is not necessarily an effective strategy for all populations. Campbell and colleagues did not show significant benefits of exercise in preventing falls in older people taking centrally acting medications or with severe visual impairment, but were able to show significant benefits from medication withdrawal [3] and occupational therapy home assessment [17] in these populations, respectively.

Multi-faceted approaches to care involve addressing more than one identified risk factor and may involve more than one professional. When more that one risk factor is addressed, it is difficult to identify which components of an intervention have been beneficial (or for that matter harmful). Trials with factorial designs can address this although they require a large number of subjects, particularly when directly comparing two interventions. Only a few studies have considered whether multiple approaches provide additive or multiplicative value to date [3, 12].

Tinetti *et al.*'s seminal study [15] in 1994 targeted the intervention to a community-dwelling population with predetermined risk factors and showed the benefits of tailored intervention. Most successful trials undertaken in the community since then have also targeted their interventions to older people at increased risk of falls, with only a few having shown benefits of interventions in relatively low risk, unselected populations [12, 13, 16].

Table 17.2a Summary of unifaceted successful interventions to prevent falls in community-dwelling older people

Population and numbers	Interventions and duration of follow-up	Author, year, country
Community dwellers recruited by local advertisement *Mean age 76.2 yrs* **N = 200**	I1: Tai Chi I2: conventional balance training C: education Intervention was for 15 weeks. Follow-up 7–20 months. **Results**: reduced risk of **multiple** falls in Tai Chi group using locally derived falls definition (risk ratio = 0.525, p = 0.01).	Wolf *et al.* 1996 [1] USA
Community-dwelling women aged 80+ from GP register *Mean age 84.1 yrs* **N = 233**	I: individually tailored programme of strength and balance training in the home. Four one hour sessions with a physiotherapist in the first two months of the study + 3×30 min walks per week. C: social visits Regular phone contact for both C and I group. One-year follow-up period **Results**: statistically significant reduction in mean number of falls between control and intervention group. Mean difference = 0.47 (95% CI = 0.04–0.9).	Campbell *et al.* 1997 [4] New Zealand
HMO enrolees with deficits in strength or balance *Mean age 75 yrs* **N = 105**	I: group-based strength and/or endurance training undertaken three times/week for six months then self-supervised exercise C: usual level of activity Physical measures reassessed at six months and diary cards for falls collected for up to 25 months post-randomization **Results**: no significant impact of exercise on the physical measures over the six month period of exercise. However, exercise reduced the risk of falling. Relative hazard = 0.53 (95% CI = 0.3–0.91).	Buchner *et al.* 1997 [29] USA
Community dwelling people discharged from hospital setting	I: occupational therapy home assessment targeted at environmental modifications and safety awareness in older people discharged from hospital (84%) or from outpatient or Day centre setting (16%)	Cumming *et al.* 1999 [5] Australia

Mean age 77 yrs N = **530**	C: usual care One-year follow-up period using monthly falls diary ***Results***: significant reduction in falls only for those people with at least one or more falls in the year prior to recruitment (relative risk = 0.64, 95% CI = 0.50–0.83). Equally effective for falls reduction in the home and outside.	Campbell *et al.* 1999 [3] New Zealand
Community dwelling people on centrally acting medications from GP registers Mean age 74.7 yrs N = **93**	2×2 factorial design. I1: gradual withdrawal of psychotropic medication I2: home based exercise programme, I3: Both C: usual care 44-week follow-up with monthly falls diary ***Results***: significant reduction in risk of falling for those in the medication withdrawal groups – relative hazard = 0.34 (95% CI = 0.16–0.74). No significant benefit from exercise in this population. Note the low recruitment rates (19%) for this trial and the fact that 47% of those in the medication withdrawal programme went back on their medications after completion of the study.	
Community population aged 75+ From GP register Mean age 80.9 yrs N = **240**	I: district nurse delivery of strength and balance training programme C: usual care One-year follow-up period with monthly falls diary ***Results***: significant reduction in the number of falls in the intervention group – indicate rate ratio = 0.54 (95% CI = 0.32–0.9).	Robertson *et al.* 2001 [9] New Zealand
Retirement village residents Mean age 79.5 yrs N = **551**	I:12 month group-based weight-bearing exercises designed to improve activities of daily living C: flexibility and relaxation groups One-year follow-up using monthly questionnaires ***Results***: significant reduction in number of falls in the intervention group – incidence rate ratio = 0.78 (95% CI = 0.62–0.99).	Lord *et al.* 2003 [8] Australia

Table 17.2a (*cont.*)

Population and numbers	Interventions and duration of follow-up	Author, year, country
Community-dwelling older people identified as at risk of falling using a standardized assessment screen *Mean age 74.9 yrs* **N = 163**	I: weekly exercise group – total of 37 classes + information on how to avoid falls C: information on how to avoid falls One-year follow-up with monthly postal surveys ***Results***: significant reduction in rate of falls in the intervention group – incidence rate ratio = 0.6 (95% CI = 0.36–0.99).	Barnett *et al.* 2003 [2] Australia
Community-dwelling older people attending 'senior citizen centres' *Mean age 73.5 yrs* **N = 338**	I: six weeks of supervised stretching, balance, endurance, coordination and strengthening exercises C: attended seminars for same period Six-month follow-up with weekly falls postcards completed ***Results***: main outcome was improvement on functional obstacle course. Significant difference in falls rate between control and intervention group at baseline. Some measures of falls outcome showed significant improvement in the intervention group during the follow-up period (22 fallers among the exercise group (15%) and 36 fallers in the control group (38%)).	Means *et al.* 2005 [10] USA
Women aged 70+ referred for cataract surgery *Mean age ~ 78 yrs* **N = 306**	I: expedited cataract surgery (four weeks after listing for surgery) C: routine surgery (average wait of 12 months after listing for surgery) One-year follow-up ***Results***: significant reduction in rate of falling in the intervention group – incidence rate ratio = 0.66 (95% CI = 0.45–0.96) but not in the number of people who fell. Statistically significant reduction in number of fractures in the intervention group 12 vs. 8 ($p = 0.04$).	Harwood *et al.* 2005 [6] UK
Community-dwelling men and women with significant visual impairment (6/24 or worse)	Factorial design I1: home safety assessment and modification programme I2: home based exercise programme +vitamin D I3: both	Campbell *et al.* 2005 [17] New Zealand

Mean age 83.6 yrs

N = **391**

C: social visits

One-year follow-up with monthly falls diary

Results: falls reduced by home safety programme – incidence rate ratio = 0.59 (95% CI = 0.42–0.83) but not by the exercise programme – incidence rate ratio = 15 (95% CI = 0.82–1.61).

Li *et al.* 2005 [7]

USA

Patient database of community-dwelling men and women aged 70+ with low levels of reported physical activity

Mean age 77.5 yrs

N = **256**

I: Tai Chi class 3×/week for 26 weeks

C: stretching 3×/week for 26 weeks

Follow-up at three, six and 12 months

Results: statistically significant difference in falls seen at the end of the six month exercise programme (38 falls in intervention group and 73 in control group, *p* = 0.007), and sustained for the six-month post-intervention follow-up. Differences in falls rate seen from approximately three months into the exercise programme.

Skelton *et al.* 2005 [30]

UK

Community-dwelling women aged 65+ with a history of three or more falls in the previous year

Mean age 72.8 yrs

N = **81**

I: weekly group-based class (individualized and tailored) + weekly home exercise

C: twice weekly home based seated exercise for 36 weeks

50-week follow-up from end of 36 week intervention with fortnightly falls diaries

Results: significant reduction in number of falls in the intervention group in the follow-up period (incident rate ratio = 0.69, 95% CI = 0.50–0.96). (Analysis not done on an intention to treat basis.)

I = Intervention, C = Control

Table 17.2b Summary of multi-faceted successful interventions to prevent falls in community-dwelling older people

Population and numbers	Interventions and duration of follow-up	Author, year, country
Community-dwelling population aged 70+ with a predetermined risk factor for falling *Mean age ~ 78 yrs* **N = 301**	I: nurse led protocol driven assessment with targeted recommendations and physiotherapy led gait and transfer training and strength and balance exercise twice a day for approximately three months C: home visits from social work students who conducted structured interviews 12-month follow-up with monthly diary **Results**: significant reduction in number of falls in the intervention group – incidence rate ratio = 0.64 (95% CI = 0.49–0.83). Also a statistically significant difference in risk factor profile between the control and intervention group at the end of the follow-up period.	Tinetti *et al.* 1994 [15] USA
Community dwellers from HMO *Mean age 73 yrs* **N = 3182**	Both groups had home assessment and falls safety hazards check I: remove/repair safety hazards and access to falls information groups including group exercise C: no repair advice or help and no group sessions 23 month follow-up period **Results**: significant reduction on chances of being a faller ($p < 0.05$). Some 6.6% fewer falls in the intervention group which was not statistically significant.	Hornbrook *et al.* 1994 [13] USA

Day et al. 2002 [12]
Australia

Community dwellers identified from electoral role
Mean age 76.1 yrs
N = 1107

Factorial design
I1: group exercise
I2: home hazard management
I3: vision management
Interventions were based on a combination of one or more of the above
C: none of above interventions
18-month follow-up period
Results: incidence rate ratio for exercise was 0.82 (95% CI = 0.7–0.97) Significant benefit seen in all combinations which included exercise. Neither home hazard management or visual interventions had any significant impact on their own. Maximum reduction in falls seen in group receiving all three intervention – incidence rate ratio = 0.67 (95% CI = 0.51–0.88).

Nikolaus, 2003 [14]
Germany

Community-dwelling population admitted to hospital and showing evidence of functional decline
Mean age 81.5 yrs
N = 360

I: comprehensive geriatric assessment and multidisciplinary diagnostic intervention in person's own home.
C: comprehensive geriatric assessment + recommendations and usual care
One year follow-up with monthly telephone contact to collect falls information
Results: statistically significant reduction in falls in the intervention group – incidence rate ratio = 0.69 (95% CI = 0.51–0.97) Intervention was most effective in those with a history of two or more falls in the previous year.

Table 17.2b (cont.)

Population and numbers	Interventions and duration of follow-up	Author, year, country
Random sample of community-dwelling HMO enrolees *Mean age 72 yrs* **N = 1559**	I1: 60–90 min nurse assessment and tailored intervention targeting risk factors for falls I2: general health promotion nurse visit C: usual care Two-year follow-up period ***Results***: significant difference in number of people falling between the targeted assessment group and the control after one year and this difference disappeared at two years. No difference in overall fall rates between the three groups.	*Wagner et al.* 1994 [16] USA
Community dwelling older people with a history of a fall in the last year or who considered themselves to be at risk *Mean age 78 yrs* **N = 310**	I: 'Stepping on' – multi-faceted group-based approach, including education, behaviour modification, strength and balance training, and occupational therapy home assessment. Two hour sessions conducted weekly for seven weeks. C: social visits 14-month follow-up period ***Results***: significant reduction in falls in the intervention group – relative risk = 0.69 (95% CI = 0.5–0.96). Subgroup analysis showed that approach was most effective in men – relative risk = 0.32 (95% CI = 0.17–0.59).	*Clemson et al.* 2004 [11] Australia

I = Intervention, C = Control.

Emergency department attendees

Although the emergency department does not represent a place of residence, it offers a defined point of access to healthcare which serves high-risk populations in terms of falls and fracture risk. Emergency department presentation is therefore a useful means for identifying at-risk populations that does not require significant resources in terms of funding and personnel. Trials involving older people presenting to the emergency department [18–20] have predominantly recruited community-dwelling older people. The successful trials involve specialist input, including access to detailed cardiovascular assessment for unexplained falls, dizziness and syncope. Table 17.3 summarizes these studies.

Residential and aged care facilities

Nursing home residents comprise the frailer end of the spectrum of older people with most having physical and/or cognitive deficits precluding independent living. As with emergency department attendees, these people represent an at-risk population for falls and fractures. Single intervention approaches for the prevention of falls have not been effective in nursing home residents. In contrast, four trials taking a multi-faceted and multiprofessional approach to prevention have been successful in this setting [21–24]. All four studies included staff education and environmental modifications. Two trials included medication review, two included provision of hip protectors and two included exercise as components of intervention. In one of the trials [22], a sub-group analysis showed that those with higher cognitive abilities benefited from the intervention whereas those with cognitive impairment did not. Table 17.4 includes the successful studies conducted in nursing home settings.

Hospital inpatients

Two recent studies have provided evidence that falls can be prevented in hospital in-patients [25, 26]. These studies differed with respect to the populations studied and the interventions offered. Haines and colleagues [25] selected patients from a sub-acute hospital and focused on exercise and education. Healey and colleagues [26] selected patients from acute and sub-acute care settings with interventions focused around management of vision, medication use and postural hypotension identified with a health screening checklist. These interventions are summarized in Table 17.4.

Quality of the research and comparability

In weighing up the evidence for effective falls prevention strategies, discerning clinicians need to evaluate the quality of published studies, and whether they are

Table 17.3 Summary of successful interventions to prevent falls in community-dwelling older people presenting via the emergency department

Population and numbers	Interventions and duration of follow-up	Author, year, country
Community-dwelling people aged 65+ presenting to ED with a fall *Mean age 78.2 yrs* **N = 397**	I: comprehensive geriatric assessment and occupational therapy home assessment C: usual care One-year follow-up with monthly dairies ***Results***: significant reduction in number of falls and number of people falling in the intervention group – odds ratio = 0.39 (95% CI = 0.23–0.66).	Close *et al.* 1999 [19] UK
People presenting to ED with non-accidental fall *Mean age 73 yrs* **N = 175**	I: dual chamber pacing for unexplained falls and shown to have cardioinhibitory form of carotid sinus syndrome C: no pacemaker inserted One-year follow-up period ***Results***: significant reduction in number of falls in the intervention group – odds ratio = 0.42 (95% CI = 0.23–0.75). No statistically significant difference in number of syncopal events but overall numbers small.	Kenny *et al.* 2001 [18] UK
Cognitively intact people aged 65+ presenting to ED with a fall and a history of a previous fall in the 12 months prior to presentation *Mean age 77 yrs* **N = 313** (data analysed on 293)	I: comprehensive geriatric assessment (medicine, physiotherapy and occupational therapy) including detailed cardiovascular investigations and targeted intervention C: usual care One-year follow-up ***Results***: significantly fewer falls in the intervention group – relative risk = 0.64 (95% CI = 0.46–0.9) but no significant difference in number of fallers.	Davison *et al.* 2005 [20] UK

I = Intervention, C = Control, ED = emergency department.

comparable in terms of the quality of design, methodology and analysis, etc. Cochrane reviews assist in this regard by providing two independent assessments of methodological quality based on 11 predetermined criteria [27]. Falls prevention interventions have been subject to two Cochrane reviews and a third revision is underway. This systematic approach provides a valuable means of viewing

Table 17.4 Summary of multi-faceted successful interventions to prevent falls in care homes and hospital inpatients

Population and numbers	Interventions and duration of follow-up	Author, year, country
RCT of consultation service to reduce falls in nursing homes *Mean age 82 yrs* **N = 482**	I: structured individual assessment with advice on prescribing, environmental concerns, and transfer and mobility skills C: usual care One-year follow-up period *Results*: statistically significant reduction in number of recurrent falls in the intervention group (mean reduction of 19%). Those most likely to benefit were those with a history of recurrent falls and those in whom the recommendations were actioned.	Ray *et al.* 1997 [23] USA
Nursing home residents in Germany (6 homes) *Mean age 85 yrs* **N = 981**	I: staff and resident education, advice on environmental modifications, strength and balance training, and hip protectors C: usual care One-year follow-up period *Results*: significant reduction in falls rate – relative risk = 0.55 (95% CI = 0.41–0.73), number of fallers – relative risk = 0.75 (95% CI = 0.57–0.98) and number of frequent fallers – relative risk = 0.56 (95% CI = 0.35–0.89) in the intervention group.	Becker *et al.* 2003 [21] Germany
Residents in one of nine residential homes *Mean age 83 yrs* **N = 439**	I: 11-week multidisciplinary intervention – education, environmental modifications, exercise, medication review and hip protectors C: usual care 34-week follow-up period. MMSE of 19 was used to divide those with higher and lower levels of cognition. *Results*: significant benefit from the intervention in those with MMSE >19. Incidence rate ratio for people with MMSE >19 was 0.61 (95% CI = 0.48–0.78) and for MMSE <19 was 1.05 (95% CI = 0.84–1.30).	Jensen *et al.* 2002 [22] Sweden
Incontinent residents in four nursing homes	I: low-intensity functionally orientated exercise and continence care provided	Schnelle *et al.* 2003 [24] USA

Table 17.4 (*cont.*)

Population and numbers	Interventions and duration of follow-up	Author, year, country
Mean age 87.5 yrs N = 190	every 2 hours between the hours of 8 am and 4 pm for five days a week for a duration of eight months C: usual care *Results*: statistically significant difference seen in incidence rate of falls but this was due to an increase in falls seen in the control group as opposed to a significant decrease in falls in the intervention group (odds ratio = 0.46 ± 0.18).	
Inpatients on a mix of acute and rehabilitation settings in UK *Mean age 81 yrs* N = 1654	I: multifactorial intervention targeted at identified risk factors including vision, drugs, blood pressure, exercise and environmental modification C: usual care Six-month follow-up following introduction of the intervention *Results*: significant reduction in risk of falling in the intervention group – relative risk = 0.79 (95% CI = 0.65–0.95). No reduction seen in control group.	Healey *et al.* 2004 [26] UK
Inpatients on three sub-acute wards in Australia *Mean age 80 yrs* N = 626	I: multifactorial intervention targeted at identified risk factors, including education, physiotherapy, occupational therapy and use of hip protectors C: usual care Patients followed up until point of discharge or death *Results*: statistically significant reduction in number of falls in the intervention group (30% fewer falls) with maximum benefits seen after 45 days of follow-up. No significant difference in the number of people falling in the control and intervention group.	Haines *et al.* 2004 [25] Australia

I = Intervention, C = Control, RCT = randomized controlled trial.

meta-analysis summary data and directly comparing randomized controlled trial findings.

A complementary methodological framework for examining quality has been developed by the Centre for Evidence Based Physiotherapy at University of Sydney – PEDro (Physiotherapy Evidence Database) [28]. This is a free web-based database containing trials relevant to physiotherapy. As well as providing summaries of research findings, PEDro provides information on the quality of research papers based on the following quality indicators:

(1) Random allocation to groups
(2) Concealed allocation
(3) Comparability of groups at baseline
(4) Blinding of subjects
(5) Blinding of therapists administering the therapy
(6) Blinding of assessors who measure at least one key outcome
(7) Measures of at least one key outcome obtained from more than 85% of the subjects initially allocated to groups
(8) Intention to treat analysis
(9) The results of between-group statistical comparisons are reported for at least one key outcome
(10) The study provides both point measures and measures of variability for at least one key outcome

The limitation of PEDro in relation to the field of falls prevention is that it does not include findings of falls prevention trials which have not involved physiotherapy or exercise

Comparability of outcomes from falls prevention trials is remarkably difficult and an agreed international taxonomy would greatly enhance the objective assessment of differing approaches to intervention. A further criticism of the literature in falls prevention is the paucity of data on costs and cost-effectiveness of different approaches to intervention. In the context of limited healthcare resources, lack of comparative effectiveness and efficiency data is a significant obstacle to objective planning, and commissioning of falls prevention services.

Little attention has been paid to measuring the health and personal costs associated with functional changes resulting from falls during longitudinal studies. This is unfortunate, as this information could be used as an economic argument to justify investing resources in falls prevention services. Several studies have shown significant differences in the functional status between control and intervention groups at the end of the trials. It is likely that by preserving function, many of the successful trials have economic benefits that have not been measured, i.e. reduced use of both formal and informal care, delays in transfers to institutional care, etc. However, without attaching a cost to the consequences of different levels of functional ability, it is difficult to make a convincing financial argument to justify investment in services.

Patient-centred care and choice

One of the many challenges facing a modern health and social care system is to provide effective treatments for a range of conditions to a diverse population. Whilst this book focuses on the assessment and prevention of falls in older people, we should acknowledge that this may be one of several problems facing older people, and the challenge remains as to how to combine effective intervention strategies in such a way as to maximize adoption and acceptability. Discrete disease-based exercise programmes for specific conditions are common and may need to be reconsidered. People with several chronic diseases may be invited to participate in more than one exercise programme and may be given potentially conflicting information. Moving from a disease-specific model to one based on physiological deficits offers a more efficient and perhaps more acceptable approach to exercise that can still accommodate necessary disease-specific education. This will require a change in culture whereby we move from a model dictated by disease and departmental expertise to one that has interventions designed around and tailored to the overall needs of the older person.

A further sequela to the concept of person-centred care is the principle of choice. In keeping with a purist approach to research, the majority of clinical trials have offered interventions in a standardized and rigid format. This is particularly true of the exercise interventions where programmes have often been either home- or group-based. Whilst entirely appropriate in order to determine the effectiveness of an intervention, it does not reflect the more pragmatic approach required to translate care from the research setting to everyday practice. If we are to maximize the potential benefits of interventions to a large population we need to offer choice in how people take up an intervention. The basic components of the intervention do not need to be changed but the approach and setting may require modification. Some people will prefer to exercise in their own home whilst others may prefer the group setting. Some people will progress quicker than others and a rigid programme may not accommodate for this. These issues are now starting to be addressed in many aspects of chronic disease management. However, more research is required to develop our understanding as to what motivates older people to take up and adhere to interventions. Choice is likely to be an important determinant but there will be other barriers and motivators which as yet are poorly understood in the area of falls and injury prevention.

Conclusion

There is now little doubt that falls are not an inevitable consequence of ageing, and that strategies can be deployed to reduce and prevent falls in a variety of populations and settings. However, care must be taken when extrapolating findings from one population to another. Interventions need to be context specific and resources channelled to areas of proven efficacy.

As yet, there is limited evidence to support falls prevention as a means of fracture prevention. This is because studies which have used falls as the primary outcome have required relatively small sample sizes for this common outcome event and have had insufficient power to detect beneficial effects on less common outcomes such as fractures. Studies of osteoporosis management as a fracture prevention strategy have been of an order of magnitude larger than falls prevention trials.

Longer term strategic planning and policy development is still required to take evidence from the research setting and apply it to larger at-risk populations. This will require co-operation among health service managers, practising clinicians, patients and researchers.

Whilst highlighting areas where evidence exists to prevent falls and injury, it is recognized that there are still gaps in research in this area requiring further academic scrutiny. Given the continuously expanding interest and developing expertise in the area, these gaps are likely to be filled over the next decade. At the same time, if existing evidence to prevent falls is systematically applied to at-risk populations then in the next decade we should start to see a reduction in fracture rates in older people attributable to interventions to prevent falls.

REFERENCES

1. S. L. Wolf, H. X. Barnhart, N. G. Kutner *et al.*, Reducing frailty and falls in older persons: an investigation of Tai Chi and computerized balance training. Atlanta FICSIT Group. Frailty and Injuries: Cooperative Studies of Intervention Techniques. *Journal of the American Geriatrics Society*, **44**(5) (1996), 489–97.
2. A. Barnett, B. Smith, S. R. Lord, M. Williams & A. Baumand, Community-based group exercise improves balance and reduces falls in at-risk older people: a randomised controlled trial. *Age and Ageing*, **32**(4) (2003), 407–14.
3. A. J. Campbell, M. C. Robertson, M. M. Gardner, R. N. Norton & D. M. Buchner, Psychotropic medication withdrawal and a home based exercise programme to prevent falls: results of a randomised controlled trial. *Journal of the American Geriatrics Society*, **47** (1999), 850–3.

4. A. J. Campbell, M. C. Robertson, M. M. Gardner *et al.*, Randomised controlled trial of a general practice programme of home based exercise to prevent falls in elderly women. *British Medical Journal,* **315**(7115) (1997), 1065–9.

5. R. G. Cumming, M. Thomas, G. Szonyi *et al.*, Home visits by an occupational therapist for assessment and modification of environmental hazards: a randomized trial of falls prevention. *Journal of the American Geriatrics Society,* **47**(12) (1999), 1397–402.

6. R. H. Harwood, A. J. Foss, F. Osborn *et al.*, Falls and health status in elderly women following first eye cataract surgery: a randomised controlled trial. *British Journal of Ophthalmology,* **89**(1) (2005), 53–9.

7. F. Li, P. Harmer, K. J. Fisher *et al.*, Tai Chi and fall reductions in older adults: a randomized controlled trial. *Journals of Gerontology. Series A, Biological Sciences and Medical Sciences,* **60**(2) (2005), 187–94.

8. S. R. Lord, S. Castell, J. Corcoran *et al.*, The effect of group exercise on physical functioning and falls in frail older people living in retirement villages: a randomized, controlled trial. *Journal of the American Geriatrics Society,* **51**(12) (2003), 1685–92.

9. M. C. Robertson, N. Devlin, M. M. Gardner & A. J. Campbell, Effectiveness and economic evaluation of a nurse delivered home exercise programme to prevent falls. 1. Randomised controlled trial. *British Medical Journal,* **322**(7288) (2001), 697–701.

10. K. M. Means, D. E. Rodell & P. S. O'Sullivan, Balance, mobility, and falls among community-dwelling elderly persons: effects of a rehabilitation exercise program. *American Journal of Physical Medicine and Rehabilitation,* **84**(4) (2005), 238–50.

11. L. Clemson, R. G. Cumming, H. Kendig *et al.*, The effectiveness of a community-based program for reducing the incidence of falls in the elderly: a randomized trial. *Journal of the American Geriatrics Society,* **52**(9) (2004), 1487–94.

12. L. Day, B. Fildes, I. Gordon *et al.*, A randomized factorial trial of falls prevention among older people living in their own homes. *British Medical Journal,* **325** (2002), 128–33.

13. M. C. Hornbrook, V. J. Stephens, D. J. Wingfield *et al.*, Preventing falls among community-dwelling older persons: results from a randomized trial. *The Gerontologist,* **34** (1) (1994), 16–23.

14. T. Nikolaus & M. Bach, Preventing falls in community-dwelling frail older people using a home intervention team (HIT): results from the randomised falls-HIT trial. *Journal of the American Geriatrics Society,* **51** (2003), 300–5.

15. M. E. Tinetti, D. I. Baker, G. McAvay *et al.*, A multifactorial intervention to reduce the risk of falling among elderly people living in the community. *New England Journal of Medicine,* **331**(13) (1994), 821–7.

16. E. H. Wagner, A. Z. LaCroix, L. Grothaus *et al.*, Preventing disability and falls in older adults: a population-based randomized trial. *American Journal of Public Health,* **84**(11) (1994), 1800–6.

17. A. Campbell, M. Robertson, S. La Grow *et al.*, Randomised controlled trial of prevention of falls in people aged 75 with severe visual impairment: the VIP trial. *British Medical Journal,* **331**(7520) (2005), 817–925.

18. R. A. Kenny, D. A. Richardson, N. Steen *et al.*, Carotid sinus syndrome: a modifiable risk factor for nonaccidental falls in older adults (SAFE PACE). *Journal of the American College of Cardiology*, **38**(5) (2001), 1491–6.

19. J. Close, M. Ellis, R. Hooper *et al.*, Prevention of falls in the elderly trial (PROFET): a randomised controlled trial. *The Lancet*, **353**(9147) (1999), 93–7.

20. J. Davison, J. Bond, P. Dawson, I. N. Steen & R. A. Kenny, Patients with recurrent falls attending Accident and Emergency benefit from multifactorial intervention – a randomised controlled trial. *Age and Ageing*, **34**(2) (2005), 162–8.

21. C. Becker, M. Kron, U. Lindemann *et al.*, Effectiveness of a multifaceted intervention on falls in nursing home residents. *Journal of the American Geriatrics Society*, **51** (2003), 306–13.

22. J. Jensen, L. Lundin-Olsson, L. Nyberg & Y. Gustafson, Fall and injury prevention in older people living in residential care facilities: a cluster randomized trial. *Annals of Internal Medicine*, **136**(10) (2002), 733–41.

23. W. A. Ray, J. A. Taylor, K. G. Meador *et al.*, A randomized trial of a consultation service to reduce falls in nursing homes. *JAMA: Journal of the American Medical Association*, **278**(7) (1997), 557–62.

24. J. F. Schnelle, K. Kapur, C. Alessi *et al.*, Does an exercise and incontinence intervention save healthcare costs in a nursing home population? *Journal of the American Geriatrics Society*, **51**(2) (2003), 161–8.

25. T. P. Haines, K. L. Bennell, R. H. Osborne & K. D. Hill, Effectiveness of targeted falls prevention programme in subacute hospital setting: randomised controlled trial. *British Medical Journal*, **328** (2004), 676.

26. F. Healey, A. Monro, A. Cockram, V. Adams & D. Heseltine, Using targeted risk factor reduction to prevent falls in older in-patients: a randomised controlled trial. *Age and Ageing*, **33**(4) (2004), 390–5.

27. L. D. Gillespie, W. J. Gillespie, M. C. Robertson *et al.*, *Interventions for Preventing Falls in Elderly People (Cochrane Review)*. The Cochrane Library, vol 2. (Chichester: John Wiley and Sons, Inc., 2003).

28. C. G. Maher, C. Sherrington, R. D. Herbert, A. M. Moseley & M. Elkins, Reliability of the PEDro scale for rating quality of randomized controlled trials. *Physical Therapy*, **83**(8) (2003), 713–21.

29. D. M. Buchner, M. E. Cress, B. J. de Lateur *et al.*, The effect of strength and endurance training on gait, balance, fall risk, and health services use in community-living older adults. *Journals of Gerontology. Series A, Biological Sciences and Medical Sciences*, **52**(4) (1997), M218–24.

30. D. Skelton, S. Dinan, M. Campbell & O. Rutherford, Tailored group exercise (FaME) reduces falls in community dwelling older frequent fallers (an RCT) [research letter]. *Age and Ageing*, **34**(6) (2005), 636–9.

Part III

Research issues in falls prevention

18

Falls in older people: future directions for research

Since the pioneering work of Sheldon in the 1960s, a great deal of research has been undertaken into falls, and there is now a considerable body of knowledge about the various risk factors and the effectiveness of a range of intervention strategies. Indeed, since the first edition of this book was published in 2001, many more studies have been undertaken, with many completed in areas identified in the first edition's chapter on future directions for research. However, as in every area of scientific study, the findings of one study pose questions for another. In this final chapter, we present a brief review of a range of research issues that need to be addressed in the future.

Epidemiology and taxonomy

Common taxonomy for reporting falls and fall-related issues

Comparability of outcomes from falls prevention trials is remarkably difficult and this relates not only to the heterogeneity of the populations selected and the approaches to intervention, but also to the way in which results are reported. A vast array of statistical tests have been used and reported in the literature, including mean, median and total number of falls, number of people falling, number of recurrent fallers, time to first fall, time to first four falls, odds ratios, relative risks, hazard ratios, incident rate ratios, etc. Number needed to treat to prevent a fall or a person falling is a potentially useful comparator, but the methods of statistical analysis and data presentation used in different studies make this information impossible to extract from some published papers.

A recent paper by Robertson and colleagues [1] addresses the issue of statistical analysis of efficacy in falls prevention trials and openly challenges some of the approaches to data analysis in published trials. It cogently argues that a statistical test needs to reflect the frequent and recurrent nature of falls that exhibit a non-normal distribution. It concludes that incident rate ratios calculated from negative binomial regression modelling are the most appropriate and parsimonious measures for falls outcome analysis.

Another recent publication from the Prevention of Falls Network Europe (ProFaNE) collaboration [2] has produced a consensus document which also makes recommendations for addressing the difficulties with comparability among published studies. Recommendations derived by international experts in the field include:

(i)   An agreed definition of a fall – 'an unexpected event in which the participants come to rest on the ground, floor, or other lower level'.

(ii) Method for collecting falls data – minimum of monthly collection of falls using falls diaries with follow-up telephone contact if required.

(iii) Data analysis – number of falls, fallers/non-fallers/recurrent fallers, falls rate per person year and time to first fall (as a safety measure).

(iv) Injury definition – number of radiologically confirmed peripheral (limb and girdle) fracture events per person year.

The adoption of common taxonomy for reporting falls and falls-related issues, such as injuries, falls efficacy scales, physical activity, disability and quality of life, would substantially contribute toward much easier appreciation and comparison of research trials. A similar taxonomy is required to help define and quantify the different approaches to interventions to prevent falls as well as an agreed methodological approach to assessing the quality and cost of complex interventions.

Understanding cross-cultural differences in fall rates

As indicted in Chapter 1, rigorous data regarding falls incidence in older people from non-White populations is limited. However, studies of fall rates in Japanese people living in Japan and Hawaii found fall rates to be only half that of populations of predominantly White people. Davis *et al.* attempted to determine whether neuromuscular performance measures and functional disabilities could account for this difference [3]. They found that Japanese women performed better in some measures (chair stands, balance, walking speed) but worse in others (strength, reaction time). It is possible that better performances in the more functional strength and balance tests that translate more directly to activities of daily living, could explain the lower risk of falls among Japanese women. Further research could identify lifestyle factors that account for cross-cultural differences in fall rates.

Furthering the understanding of balance and associated falls risk factors

Studies on human balance and related sensorimotor systems

Further studies are required to enhance our understanding of human balance. In particular, work is needed to elucidate whether impairments in vestibular function that lead to a reduced sense of the upright and/or unstable retinal images during head movements are significant causes of falling in older people. Contributions from the vestibular system to turning, stepping and gait also need clarification. There is a clear need for the findings of laboratory studies to be tested in larger community samples where feasible.

Transient risk factors

As indicated in Part I of this book, most headway into identifying risk factors for falls has been in the area of chronic conditions. New studies are required to tackle the more difficult areas of transient falls risk factors. The main areas that require attention in this regard are cardiovascular conditions, including orthostatic hypotension, cardiac arrhythmias and disorders of vestibular function. This may best be achieved by integrated approaches to the investigation of dizziness and syncope. However, before any real progress can be made in this area, a clearer consensus is required regarding the very definitions of these terms. As discussed in Chapter 6, progress towards a more complete understanding of dizziness is considerably hampered by inconsistent definitions across the literature [4].

Medication effects on balance

Another area which has received only limited attention is evaluation of the mechanisms underlying loss of balance in response to certain medications. One study has reported a dose-dependent increase in sway in response to psychoactive medication use [5]. However, further work is required to assess how different medications impair stability when performing more complex tasks, the duration of effects after a single dose and whether effects are maintained over longer term administration.

Neuropsychological risk factors

In recent years, many investigators have included neuropsychological assessments in studies of balance control and in screening batteries for predicting falls [17]. These have shown that the attentional demands of balance control vary depending on the complexity of the postural task, the nature of the secondary task, the age of the individual and their balance abilities. While poor performance in these tests may indicate general cognitive decline, they provide interesting insights into the causes of falls.

The issue of fear of falling has received considerable attention in the past few years. Balance confidence and falls efficacy measures have been shown to be associated with objectively assessed measures of balance or falls. Interestingly, no studies have found that fear of falling is an independent risk factor for falls after adjusting for impaired balance and/or reduced physical functioning. This issue requires further attention in research studies.

Development of evidence-based falls assessment tools

Many falls risk assessment tools used in community, hospital and residential care settings have not been formally validated. Further studies are required to validate a range of simple screens and more comprehensive assessment tools, so as to enable the accurate identification of falls risk factors and to target interventions accordingly.

Efficacy of approaches to intervention

Falls prevention strategies in population sub-groups

Chapter 6 outlined the many medical conditions that predispose older people to falling. Studies identifying mechanisms of improving physical functioning are required in these population sub-groups. Initial intervention studies that aimed at preventing falls in older people with dementia have not been successful, despite well planned and executed studies [6]. Further development of intervention programmes for this patient group incorporating specific dementia-specific risk factors may be required. Interventions for other high-risk groups, such as people with a stroke, Parkinson's disease and those who have suffered a hip fracture, are also required.

Intensity and type of exercise intervention programmes

Further work is required to identify the most effective exercise interventions for improving physical functioning and preventing falls in older people. Grouped results from the FICSIT studies [7] indicated that interventions that addressed strength alone did not result in a significant reduction in falls, whereas programmes that included a balance component achieved reductions in fall rates. Further studies have indicated that effective exercise programmes comprise a combination of challenging and progressive balance exercises performed in weight-bearing positions that minimize the use of the upper limbs for support. However, as the older population comprises a diverse group in relation to physical functioning, there will be no single effective exercise prescription. Specific studies are required to identify exercise components that are effective in maintaining balance, strength, coordination and the ability to carry out functional activities, in both the more vigorous, independent older population and in frailer groups.

Interventions for maximizing vision

Simple intervention strategies such as expedited cataract surgery have now been shown to reduce fall rates in older people [8]. Optical interventions also have the potential to improve contrast sensitivity, stereoacuity and depth perception in addition to visual acuity in this group. No studies have examined the benefits of providing optimal glasses for distance vision, despite the finding that multifocal glasses present an important risk factor for falls in older people [9] and that this group may benefit from improved distance vision in situations that present a postural threat (e.g. walking on stairs and in unfamiliar outdoor settings). As poor vision in one eye elevates the risk of both falls [10] and fall-related fractures [11], strategies to maximize vision in both eyes may also be particularly beneficial in preventing falls.

Psychoactive medication withdrawal

As indicated in Chapter 7, the role of many medications as risk factors for falls may have been overstated. In many cases, it appears that medication use has simply been a marker for the medical conditions for which they were prescribed. The psychoactive medications, however, have been consistently shown to be significant and independent risk factors for falls. In a well designed study, Campbell *et al.* [12] found that it is possible to reduce falls by withdrawing psychoactive medications. However, they experienced great difficulty in recruiting older users of psychoactive medications into the study. Further, it proved difficult to modify psychoactive medication use in the minority who did participate. Further work is required to identify alternatives to pharmacological treatment of sleep disorders and anxiety in older people. As benzodiazepine withdrawal, in particular, has been shown to be difficult, strategies for preventing initial use of these medications would be important to identify. To be successful, such strategies would need to be seen as an acceptable alternative to medication use by older people, their doctors and other health professionals.

The role of vitamin D in preventing falls

As indicated in Chapter 12, vitamin D insufficiency is common in older people, particularly those who are housebound or who reside in nursing homes. Recent studies have found that vitamin D supplementation can reduce postural sway and improve strength, and there is some evidence that vitamin D may reduce the risk of falls [13]. Further work is required to determine if routine vitamin D supplementation in the form of an oral tablet or increased exposure to sunlight can prevent falls in at-risk older people.

Identifying optimal shoe designs

Chapter 13 synthesized the available information from studies undertaken to date. There is little doubt that high heeled shoes constitute an unnecessary falls risk factor for older women [14]]. Other posited hazardous and safe shoe characteristics still require evaluation in appropriate experimental and prospective epidemiological studies. In particular, the following areas require investigation: heel collar height, tread patterns and sole hardness. Further, studies are required to determine whether there is one optimal shoe type for older persons for all circumstances or whether there are shoe characteristics that are particularly suited to certain conditions. For example, it needs to be determined whether a shoe that is appropriate for wearing indoors is also appropriate for wearing outdoors. Studies are also required to identify the shoe characteristics that maximize balance in situations that predispose people to falls, such as wet and slippery floors, and uneven and icy surfaces.

Preventing falls in institutions

The major falls risk factors for older persons in hospitals and nursing homes have been identified. Evaluation of multidisciplinary, multifactorial assessment and intervention programmes addressing these risk factors have produced mixed results, and further evaluation of the effectiveness and cost-effectiveness of such interventions, is required. The efficacy of specific interventions, such as patient movement alarms, alterations to bed heights and use or non-use of bedrails, also needs to be determined. Furthermore, staffing issues need to be fully evaluated to determine whether modifications to timetabling of nursing and support staff can increase vigilance, and identify potential hazards in the institutional environment.

Falls prevention trials with fracture as the outcome

As yet, there is limited evidence to support falls prevention as a means of fracture prevention. This is because studies which have used falls as the primary outcome have required relatively small sample sizes for this common outcome event, and have had insufficient power to detect beneficial effects on less common outcomes such as fractures. An appropriately powered trial is required to determine whether fracture prevention can be achieved by interventions to prevent falls.

Determining the best intervention strategies

There are now encouraging findings from well planned and executed studies which indicate that many falls are preventable. However, further work is still required to determine which interventions are the most effective and whether some intervention components may actually cause harm. This evidence will only be provided by randomized controlled trials, particularly those with factorial designs, and meta-analyses.

Understanding falls prevention from an older persons perspective – barriers and motivators to uptake of interventions

Regardless of the intervention modality for preventing falls, a crucial factor is compliance. There is a growing body of knowledge of factors related to adherence to exercise. Further work is required to determine if similar factors also predict poor compliance to other interventions, such as medication withdrawal, use of hip protectors and adoption of home safety modifications. More work needs to be undertaken to maximize the uptake of interventions that have been shown to be successful.

Effectiveness and cost-benefits of applying the existing evidence

Population interventions

As the causes of falls are multifactorial and the older population a diverse one, there is likely to be no single formula for preventing falls. Strategic planning and policy development is required to translate evidence from the research setting and apply it to relevant at-risk populations. This will require co-operation among health service managers, practising clinicians, patients and researchers. Interventions need to be conducted as public health initiatives, not just as demonstration projects, to identify programmes that are acceptable to older people in the long term. Such work should also address cost-effectiveness and strategies for overcoming barriers to participation.

Evaluation of falls clinics

The last ten years have seen the advent of falls clinics [15, 16]. These have been devised on an individual basis with no two clinics alike. The main models, however, have included: (i) clinics which use a standardized protocol for the medical management of falls; (ii) clinics which involve the contributions of relevant health professionals, including medical specialists, physiotherapists, occupational therapists and podiatrists; and (iii) clinics which use tests for identifying those at risk of falling and the underlying impairments, with intervention strategies targeted to identified deficit areas. These clinics still require evaluation with respect to their effectiveness and cost-effectiveness compared with usual care.

Conclusion

Falls and fall-related injury are likely to be major healthcare problems for older people for the foreseeable future. Consequently, the identification and implementation of effective falls prevention strategies will remain an important public health priority. Much has been learned about risk factors for falls and fractures in recent years, but further work remains to be done to fully understand the role of certain medical, physiological, psychological and environmental factors in predisposing older people to falls. Currently, known effective interventions include exercise, expedited cataract surgery, psychoactive medication withdrawal, occupational therapy interventions and targeted multifactorial interventions. Further progress will be made if large randomized controlled trials and population interventions are conducted that can confirm the effectiveness of these interventions and examine other interventions suggested from observational studies.

REFERENCES

1. M.C. Robertson, A.J. Campbell & P. Herbison, Statistical analysis of efficacy in falls prevention trials. *Journal of Gerontology*, **60** (2005), M530–4.

2. S.E. Lamb, E.C. Jørstad-Stein, K. Hauer, & C. Becker, Development of a common outcome data set for fall injury prevention trials: the Prevention of Falls Network Europe Consensus. *Journal of the American Geriatrics Society*, **53** (2005), 1618–22.

3. J.W. Davis, M.C. Nevitt, P.D. Wasnich & P.D. Ross, A cross-cultural comparison of neuromuscular performance, functional status, and falls between Japanese and white women. *Journal of Gerontology*, **54** (1999), M288–92.

4. P.D. Sloane & J. Dallara, Clinical research and geriatric dizziness: the blind men and the elephant. *Journal of the American Geriatrics Society*, **47** (1999), 113–14.

5. Y.J. Liu, G. Stagni, J.G. Walden, A.M.M. Shepherd & M.J. Lichtenstein, Thioridazine dose-related effects on biomechanical force platform measures of sway in young and old men. *Journal of the American Geriatrics Society*, **46** (1998), 431–7.

6. F.E. Shaw, J. Bond, D.A. Richardson *et al.*, Multifactorial intervention after a fall in older people with cognitive impairment and dementia presenting to the accident and emergency department: randomised controlled trial. *British Medical Journal*, **326** (2003), 73–5.

7. M.A. Province, E.C. Hadley, M.C. Hornbrook, *et al.*, The effects of exercise on falls in elderly patients. A preplanned meta-analysis of the FICSIT trials. Frailty and Injuries: Cooperative Studies of Intervention Techniques. *Journal of the American Medical Association*, **273** (1995), 1341–7.

8. R.H. Harwood, A.J. Foss, F. Osborn *et al.*, Falls and health status in elderly women following first eye cataract surgery: a randomised controlled trial. *British Journal Ophthalmology*, **89** (2005), 53–9.

9. S.R. Lord, J. Dayhew & A. Howland, Multifocal glasses impair edge-contrast sensitivity and depth perception and increase the risk of falls in older people. *Journal of the American Geriatrics Society*, **50** (2002), 1760–6.

10. S.R. Lord & J. Dayhew, Visual risk factors for falls in older people. *Journal of the American Geriatrics Society*, **49** (2001), 508–12.

11. D. T. Felson, J. J. Anderson & M. T. Annan, Impaired vision and hip fracture. The Framingham study. *Journal of the American Geriatrics Society*, **37** (1989), 495–500.

12. A. J. Campbell, M. C. Robertson, M. M. Gardner, R. N. Norton & D. M. Buchner, Psychotropic medication withdrawal and a home based exercise programme to prevent falls: a randomised controlled trial. *Journal of the American Geriatrics Society*, **47** (1999), 850–3.

13. H. Bischoff, H. Stahelin, W. Dick *et al.*, Effects of vitamin D and caclium supplementation on falls: a randomized controlled trial. *Journal of Bone and Mineral Research*, **18** (2003), 343–51.

14. A. F. Tencer, T. D. Koepsell, M. E. Wolf *et al.*, Biomechanical properties of shoes and risk of falls in older adults. *Journal of the American Geriatrics Society*, **52** (2004), 1840–6.

15. G. P. Wolf-Klein, F. A. Silverstone, N. Basavaraju *et al.*, Prevention of falls in the elderly population. *Archives of Physical Medicine and Rehabilitation*, **6** (1988), 689–91.

16. K. D. Hill, J. M. Dwyer, J. A. Schwarz & R. D. Helme, A falls and balance clinic for the elderly. *Physiotherapy Canada*, **46** (1994), 20–7.

17. M. Woollacott & A. Shumway-Cook, Attention and the control of posture and gait: a review of an emerging area of research. *Gait and Posture*, **16** (2002), 1–14.

Index

Lightning Source UK Ltd.
Milton Keynes UK
UKOW07f2303270817
308029UK00004B/55/P